www.harcourt-international.com

Bringing you products from all Harcourt Health Sciences companies including Baillière Tindall, Churchill Livingstone, Mosby and W.B. Saunders

- ● **Browse** for latest information on new books, journals and electronic products

- ● **Search** for information on over 20 000 published titles with full product information including tables of contents and sample chapters

- ● **Keep up to date** with our extensive publishing programme in your field by registering with eAlert or requesting postal updates

- ● **Secure online ordering** with prompt delivery, as well as full contact details to order by phone, fax or post

- ● **News** of special features and promotions

If you are based in the following countries, please visit the country-specific site to receive full details of product availability and local ordering information

USA: www.harcourthealth.com

Canada: www.harcourtcanada.com

Australia: www.harcourt.com.au

Baillière Tindall   CHURCHILL LIVINGSTONE   Mosby   W.B. SAUNDERS

Meeting the Health Needs of People who have a Learning Disability

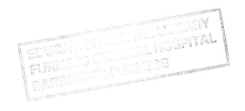

For Baillière Tindall

Commissioning Editor: Sarena Wolfaard
Project Manager: Jane Dingwall
Design Direction: George Ajayi

Meeting the Health Needs of People who have a Learning Disability

Edited by

Jeanette Thompson MA BSc(Hons) RNMH DipN(Lond) CertEd ITEC
PGDip(HSSM) DipMan
Lecturer, Learning Disabilities Nursing, University of York, UK

Sharon Pickering MSc BSc(Hons) BA(Hons) RGN DipN(Lond) PGDip(HSSM)
Project Manager, NHSE Trent, UK

Foreword by

The Healthy Living Group, York

Prologue by

Oliver Russell MA BM BCh DPM FRCPsych
Reader in Psychiatry, Norah Fry Research Centre, University of Bristol, UK;
Chair of Trustees, British Institute of Learning Disabilities

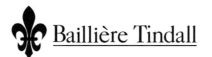
Baillière Tindall

EDINBURGH LONDON NEW YORK PHILADELPHIA ST LOUIS SYDNEY TORONTO 2001

BAILLIÈRE TINDALL
An imprint of Harcourt Publishers Limited

© Harcourt Publishers Limited 2001

♣ is a registered trademark of Harcourt Publishers Limited

The right of Jeanette Thompson and Sharon Pickering to be identified as editors of this work has been asserted by them in accordance with the Copyright, Designs and Patents Act 1988

First published 2001

ISBN 0 7020 2532 1

British Library Cataloguing in Publication Data
A catalogue record for this book is available from the British Library

Library of Congress Cataloging in Publication Data
A catalog record for this book is available from the Library of Congress

Note

Medical knowledge is constantly changing. As new information becomes available, changes in treatment, procedures, equipment and the use of drugs become necessary. The editors, contributors and the publishers have taken care to ensure that the information given in this text is accurate and up to date. However, readers are strongly advised to confirm that the information, especially with regard to drug usage, complies with the latest legislation and standards of practice.

The
publisher's
policy is to use
**paper manufactured
from sustainable forests**

Printed in China

Contents

List of contributors   xiii

Foreword   xv

Prologue   xvii

Preface   xxi

Section 1: Context of health   1

1   Future directions—initiatives and agendas   3
    John Brown

    Introduction   3
    The Conservative legacy   4
    Policy across the United Kingdom   7
    Changing agendas   14
    Future direction   18
    Further reading   20
    References   21

2   Concepts of health and disability   24
    Marc Saunders

    Introduction   24
    Defining health   24
    Health as an evolutionary concept   28
    Pluralist perspectives of health   30
    Modern constructs of health and their influence on health education and
      health promotion   32
    Attitudes to disability, learning disability and the superimposition of health
      and ill health constructs   34
    Health and quality of life   36
    Conclusion   38
    Further reading   39
    References   39

3   Influences on health   41
    Mavis Arevalo

    Introduction   41
    Genetic inheritance and biology   42
    Age and generation   43
    Sex and gender   44
    Socialization and lifestyle   47
    Race, ethnicity and culture   48
    Social class   51
    The education system   54
    Occupation, work environment and unemployment   58
    Access to healthcare   59
    Conclusion   60
    Further reading   61
    References   61

4   Health needs of people who have a learning disability   63
    Steve Turner

    Introduction   63
    Down's syndrome   65
    Fragile X syndrome   71
    Health problems not related to cause of learning disability   72
    Risk factors and lifestyle   77
    Implications for practice   81
    Conclusion   82
    Further reading   82
    References   83

Section 2: Strategies for identifying health needs   89

5   The public health agenda   91
    Jeanette Thompson and Sharon Pickering

    Introduction   91
    What is public health?   92
    Health inequalities and the underlying causes of ill health   95
    Promoting positive health   101
    Building community participation   103
    Developing skills in public health   108
    Conclusion   110
    Further reading   110
    References   111

6   The assessment of health needs   113
    Elizabeth Newbronner

    Introduction   113
    Health needs and health needs assessment   113
    Health needs assessment in practice   115
    Conducting a health needs assessment   116
    Further reading   123
    References   124

7   Health promotion with people who have a learning disability   126
    Philomena Shaughnessy and Susan Cruse

    Introduction   126
    Problems with access to and availability of health promotion   126
    Overcoming barriers to health promotion   129
    Promoting health – setting the scene   132
    The elements of health promotion   132
    Approaches to health promotion   133
    The importance of self-efficacy   136
    Assessing the need for health promotion   137
    Designing and implementing appropriate health promotion   144
    Health promotion and healthy alliances   147
    Evaluation of health promotion   150
    Conclusion   153
    Further reading   154
    References   155

8   Accessing health information   158
    Nicola Taylor with Susan Smithurst

    Introduction   158
    How did we start out?   159

Why do this research?
Formation of the Acorn Group
How did we run the group?
What is information? 162
Using different ways to give information 164
Where are we now? 165
Practicalities in accessing information 166
Recommendations 167
References 168

Section 3: Meeting health needs 169

9   Being well and my well-being 171
    Anya Souza with Paul Ramcharan

    Introduction 171
    Health and staying healthy 171
    Illness and getting well 175
    When is health not health and illness not illness? 177
    Conclusion 178
    References 178

10 Self-concept and people who have learning disabilities 179
    Mark Statham and Diane Timblick

    Introduction 179
    The implication of legislation 180
    Issues of self-concept 181
    Construction of group identities 190
    Conclusion 192
    Further reading 193
    References 193

11 Valued occupation for people who have a learning disability 195
    Caroline Heason, Lynne Stracey and Dommie Rey

    Introduction 195
    Historical perspectives 197
    Defining valued occupation 198
    Concepts of health and occupation 200
    Ethical dilemmas 201
    Risk in valued occupation 202
    Psychosocial aspects of health and occupation for people who have
        learning disabilities 203
    Cultural diversity and valued occupation 203
    Service options and Partnerships in Action 204
    Discussion 206
    Towards enabling valued occupation for people who have
        learning disability 207
    Conclusion 209
    Further reading 210
    References 210

12 Sexual health 211
    Damian Dunn

    Introduction 211
    What is sexual health? 211
    Sexual health and rights 213
    Who are we talking about? 214
    How do we assess need? 215

What helps people stay sexually healthy?   218
Factors which influence decisions about health   220
The health action model   224
Effective health promotion interventions   225
Evaluating health promotion   228
Legal and ethical issues   229
Conclusion   232
Further reading   233
References   233

13 Mental health   235
    Steve Moss and Pauline Lee

Introduction   235
Defining mental illness   235
Risk factors for mental illness   236
Prevalence of mental health problems   238
Psychiatric disorders and challenging behaviour   238
Assessment of mental health problems   240
Case recognition   249
Mental health problems across the lifespan   250
Treatment   254
Conclusion   258
Further reading   259
References   259

14 Life transitions and personal change   264
    Jeanette Thompson and Sharon Pickering

Transition and change   265
Personal change   266
Life events   267
Reactions to personal change   274
Personal meaning of transitions   275
Coping with change   276
Analysing life transitions   278
Models for managing transitions and change   280
Implications for service delivery   281
Conclusion   281
Further reading   281
References   282

Section 4: Developing partnerships

15 Supporting the supporters – some reflections on family caregiving   287
    Gordon Grant

Introduction   287
Theoretical perspectives and family care   288
Formal and informal care relations and healthcare: practice issues   294
Discussion   301
Further reading   302
References   303

16 Working with communities   306
    Angela Butcher with Jeanette Thompson and Sharon Pickering

Introduction   306
The concept of community: a sense of belonging   307

Strategies for developing inclusive communities and increasing
    community participation   310
Conclusion   317
Further reading   318
References   318
Useful addresses   319

17 Interprofessional and multi-agency working   320
   Peter Mathias and Tony Thompson

Why we need to work across professional and organizational boundaries   320
The realities of interprofessional working   324
Effective teamwork   328
The interface between support systems   329
The framework for strengthening and supporting the helping systems   331
Further reading   334
References   335

Index   337

Contributors

Mavis A D Arevalo, Senior Lecturer, School of Human and Health Sciences, University of Huddersfield, Huddersfield, West Yorkshire

John Brown, Director, Centre for Inter-professional Studies in Health and Social Care, Department of Social Policy and Social Work, University of York

Angela Butcher, Occupational Therapist, Community team for people who have learning disabilities, The Martyn Long Centre, Horsham, West Sussex

Susan Cruse, Health and Wellness Manager, Smithkline Beecham Pharmaceuticals, Welwyn, Hertfordshire

Damian Dunn, Project Coordinator, PMS Pilot Project for Homeless People and Traveller Families, York NHS Trust, York

Gordon Grant, Professor of Cognitive Disability, School of Nursing and Midwifery, University of Sheffield, Samuel Fox House, Northern General Hospital, Sheffield

Caroline Heason, Oxford Community Team Manager, Oxford City CTPLD, Oxford

Pauline Lee, Head of Psychology for Learning Disability, East Cheshire NHS Trust

Peter Mathias, Manager of City and Guilds Affinity, London

Steve Moss, Senior Lecturer, Institute of Psychiatry, London

Elizabeth Newbronner, Partner, Acton Shapiro, Consultants in Primary and Community Care; Visiting Senior Research Fellow, Department of Health Studies, University of York

Sharon Pickering, Project Manager, NHSE Trent, Sheffield

Paul Ramcharan, Senior Lecturer, Department of Mental Health and Learning Disabilities, School of Nursing and Midwifery, University of Sheffield

Dommie Rey, Clinical Specialist in Occupational Therapy, Oxford City CTPLD, Oxford

Marc Saunders, General Manager, Wolverley Services, North Warwickshire NHS Trust

Philomena Shaughnessy, Senior Lecturer, Division of Post Registration Nursing, Faculty of Health and Human Sciences, University of Hertfordshire, Hatfield

Susan Smithurst, Postgraduate Researcher, School of Health Policy and Practice, University of East Anglia, Norwich

Anya Souza has worked in self advocacy organisations and with other organisations run by and for people who have learning difficulties. Anya has made a number of media appearances discussing issues that affect the lives of people who have learning difficulties

Mark Statham, Senior Lecturer, Thames Valley University, Reading

Lynne Stracey, Clinical Specialist in Learning Disability Nursing, Oxford City CTPLD, Oxford

Nicola Taylor, Client, Adult Training Centre, Sprowston, Norfolk

Jeanette Thompson, Lecturer, Learning Disabilities Nursing, University of York

Tony Thompson, Director of Practice Development, Ashworth Hospital Authority, Ashworth Centre, Liverpool

Diane Timblick, Lecturer Practitioner, Oxford Brookes University, Oxford

Steve Turner, Research Fellow, Centre for Social Research on Dementia, Department of Applied Social Science, University of Stirling

Foreword

The following Foreword has been written by a group of people who have under-taken a Healthy Living course in York and these are their reflections on how important it is to know about their health.

We have been meeting together as a group, of three men and three women, for 7 weeks to look at things to do with our health. While we have been doing this we have learnt a lot of things about our health and about the people who help us with this. The useful things we have learnt from all of these sessions are that we have been shown how to dial 999 and when we are living more independently this could save someone's life. The chance to practise this means we know what to expect when we use this number. We were told things about our personal health and relationships that no one else had discussed with us. Although we found these sessions difficult at first, by the end of the course they made more sense to us and we feel that these sessions will help us to understand our relationships better in the future. We already knew some things about healthy eating but we now understand more about why we need to eat healthy food.

The sessions gave us a chance to meet with our friends and learn new things about our bodies and feelings and we really enjoyed it. Even though we know these things now it is still hard for us to have control over the things that affect our health. One of our group lives in a group home and does not have the chance to say what he would like to eat. Some of us are not allowed to make our own appointments when we go to the doctors. When we do go to the health centre the doctors and nurses use long words and sometimes talk to our carers rather than to us. Lots of times people do not spend long enough explaining things to us so we can understand them. We know all of these things are getting better, but they still have a long way to go; this is why a book for professionals about our health needs is important. To help us use what we have learnt when we go to the doctor or nurse we are going to do another course on assertiveness.

Healthy Living Group, York

Prologue

The enjoyment of good health is the key to a good quality of life. While we recognize that some people who have a learning disability have good health and enjoy life to the full we know that the lives of many other, often equally disabled, people are diminished by poor health, frequent illness, and lack of accessible healthcare. At the beginning of the 21st century, with scientific knowledge moving rapidly forward, dramatic advances being made in the treatment of disease, and the human genome decoded, it is not unreasonable to ask that more attention should be given to the health needs of people who have a learning disability. They may not always be able to articulate their needs, or describe their symptoms or express their pain but our responsibilities as health professionals are clear: we need to be able to plan and deliver high quality healthcare that is well targeted, evidence-based and effective.

The publication of this book is timely. Firstly, because people who have learning disabilities are themselves voicing their concerns about the inadequacy of the health services they are being offered (during the past few months members of self-advocacy groups have related to me some really dreadful experiences with health service provision). Secondly, because these concerns are being mirrored by family carers; their complaints about the inadequacies of healthcare for their sons and daughters are compelling. Thirdly, on a more positive note, because we are witnessing an encouraging surge of interest in healthcare issues among health and social care staff who really want to make a difference in the lives of people with a learning disability. Lastly, this book will be appearing soon after the publication of major policy reviews from the Scottish Executive, from the Department of Health and from the National Assembly for Wales. These statements of government policy reflect some common themes – person-centred planning, enabling people with a learning disability to have more control over their lives, ensuring that mainstream NHS providers recognize the need to provide good quality healthcare for people who have a learning disability and reducing health inequalities.

HEALTHY LIFESTYLES

The NHS Plan encourages the promotion of healthy lifestyles. But maintaining good health depends in the first instance on being able to make informed choices about key issues such as lifestyle, diet and living environment. Making informed choices is not easy for people who have a learning disability and are often poorly informed about the choices open to them, and when they do find what they want many discover that they are unable to access their preferred option. Most non-disabled people have a high degree of choice over where they live but many people who have learning disabilities are given little choice and often have to accept some form of congregate living. While most of us are educated about what constitutes a healthy lifestyle, people who have learning disabilities may not be given the information needed to make wise choices nor possess the financial resources to purchase the most nutritious foods. A reduction of inequalities in health cannot be achieved without dealing with the fundamental causes – poverty, social exclusion, low educational attainment, discrimination, and the lack of a job. Poverty, poor quality diets and overcrowded environments do not provide the basis for a healthy lifestyle.

RECOGNIZING ILL HEALTH

Of course, enjoying a healthy life goes beyond having a healthy lifestyle. It also involves being able to recognize ill health and having access to good quality healthcare. Understanding the significance of symptoms is often not easy. For example, a sensation of feeling generally unwell may, on the one hand, be the advance warning of serious illness but, on the other hand, such symptoms may reflect some trivial and temporary imbalance in bodily function. For example, feeling tired or debilitated might be an advance sign of a loss of thyroid function, of chronic anaemia or possibly more seriously heart disease or cancer. Such symptoms might equally well signify the onset of depression. Access to sound diagnosis is vital to maintaining good health.

ACCESSING DIAGNOSIS AND TREATMENT

Being able to get a diagnosis and treatment depends on being able to access services that are available. Accessing healthcare may be a problem for some people who have a learning disability. Many people who have learning disabilities will require accessible information and support if they are to engage with healthcare services. They may face barriers in navigating access to the services and support they need. Family carers, social care providers, and support personnel are powerful gatekeepers to healthcare and may unwittingly block access to healthcare. They may not be aware of the significance of their role in enabling service users to gain access to health services. In particular people who have learning disabilities from black and ethnic minority communities may have difficulties in accessing appropriate care for a variety of reasons including language difficulties and cultural misunderstanding.

IMPROVING HEALTHCARE

Among the recommendations of the recent report of the Scottish Executive are a number of initiatives to enhance healthcare. Health boards are encouraged to offer regular health checks. Larger primary care centres are asked to consider choosing a GP with lead responsibility for managing and co-ordinating primary health care for people with a learning disability. The report also calls for a named learning disability nurse for each practice and for health assessments to be undertaken in primary care. In parallel with the report from Scotland recently published, government policy for England calls for similar initiatives, including the nomination of health facilitators to support people who have learning disabilities to access the health they need, with health action plans to monitor how their needs are being met.

New service philosophies, such as normalization, have put great emphasis on the rights of people who have a learning disability to make choices and to speak for themselves. New ways of construing health needs are forcing us to revise some of our traditional approaches. New policies from our governments demand that we make changes. Many problems remain but this book strengthens the evidence base and throws light on how to meet the healthcare needs of people who have a learning disability more effectively.

Oliver Russell

Preface

When starting the process of writing a book you are inevitably driven by your belief that you have something to say that perhaps everyone is not yet thinking about. This book was no exception. Almost three years ago now we had the idea that it would be sensible, if not extremely useful, to integrate the knowledge base that typifies learning disability services with that which is common in parts of primary care. In doing this it was hoped that both learning disability practitioners and primary healthcare professionals would be better equipped to meet the health needs of people who have a learning disability. This agenda is even more relevant in the context of the forthcoming White Paper on learning disability services.

This overall goal was important to us as a consequence of the changing knowledge base that we held regarding the health needs of this part of the population. This was further reinforced by our commitment to the use of generic services. The problem was that without some integration of these two knowledge bases this goal was highly unlikely to reach fruition. Nowhere was this more obvious than in the chapter focusing upon the new public health agenda— this chapter was the most difficult of all chapters to find an author for and in the end we trusted in our own knowledge base, some diligent reading and the expert advice of Val Buxton, Kate Billingham and Sue Carmichael. To each of these people we are extremely grateful.

Another aspect of this text that was extremely important to us was that it would not be written purely by professionals but that it would also allow for valued opportunities and experiences for people who have a learning disability. To this end two of the chapters have been written by people who have a learning disability. Both of these chapters provide valuable insights into those things that we as professionals and service providers need to consider in the context of service development and delivery. In addition, the front cover for this text has been based upon a design by Anya Souza. These contributions add greatly to the overall value of this text in creating positive opportunities and positive identities for the people who we work with and alongside.

We hope you enjoy this text and find some way for it to influence the service we provide to people who have a learning disability.

Jeanette Thompson
Sharon Pickering

Note : ⌒ or ⌒ appears in the margin throughout and denotes cross-references to other chapters in the book.

1 CONTEXT OF HEALTH

This section sets the scene for the book by exploring a number of the underpinning issues that the reader needs to consider. It begins by exploring current issues within the four countries of the United Kingdom and identifies some of the differences in relation to the position within each area. In addition, and perhaps crucially, this section introduces the reader to the concepts of health and disability. Whilst this section utilizes much of the contemporary literature in relation to the nebulous concept of health, it also strikingly integrates these with concepts of the social construction of disability and relates all these issues to people who have a learning disability. Subsequently this section considers the influences upon health, a subject that may be well understood by many people but one that is not always articulated in the context of people who have a learning disability. Finally this section considers the health needs of people who have a learning disability. The picture created by all these chapters together provides the baseline from which the remainder of the book evolves.

SECTION CONTENTS

1 **Future directions – initiatives and agendas**
   John Brown

2 **Concepts of health and disability**
   Marc Saunders

3 **Influences on health**
   Mavis Arevalo

4 **Health needs of people who have a learning disability**
   Steve Turner

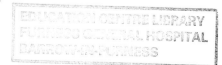

Future directions – initiatives and agendas

John Brown

KEY ISSUES

- Policy context
- Devolution
- Partnership
- Changing contexts of service delivery
- Workforce development

INTRODUCTION

In May 1997 the Labour Party was returned to government after a period in opposition stretching back to 1979. This period of 18 years was marked by the Conservative administration developing and promoting radical changes in the scope and function of state-run welfare provision. In the arena of health and social care the emphasis upon the mixed economy of welfare led to the introduction of the internal market, the vigorous pursuit of community care and the espousal of the benefits of the independent sector, in particular privately sponsored and run initiatives. Changes such as these were accompanied by a set of values, language and policy infrastructure that led to services for those who have a learning disability, as with other user groups, undergoing fundamental change. This change provided a crucial legacy for the incoming Labour administration as it introduced its own policy directives. These changes were further compounded by the impact of devolution and the influence of this upon strategy development in the United Kingdom.

The learning disability document *'Signposts for success'* (NHSE 1997a), although published in the first few months of the Labour administration, was very much a document that reflected the achievements and issues of the previous government. It was not until 1999 that the governments of some of the four United Kingdom countries embarked upon a consultation process to inform the drawing up of their own learning disability strategies. A key issue that appears to be emerging from each of these areas of work is the need to focus upon the health needs of people who have a learning disability. This can be particularly considered from the context of inclusion, equality of access, fairness and equity. The evolving policy setting that provides the context for these initiatives also provides the focus for this chapter. Throughout, the emphasis is upon education and training with particular consideration of the roles and responsibilities of professional bodies within the emergence of new organizations that will increasingly set the agendas that the professions have to address.

The chapter is organized into three main sections. The first section provides a synopsis of some of the key trends and elements that the Labour administration inherited from the previous government. Devolution is one of the major constitutional reforms of the Labour administration and as such has a significant impact upon the delivery of health and social care to a small constituent group of the general population, i.e. people who have a learning disability. It is for this reason that an overview of learning disability policy in each of the four United Kingdom countries is presented in the second section. Finally, the third section considers the changing policy context, and agendas, in which education and training programmes are being designed and implemented. This is important in that the agendas being created within this context will have significant implications for the way in which both services are delivered and both health and social care professionals are educated.

THE CONSERVATIVE LEGACY

When the Labour administration was returned in May 1997 it set itself a number of timetables. A clear commitment to holding public spending to Conservative levels for the first 2 years indicated that little would change in the immediate future for a wide range of service provision, including health and social care. Exceptions were only in limited cases; for example, meeting election manifesto promises over 'education, education and education' and where there were 'immediate' political concerns, such as meeting heavy winter demands on health services and addressing the increasing demands over nurses' pay and conditions. While examples such as these occupied the centre stage for the media, the government also made announcements on the future structure of health and social care provision for when the commitments to Conservative spending levels expired.

An unpublished literature review identified a range of trends and issues with staffing implications in learning disabilities that the evolving health and social care agenda had to address (Brown et al 1999).

Trends

Developments over the last 30 years have led to a number of changes that have a significant impact upon service delivery and the training and education of the workforce. The most crucial of these has been the increasing autonomy of the person who has a learning disability, both in relation to the care and support that they receive and the planning and delivery of services. When considering the composition of the workforce, the specialist nurse practitioner in learning disabilities is currently *the* main professional resource available to both the health and social care arena. This relates to both numbers available and the range and diversity of skills that they bring to the user group. As such, therefore, on occasions this chapter will focus upon learning disability nurses. This is not to undermine the contribution of any other nurse or other health or social care professional in relation to meeting the health needs of this population but reflects their current position within the workforce.

Working within the current context of care delivery for people who have a learning disability, the specialist nurse practitioner increasingly has to work across a range of settings in both the statutory and independent (voluntary and private) sectors. In doing this the learning disability workforce has accepted the view that people who have a learning disability have social care rather than health needs. Recent literature has, however, clearly refocused the debate to include the healthcare needs of the population in order to support the effective meeting of their social care needs. It is the speed of these changes in service delivery that is responsible for creating the specific problems regarding educational preparation for both specialist and generic professionals. These developments have not always been without controversy. At the same time, debates around such developments have reflected, and contributed to, clearly discernible trends:

- The changing expectations of users and families and other informal carers to be actively involved in decisions that impinged upon their quality of life. It is no longer possible to ignore the views and feelings of those for whom support and care are being provided.

- The increasing weight of evidence that this group has distinct healthcare needs that necessitate specialist health input. Although the evidence is often not immediately comparable and can be focused upon very specific aspects of health, there is, across all four countries, data available that indicates the necessity of recognizing the specific health needs associated with having a learning disability.

- The continuing reliance upon the independent sector, especially private provision, to offer both residential and nursing accommodation. The independent sector is replacing the statutory sector as the main provider of this form of care.

- Within the residential/supported living sector, specific issues emerge regarding skill mix. Care delivery in these settings is often mediated through non-professionally qualified team members. This raises specific issues for nurses and other qualified professionals working in this environment and requires specific skills to ensure its success.

- The blurring of professional boundaries is continuing to gather momentum, particularly as new patterns of service design and delivery are creating changing expectations over both role and function of practitioners and the way in which they relate to both the service user and to their professional colleagues. This is important in the context of the partnership agenda which is outlined in much of the current policy.

- The emerging role of primary care as a possible fulcrum around which services in the community revolve. Primary care has new, albeit still embryonic structures that will inevitably impinge upon and possibly change the way in which both health and social needs are recognized and acted upon.

- The continuing issues around the closure of long-stay learning disability hospitals. Although hospital closure has been a distinctive part of policy across the UK for some time it is still necessary to create a momentum for closure that has a greater resonance in some of the four countries than in others.

- The promoting of partnerships between main stakeholders in order to create an integrated service that benefits the user. In spite of the many difficulties and obstacles to joint working, various local initiatives have shown that it can be achieved, even at a time when organizational structures and administrative responsibilities are undergoing considerable change.

From these trends a number of issues emerge that inform future directions in specialist nursing practice in learning disability together with implications for both generic professionals and care workers.

Issues

Increasing refinement of workforce planning has begun to distinguish between three distinct types of worker in learning disabilities, each with their own particular requirements and agendas.

The specialist practitioner

■ Consolidating and developing understanding of the health needs of this population built upon a rigorous evidence base.

■ Developing clinically effective and evidence-based interventions to meet these needs.

■ Ensuring that changing patterns of service design and delivery do not result in the loss of the specialist skills of the learning disability nurse to the user, irrespective of the setting in which those skills are practised.

■ Clarifying career profiles across health and social care that recognize cross-sector mobility.

■ Incorporating in education and training the full range of responsibilities that different sectors expect from a qualified practitioner, especially with regards to management and leadership abilities.

■ Promoting developments that enhance the ability of users to access health and social care services.

■ Facilitating learning disability nursing involvement in local, regional and national initiatives that ensure the specialist nurse practitioner is proactive rather than reactive to policy developments which impact upon the user's quality of life.

■ Developing interprofessional relationships across the health and social care spectrum that promote the needs of the users within the changing patterns of service delivery, especially in the primary care setting.

The generic worker

■ Developing sensitivity to the health and social care needs of those who have a learning disability.

■ Promoting awareness of how to incorporate specialist practice within an often wide and diverse user base within the community.

■ Ensuring familiarity with the often different expectations and practice context associated with the statutory and independent sectors.

■ Identifying constraints and ways to respond that facilitate the effective delivery of specialist practice to the user.

The care worker

- Recognizing the primacy of promoting the involvement of the user in decisions that influence the quality of their life.
- Preparing to work in a team where the delivery of specialist services is a integral part of care management.
- Fostering an awareness of issues around meeting the healthcare needs of those who have a learning disability.

For all staff working in learning disabilities the extent to which such issues influence their preparation and practice depends very much upon the local situation and, in particular, the history of services through which current thinking is filtered. This is especially the case when considering services in each of the four United Kingdom countries.

POLICY ACROSS THE UNITED KINGDOM

Across the four UK countries policy and associated issues vary depending upon their particular history as to the relationship between health and social care organizations and their respective responsibilities for the design and delivery of services for those who have a learning disability. Each country has a distinct history and tradition that is reflected in the way that its services have evolved and that, at times, can make direct comparison of any particular initiative difficult. Often there is an imbalance in the volume of material available between the four countries which, as a recent UK-wide focused article illustrates, can lead to a preponderance of English material (Ayer 1997). One Scottish commentator has argued that 'Although (policy documents may) address strategy in England they do highlight priorities which "commissioners" and "providers" in Scotland should consider' (Espie 1998). Comparative academic commentary between the four countries is limited. Nonetheless, it is possible to discern common concerns and similar issues.

Northern Ireland

In Northern Ireland since 1973 health and social services have been organized into a single management framework that oversees four health and social services boards. Research has indicated that the community care policy promoted through these boards could lead to an improved quality of life for those moved into the community from long-stay hospitals while also costing slightly less than hospital-based provision (Donnelly et al 1994). At the same time, this research identified a number of significant problems associated with an integrated structure of health and social care provision that were subsequently incorporated into a major review of learning disability services in Northern Ireland (DHSS 1978).

Published in 1995, the *'Review of policy for people with a learning disability'* looked at developments since publication of 'the 1978 statement' (DHSS 1995). Reaffirming commitment to that document's principles of prevention and normalization (subsequently called 'inclusion'), a number of achievements over the review period were identified:

- Targets set for a reduction in the number of learning disability hospital places had been met and those set for the 1992–97 Regional Strategy were on schedule.

- The reduction in the number of hospital places had enabled the boards to achieve significant improvements in hospital care.

- Bridging finance used for community care development had been beneficial.

- Targets for residential accommodation in the community had been met (and exceeded) although not necessarily within original timetables.

- Day-care facilities had expanded in line with targets although day-care services remained under pressure.

These achievements, however, were also associated with a number of difficulties:

- Health promotion and education had not had a high profile.
- Proper planning of services was hampered by lack of appropriate data.
- Choice was restricted owing to a limited mix of accommodation.
- Community 'mental handicap' teams were not working well in practice.
- The flow of resources was inadequate to maintain the shift in service provision.
- Primary healthcare was failing to meet the totality of needs of people who have a learning disability.

From this analysis a number of 'critical issues' were identified:

- The future of long-stay beds and the outcomes for those discharged.

- A fundamental shift in resources to meet the full range of community care services required by those who have a learning disability.

- The development of health promotion and prevention.

- Improving access to facilitate inclusion.

- Recognizing carers' needs in the assessment process.

- Consideration of the minimum qualification and professional skill mixes required in non-hospital settings along with the need to prepare hospital staff to work in the community (DHSS 1995).

These points identified and discussed in the review have formed the basis for a Regional Strategy for the 5-year period 1997–2002. Two targets are identified (DHSS 1997).

1. Each board and trust should develop a comprehensive range of supportive services for people who have a learning disability and their carers. The overall objective is that, by 2002, long-term institutional care should no longer be provided in traditional specialist hospital environments.

2. As an integral feature of the comprehensive services, specialist provision should be linked to community-based care and treatment which should reduce the number of adults who have a learning disability admitted to specialist hospitals by 50% and the number of children, other than in exceptional cases, to zero by 2002.

These targets are tied to 11 action areas:

1. Better information about people who have a learning disability
2. Reallocation of resources
3. Monitoring of residential placements
4. Development of respite care services
5. Availability of advocacy and empowerment services
6. Clear hospital discharge policy and procedures
7. Better information for people who have a learning disability and their families and carers
8. Availability of a comprehensive service for children with complex disabilities
9. Development of specialist provision for adults with complex needs
10. Review of the composition and role of community learning disability teams
11. The promotion of cross-professional education and development.

With the 1999 publication *Fit for the future – a new approach* containing no explicit reference to learning disabilities, these action areas and the two targets provide the current basis and focus for developing services in Northern Ireland (DHSS 1999). The emphasis is very much upon moving away from dependence on long-stay hospital accommodation as the mainstay of provision and ensuring that, at the same time, there is a corresponding increase in community services and facilities. A similar situation can be found in Scotland.

Scotland

In Scotland the 1988 document *Scottish Health Authorities review of priorities for the eighties and nineties* (SHARPEN) identified people who have a learning disability as a priority group (Scottish Office 1988). Promoting services to meet the needs of this priority group was organized through 15 health boards that in 1995 were replaced by 18 area health boards. In 1996, unitary local government authorities were introduced to replace the existing two-tier authorities. Together these two changes have had an impact upon the move away from long-stay hospital provision into the community that was outlined in a review of long-stay hospitals published in 1993 (Scottish Home and Health Department 1993).

This is illustrated by a recent evaluation of the Greater Glasgow Joint Learning Disability Project. Here the health board initially established a partnership with one social work authority only to find itself, following local government reorganization, dealing with six social work authorities each with an expanded remit to include housing (Dalrymple 1999). The challenge that this posed is compounded by a situation where, historically, the move into the community and reduction of long-stay hospital places has been slower in Scotland than the rest of the UK (Dalrymple 1999). The pressure that this created to up-date the 1993 paper led to a review of policy for learning disabilities (Scottish Office 1998a) that has been accompanied by publication of a 'position statement' on learning disabilities nursing in Scotland (Scottish Office 1999).

The position paper states that 'Developments (from institutional to community care) are often unplanned and are lacking in a strategic direction or coherence' (Scottish Office 1999). The call is made for an integrated approach from health, social work, education and housing to service design and delivery as no one agency can deliver the vision for integrated, as opposed to segregated, care. Similar concerns to the Northern Ireland action areas are identified although, given the specific focus of the position statement, greater emphasis is given to the contribution of the learning disability nurse specialist.

The distinctive contribution is seen as being derived 'from their focus on positively influencing behaviour and lifestyle' (Scottish Office 1999) with an emphasis upon working in partnership with the individual to improve their personal autonomy and promote positive health. In particular, six key areas of activity are identified:

1. Child health
2. Meeting health needs
3. Working in partnership with the independent sector
4. Working in partnership with local authority social work departments
5. Meeting the needs of those who present a challenge to the services
6. Planning and development

Central to all these activities is the recognition that expectations of both carers and clients/users have changed dramatically and that they have to be involved in processes and procedures that directly impinge upon their lives. This is found also in the Northern Ireland document (DHSS 1997) and has been an integral aspect of developments in Wales.

Wales

Although administratively linked with England until devolution in 1999, Wales has, since 1983, had a distinctive policy for learning disability in the All Wales Strategy (AWS) that has provided clear guidelines about the responsibility at local and county level (Welsh Office 1983). The AWS was built around the three principles originally outlined in the Jay Report:

1. The right of those who have a learning disability to normal patterns of life in the community.
2. The right to be treated as individuals.
3. The right to additional support if required to pursue their maximum potential (DHSS 1979).

The AWS clearly recognized the important role and contribution of the voluntary sector together with that of informal carers and was among the first to consider ways in which the consumer could be meaningfully involved in decisions that affected them (All Wales Advisory Panel 1991, Donovan & Allen 1986).

Recent evaluation of the AWS has indicated that problems encountered in the other UK countries in coordinating services have also been found with the AWS (Welsh Office 1994). For example, even though investment is made in local authority services it does not mean that hospital closure automatically follows (Felce et al 1998). Timing and momentum are crucial. Similarly, preparation of staff and attitudes is crucial as services evolve and develop. In addition, work undertaken in Wales indicated significant health needs amongst the learning disability population (Welsh Office 1983, 1996). The Chief Nursing Officer for Wales responded to this changing context by producing a 10-point action plan for learning disability nursing (Chief Nursing Officer for Wales 1997):

1. Promote more healthy lifestyles.
2. Ensure care programmes are collaboratively planned and evaluated.
3. Develop knowledge and skills through appropriate clinical supervision.
4. Involve service users in the development of the nursing curricula.
5. Provide access to the range of information for service users and their carers to make informed choices.
6. Work with multiagency colleagues.
7. Identify the true costs of meeting identified needs, including the 'direct care' nursing component.
8. Identify and publicize good learning disability nursing practice across Wales.
9. Develop mechanisms to improve links between learning disability services and general health services.
10. Be involved in setting up appropriate response services for those with additional needs.

This emphasis upon identifying skills appropriate to the learning disability nurse as services develop in response to current philosophies of care can also be found in England where work is under way to determine the skills required within the whole of the learning disability workforce.

England

In England there is commitment to community care and recognition, as in the rest of the UK, of the importance of providing services that place the user central to service delivery (DoH 1997a). Whilst wide variations in the patterns of collaboration can be found between the NHS and local government (Nocon 1994), it is possible to begin to identify key principles that underpin the delivery of coordinated services to the user that enhance quality of life irrespective of the particular structure through which they are delivered. For example, an initiative promoting a joint partnership between health and social services in London illustrates the importance of (Lewisham, Southwark and Lewisham Health Authority/Lewisham Social Services 1998; see also DoH 1998e):

- shared values; commitment to making the initiative work
- willingness to be innovative on behalf of users
- identifying and using all available potential sources of funding
- adopting a comprehensive approach that recognizes the importance of diversity in learning disabilities, e.g. ethnicity.

Such principles of joint working can also underpin the promotion of ever closer working together between sectors that the government has begun to establish through pilot schemes for Health Action Zones together with Health Improvement Programmes (DoH 1997a). Each of these provides the opportunity to design and deliver services in ways that break away from traditional assumptions and patterns. Whether this happens remains to be seen.

With Health Action Zones focused primarily upon deprived areas, the emphasis is upon minimizing, if not actually eradicating, health inequalities based upon broad social disadvantage. Built upon notions around 'social exclusion', it is noticeable that this concept does not have to include learning disabilities (DoH 1999a). As the remit includes, but goes much wider than, primary care with consideration being given to the interrelationship between health, housing, education and employment, the findings from such pilot schemes could have profound implications for all learning disability nurses and other professionals working across boundaries and barriers.

Similarly, the introduction of Health Improvement Programmes highlights one of the key areas of activity that should involve the learning disability specialist and which has a clearer focus in the health promotion White Papers *Our healthier nation* and *Saving lives* (DoH 1998a, 1999b). With the emphasis upon public involvement in influencing local programmes, there is the possibility of involving people who have a learning disability in such a process, especially as consultation for a new NHS Charter specifically identifies using advocates for those who have communication problems (DoH 1998b), a scenario that indicates real rewards for people who have a learning disability (Ramcharan et al 1997). The challenge for all those working in learning disability services, particularly in relation to meeting the health needs of this client group, is to maximize those opportunities, particularly in a context in which they are not specifically mentioned in recent White Papers (DoH 1998a, 1999b).

Against this backdrop of potentially profound policy change, the available literature has yet to reflect how learning disability professionals are adapting to the evolving situation. In the past, learning disability nurses have exploited their position on the margins of nursing and away from the mainstream (a usual position occupied by all learning disability practitioners irrespective of their profession) to promote new and, for some, novel ways of working (Trecare NHS Trust 1998).

There is evidence of pioneering work in developing joint and shared training developments, primarily with social work (Brown 1994a) and occupational therapy (Weinstein 1995). Innovative ways of delivering support and care, often in the context of 'normalization' initiatives (Towell & Beardshaw 1991), have been introduced. In addition, there have been lessons from multidisciplinary team work (Ovretveit 1994) as well as work on 'multiskilling' (Smith 1999). Such work is, and has been, vitally important yet in many ways this has not been sufficient to establish the professional credibility of the learning disability nurse. All too often, it is difficult to shake off the legacy of the past where the specialist skills required to provide high-quality support and care were often not apparent to a wide range of commentators (Brown 1994b, DHSS 1972, DoH 1995, RCN 1964).

The publication of *Signposts for success* and other similar documents (e.g. NHSE 1999) does, however, begin to establish the specialist health skills required from those involved with people who have a learning disability, whether a nurse or other professional. In reality, these skills are those practised by the learning disability nurse specialist for, as the Jay Committee recognized two decades ago (DHSS 1979), there is no other professional group active in this area in sufficient numbers to offer and deliver the skills required. These skills are many and various. Fundamentally, they revolve around providing continuity of care, providing routine health checks (which can be anything but routine in the skills required), health education and promotion, providing specialist support for those with physical and sensory deprivation and the assistance to use services (DoH 1996a).

The English National Board for Nursing, Midwifery and Health Visiting identifies four key areas of learning disability nursing in which specific skills can be clustered (ENB 1999):

1. Meeting the healthcare needs of people who have learning disabilities.
2. Undertaking leadership roles within learning disability nursing.
3. Assisting people who have learning disabilities to develop self-advocacy skills.
4. Working in the independent sector.

It is important that the skills associated with these areas are in the public domain as they legitimize the necessity for specialist health input at a time when it is vitally important to promote the case for such specialized skills, together with the case for appropriate staff preparation. Not only are there the developments within health and social care (the traditional arena for the nurse specialist) but there are also debates in other areas that could impinge indirectly upon the resources available for learning disabilities and the profile that they have on the policy agenda.

This is especially the case in the area of employment initiatives which could have ramifications far beyond this immediate area in the way it helps to establish the position of learning disabilities with other groups representing the interests of people who have a disability. It cannot be assumed that others who have a disability are necessarily sensitive to the specific needs of those who have a learning disability.

The disability lobby

Within the first 18 months of the Labour government plans were announced for the establishment of a Disability Rights Commission (DoH 1998c) together with the establishment of a Disability Rights Task Force (DoH 1997b). Such initiatives are an integral part of the government's White Paper on welfare reform and, in particular, the relationship between benefits and employment. It is clear that the employment as well as related education needs of the disabled have a greater prominence than has been the case in recent years, even allowing for the passing of the Disability Discrimination Act 1995. What is not at all certain, however, is how those who have a learning disability will fit into the emerging political discourse on disability.

In the 1990s it was possible for books purporting to review and analyse the experience of all those who have a disability to ignore learning disabilities (Barnes 1994). Even in more recent publications there is an in-built leaning towards those who have a physical disability (Corker & French 1998). It appears that learning disability can be subject to the same prejudice and discrimination from within the politically active sections of the disability community as it experiences from the wider society – a form of 'double jeopardy'.

In the policy arena it cannot be assumed that the disability lobby, just as it is beginning to have an impact upon debate, will necessarily view learning disabilities as an integral part of its activities or even as a possible ally. In fact, it may well see learning disabilities as a potential rival for scarce resources and government favour.

Against this backdrop of policy developments, the immediate context in which staff are prepared for practice is itself undergoing profound changes.

CHANGING AGENDAS

The introduction of the NHS and Community Care Act 1990 signalled a dramatic change in the context in which issues around health and social care were raised and addressed. Emphasis upon the internal market and the process of commissioning and purchasing raised issues that underpin recent policy documents published in each of the four UK countries (DHSS 1999, DoH 1997a, Scottish Office 1998b, Welsh Office 1998). Of particular significance is the emphasis upon redefining responsibilities that is illustrated in the proposals for primary healthcare.

Evolving professional relationships

With developments under way for a radical reshaping of primary care, the relationships between the different professionals working in the new primary care structures become crucial. A recent report from the Health Services Select Committee on the relationship between health and social care lambasts the professionals for failing to work together in ways that promote the well-being of service users (House of Commons Health Select Committee 1999a). This is reinforced in the findings of subsequent reports from the Committee where the introduction of primary care groups in England (House of Commons Health Select Committee 1999b) and staffing issues in the NHS (House of Commons Health Select Committee 1999c) are considered.

General practitioners, along with nursing colleagues, clearly face a period of considerable change and uncertainty. This has been further heightened by the introduction of Personal Medical Services (PMS) where general practitioners can become salaried employees of the NHS rather than necessarily retaining their current self-employed status (Health Act, 1999). The significance of such a development is that there no longer has to be the expectation that leadership within general practice necessarily will be the prerogative of medical practitioners. Indeed, 'for the first time, nurses will be able to lead in the delivery of primary care services, including employing GPs' (DoH 1997c, p. 1). Admist such potentially momentous changes to the way that established practice, and expectations, are approached there is the possibility that learning disabilities is not seen as an urgent priority. This is a real danger.

There is anecdotal as well as published evidence, however, that general practitioners often fail to appreciate the specific needs of people who have learning disabilities (DHSS 1995). In many ways there is little reason to expect their attitudes to be any different from members of the public given the paucity of exposure to learning disability in their training (Ovretveit et al 1997). Overall, this lack of awareness can be a major concern (NHSE 1999). Where there is considerable pressure upon all professionals involved with primary care, it cannot be assumed that learning disabilities will be at the forefront of concerns for those directly affected by change, especially if they are not appreciative of specific issues around this area (DoH 1995), particularly as both health visiting and district nursing have recently been under the spotlight (Audit Commission 1999, DoH 1999c). Such uncertainty is mirrored in developments affecting the regulatory bodies.

Regulatory reviews

The regulatory bodies across the professions in health and social care are facing considerable changes in their structure and function. Over the last 2 years a number of proposals have been announced and initiatives introduced that will change the professional landscape.

In social work, the Central Council for Education and Training in Social Work (CCETSW) is to be replaced by the General Social Care Council and, in a new development for social work, will eventually have a regulatory function through a register of qualified practitioners (DoH 1998d, House of Commons 2000a). Trends indicate that just as services are being integrated and structures are converging, professional registers could well be moving to a situation where they complement each other, making eventual amalgamation under a common organizational and administrative umbrella a real possibility.

The Council for the Professions Supplementary to Medicine is to be replaced by a new Council for Health Professions (Health Act 1999, NHSE 2000b), a title that indicates that professions such as physiotherapy and the like are no longer viewed as necessarily 'supplementary' or 'allied' to medicine. At the same time, the new title is sufficiently broad that it does not in theory preclude other professions involved in healthcare also being included at some future date.

Nursing is also to undergo potentially significant change with the government accepting the main recommendations of a consultation exercise from JM Consulting to replace the UKCC and four national boards (DoH 1999c, NHSE 2000a). Of the small number of recommendations from this exercise rejected by the government, probably the most important was to remove health visiting as a specialized area of nursing activity. The retention of health visiting has potentially important implications for the work of learning disability nurses in the community as different nursing specialisms begin to realign themselves relative to each other and to other professions.

On a broader level the fact that nursing constitutes the largest occupational group within the NHS workforce (DoH 1994) has a potential resonance in the debates over 'integrated workforce planning' that to date has not been possible to consider. Actively promoted in government documents (DoH 1996b) and Executive Letters (DoH 2000b, NHSE 1996, 1997b), integrated workforce planning has increasingly been seen as difficult to achieve, not least because of the difficulties in adequately allowing for the complexity of the variables influencing this process, such as recruitment and retention and medical workforce planning.

This one decision, probably more than any other, indicates the seriousness with which the government is pursuing its health agenda. An integral part of this is clearly looking very closely at the work of the professions, especially in the area of regulation and accountability. In many ways, the present government has picked up the mantle left by the Conservatives who set out to 'control health professions' (Harrison & Pollitt 1994).

On the same day that the response to JM Consulting was made public, the Secretary of State announced to a delegation of senior nurses that nurse education was to stay in the higher education arena (Butterworth 1999). This was the resolution of a furious debate, sparked by comments from the Secretary of State, over whether the integration of nursing into higher education in 1996 had been an appropriate initiative. Although the status quo appears to have prevailed the debate has had the effect of subtly changing the context in which nurse education is delivered through higher education institutions. In particular, it has begun to alter the balance between higher education and the nurse education commissioners.

Accreditation

Traditionally there has been a tension between service and education in nursing (Owens & Glennerster 1990). In recent years, higher education institutions (HEIs) have entered the equation with former Colleges of Health/Nursing being integrated into HEI.

When, in 1988, the former schools of nursing became colleges of health/nursing they became either affiliated or associated to local HEIs. While some sought full integration into their local HEI, and there were already a number of long-established degree programmes offered by a small number of universities, it was not until the full integration of colleges into HEIs in 1996 that higher education became a major player in the provision of nurse education. Arguments that integration had led to Project 2000 students not being 'fit to practise' along with concerns about 'value for money' were nothing new. A government report in the early 1990s, just as Project 2000 was beginning to gain momentum, had raised such issues long before the move into higher education (National Audit Office 1992). That the issue was raised at the beginning of the year 2000, and in the terms used with claims that nurse preparation was an 'apprenticeship' and by implication not a first degree subject, probably highlighted the fact that the integration process had itself caused difficulties.

Although there has been no systematic survey at either national or regional level of the integration exercise, there is limited, and often anecdotal, evidence from around the UK that the exercise has met with varying degrees of success. Integration has been interpreted in a variety of ways, with former colleges being autonomous organizational entities within a university through to their being incorporated into a faculty structure where nursing is but one part of a range of health-related activities. Irrespective of the structure, there is no denying that the influx of NHS contract monies has been welcomed by universities experiencing ever-present funding difficulties. The political questioning of the location of nurse education in HEIs is a timely reminder that the NHS expects a return on its investment.

It also signals to commissioners and purchasers that, for some forms of nurse education and training, higher education may not be the most appropriate setting. The development and increasing adoption of national and regional credit-based initiatives where, for example, the local trust designs and delivers its own modules that are accredited and validated by the local university, is one potential way forward (Humberside and Yorkshire Credit Award Scheme 1999). The emphasis is very much upon the employer getting what they want by doing it themselves. Such a development uses universities in a totally different way. In many ways this signals the increasing emphasis upon employer-determined training rather than profession-led education that the introduction of National Vocational Qualifications heralded at the beginning of the decade (Smither 1994).

The expanding number of players in the education of the health and social care workforce

All this adds to the pressures upon nurse educationalists. Senior nurse managers now have to address not just the NHS agenda but also the higher education agenda. Both of these agendas are themselves undergoing radical change. In the NHS, along with the developments outlined above, there is the evolving role of education consortia (initially called education and training consortia) (NHSE 1997b) through which contracts are negotiated for nurse education. In higher education there is the impact of the Dearing Report (DfEE 1997a) as well as anticipated implications of the Betts Committee investigating a number of issues including contracts and employment, and the relationship between pre- and post-1992 universities.

Against these broad developments which are influencing the parameters within which programmes are designed and delivered, there are immediate pressing concerns: making sure that modules are flexible, providing high-quality placements across settings, while offering a comprehensive range of accessible programmes (Brown 1998).

In addition, the introduction of national training organizations (NTOs) to establish and promote occupational standards across the whole spectrum of training (DfEE 1997b), including both health and social care, has important implications throughout the statutory and voluntary sectors and especially for the professions (DoH 1998f). Although it is still early days in their functioning, difficulties are already emerging between the UK NTOs and those located in each of the four countries. This is but one aspect of the work of NTOs that could impinge upon learning disabilities.

With the lead for learning disabilities located in the social care NTO (or TOPSS, Training Organization for Personal Social Services) there is a clear need to consider the interface between TOPSS and Healthwork, the health NTO, so that the health needs of the users are not ignored or, at worst, lost. This is a salutary reminder of the importance of remembering, amidst the drive into the community that characterized the late 1980s through to the mid-1990s (Means & Smith 1999), that people who have learning disabilities often have particular and specific health needs that have to be met. Initial work has, not surprisingly, addressed broad workforce concerns.

Towards the end of 1999 TOPSS announced its intention to establish a clear strategy for the social care workforce (TOPSS 1999a). This was accompanied by a specific discussion paper on the learning disability workforce (TOPSS 1999b). Great emphasis was placed upon those staff working in the private residential sector, of whom it was estimated that some 80% had no qualification or adequate preparation to work with those who have a learning disability. This signals a clear intention to shift the historic focus upon professional staff across to all categories of staff, a trend reinforced by initiatives such as the Learning Disability Awards Framework (LDAF) that seeks, initially, to provide 'pathways' through the emerging National Qualifications Framework for non-professionally qualified staff (LDAF 2000).

At the same time, the private residential sector is increasingly providing employment opportunities for the qualified specialist nurse practitioner in learning disabilities as the sector as a whole becomes the mainstay of residential provision. However, this is accompanied, as with other user groups in the independent sector, by a situation where the great majority of staff providing direct care have received little or no training (TOPSS 1999a).

The regulation of the independent sector will move away from direct local authority control (DoH 1998e) and clearer guidance has emerged on the internal management and responsibilities of residential and nursing homes (DoH 1999d). Taken together, it is clear that the nursing profession as a whole cannot ignore the independent sector as it addresses issues raised by its own future direction in both preparation and practice.

Nurse preparation and practice

In 1999 two complementary reports were published that will probably prove to be seminal in shaping the direction of nursing in the immediate future. The first, *Making a difference* (DoH 1999e), outlined the overall context in which nurse preparation, practice and career progression will take place. The second, *Fitness for practice* (UKCC 1999), provided consideration of the specific detailed content to be placed within the context identified by the Department of Health.

In *Making a difference*, four career 'ranges' are identified. Ranges Two and Three coincide with preregistration and postregistration levels respectively. Range Four relates to the new 'nurse consultant' post, introduced to help stem problems in retention as well as to recognize the evolving role of the nurse practitioner in areas once seen as the prerogative of the medical practitioner. It is Range One, however, in which possibly the most radical changes are proposed. This is seen as embracing NVQs Levels 1–3 with Level 3, in certain circumstances, being used to fast-track past the Common Foundation Programme (CFP) straight on to a specialist branch programme. It is also expected that the NVQ programme will be offered by further education, which could also embrace responsibility for the CFP.

Such a development reflects the necessity of nursing undertaking a major rethink of its position on vocational qualifications and incorporating them within the framework of nursing progression, with crucial implications for learning disabilities with initiatives such as LDAF. At the same time, the reopening of the debate over the location of nurse education in higher education only months after it appeared to be resolved indicates that the discussion is far from over. Similarly, *Fitness for practice* has implications for the specialist nurse practitioner in learning disabilities. With the report prepared within 12 months, the UKCC Commission stated that there was insufficient time to consider whether the present four branch programmes – learning disabilities, mental health, adult and children – were still an appropriate division of activity. Established initially in 1919 with the Nurses Registration Act, the four branches, with changes in terminology, have remained the basis of specialist training at the preregistration level ever since. In the present climate, no branch programme can assume that it is immune from fundamental change, including possible realignment and extinction.

FUTURE DIRECTION

Taken together, the Department of Health and UKCC reports indicate that there are major changes about to embrace nursing as a whole. Such changes are taking place within a fresh legislative approach to the health and social care agenda.

Proposals around social care (DoH 2000c), together with calls in the NHS Plan to establish integrated 'Care Trusts' where 'social services would be delivered under delegated authority from local councils (to the NHS)' (DoH 2000a, p. 73) underpinned the Health and Social Care Bill published at the end of 2000 (House of Commons 2000b). Here the accompanying press release spoke of Care Trusts taking responsibility '...for *all* local health and social care... (providing a) one stop shop, including social care *and other local authority related services, such as housing*' (DoH 2000f p. 2, emphasis added). With such a potentially radical shake-up of organisational boundaries it was no surprise that in discussing a strategy for the allied health professions comments were made that 'this will require changes to traditional patterns of working' (DoH 2000d, p. 15).

The challenge for learning disability nurses is to ensure that these changes do not disadvantage the user who has learning disabilities. At the same time, it is imperative that sight is not lost of specific areas of activity that, along with a new White Paper for learning disability (DoH 2000e), will inform the direction that learning disability nursing takes in the future. These include six initiatives to inform the educational and training dimensions of the specialist, generic and care worker across the four UK countries:

1. Healthcare needs: collecting valid and reliable data that enable the profiling of needs in ways that address issues around the necessity for specialist *and* generic services and associated professional support.

2. Skills development: clarifying the skills required of learning disability nurses in a variety of settings at pre- and postregistration levels.

3. Workforce profiles: establishing a database of deployment that enable the tracing of career paths across sectors, together with accompanying roles and functions, that can inform both pre- and postregistration courses together with debates over integrated workforce planning.

4. Access pathways: clarifying the paths for the user through evolving patterns of service delivery, especially in health, and the contribution of the specialist practitioner to identifying and developing integrated care pathways through provision.

5. Partnership initiatives: collecting evidence that is both rigorous and systematic to enable the replication of successful joint service development that best meets the needs of the user in ways that reflect current national thinking in each of the four countries.

6. Service provision maps: identifying emerging infrastructures of services that enable both purchasers and providers to locate the work of the learning disability nurse practitioner so that their specific skills remain available to users.

The response to each of these areas has to address the type of policy agendas and initiatives outlined throughout the chapter. In considering the relevant policy agendas, it is necessary to think across boundaries and to anticipate the impact of developments in areas as diverse as housing, health, social care, education, employment, police and the criminal justice system upon the health needs of people who have a learning disability. Without such an approach, the achievements of the last three decades could be undermined, if not lost. Should this occur, the quality of life available to people who have a learning disability will be seriously compromised.

FURTHER READING

The majority of references for this chapter are government reports, consultation documents and White Papers. In recent years there has been a veritable avalanche of documents announcing government intentions. Finding your way around can be difficult and time consuming. The following suggestions are intended to provide an introduction to key topic areas. These can be followed up in greater detail using the references listed for the chapter.

National Health Service Executive 1997 Signposts for success in commissioning and providing health services for people with learning disabilities. Department of Health, London
Still one of the best introductions to policy issues and learning disabilities. Usually abbreviated to Signposts for success, or just Signposts, this provides a comprehensive and accessible guide to good practice in health services, both general and specialist, as well as service redevelopment.

Department of Health 1997 The new NHS: modern, dependable. Cm 3807. The Stationery Office, London
For a succinct introduction to Labour policy on all aspects of the NHS, the White Paper published within a few months of their election victory in 1997 provides general information about initiatives directly relevant to learning disabilities as well as other user groups.

Department of Health 2000 The NHS plan – a plan for investment; a plan for reform. Cm 4818. The Stationery Office, London
Essential background reading to new patterns of responsibilities within health and social care.

House of Commons Health Select Committee 1999 The relationship between health and social care. First report, HC 74-1. The Stationery Office, London
For a more detailed consideration of the difficulties involved with promoting partnership, this review carried out by the all-party House of Commons Health Select Committee is possibly the most thorough currently available.

Department of Health 1999 Making a difference: strengthening the nursing, midwifery and health visiting contribution to health and healthcare. Department of Health, London

United Kingdom Central Council for Nursing, Midwifery and Health Visiting 1999 Fitness for practice (the Peach Report). UKCC, London
The debate over workforce planning is at the heart of current NHS concerns. Central to this debate is the future of nurse education and training which is being taken forward on the basis of these two complementary documents.

Although neither refers directly to learning disabilities, the discussion they contain about future directions and the way that government develops the arguments will have a profound impact upon the future of learning disability nursing.

Training Organization for Personal Social Services (England) 1999 Modernising the social care workforce – the first national strategy for England: supplementary report on learning disabilities. TOPSS, London

Finally, to gain appreciation of the issues around staffing services for people with learning disabilities in the independent sector, this discussion document illustrates some of the concerns that will inform future strategy initiatives. It provides clear examples of the paucity of data available upon which to base strategic decisions. Crucially, it gives a solid introduction to the concerns of policy makers as educational initiatives have to address new agendas associated with workforce planning.

REFERENCES

All Wales Advisory Panel 1991 Consumer involvement and the All Wales Strategy. Report from the Consumer Involvement Sub-Group. All Wales Advisory Group, Cardiff

Audit Commission 1999 A review of district nurse services in England and Wales. The Stationery Office, London

Ayer S 1997 Services for people with learning disabilities in the UK. In: Gates B, Beacock C (eds) Dimensions of learning disability. Baillière Tindall, London, pp 264–293

Barnes C 1994 Disabled people in Britain. Hurst, London

Brown J 1994a The hybrid worker. SPSW Publishing, York

Brown J 1994b Analysis of responses to the consensus statement on the future of the specialist nurse practitioner in learning disabilities. Department of Health, London

Brown J 1998 The NHS perspective. Health Professions Committee of the Committee of Vice-Chancellors and Principals. Unpublished presentation

Brown J, Churchill J, Thompson J 1999 Learning disabilities: a policy paper. UKCC, unpublished

Butterworth T 1999 Report of a meeting with Secretary of State for Health and Social Services. e-mail distributed 9 February 1999

Chief Nursing Officer for Wales 1997 Caring for the future: the nursing agenda learning disability nursing action plan. CNO (97)4. Welsh Office, Cardiff

Corker M, French S 1998 Disability discourse. Open University Press, Buckingham

Dalrymple J 1999 Deinstitutionalisation and community services in Greater Glasgow. Tizard Learning Disability Review 4:13–23

Department for Education and Employment 1997a Higher education for a learning society (the Dearing Report). The Stationery Office, London

Department for Education and Employment 1997b A guide to achieving NTO status: promoting sector skills. Department for Education and Employment, London

Department of Health 1994 The challenges for nursing and midwifery in the 21st century. Department of Health, London

Department of Health 1995 Continuing the commitment: the report of the Learning Disability Nursing Project. Department of Health, London

Department of Health 1996a Learning disability: meeting needs through targeting skills. A guide to learning disability nursing for health and social care commissioners, GP fundholders, NHS trusts and the independent sector. Department of Health, London

Department of Health 1996b The National Health Service: a service with ambitions. Cm 3425. The Stationery Office, London

Department of Health 1997a The new NHS: modern, dependable. Cm 3807. The Stationery Office, London

Department of Health 1997b Disability rights task force established. Ministerial statement, 3 December. Department of Health, London

Department of Health 1997c New pilots will improve quality in primary care services. Press Release 97/416. Department of Health, London

Department of Health 1998a Our healthier nation: a contract for health. Cm 3857. The Stationery Office, London

Department of Health 1998b The new NHS charter: a different report (the Dyke Report). The Stationery Office, London

Department of Health 1998c Promoting disabled people's rights: creating a Disability Rights Commission fit for the 21st century. The Stationery Office, London

Department of Health 1998d Social worker training to be replaced. Press release 98/415. Department of Health, London

Department of Health 1998e Partnership in action: new opportunities for joint working between health and social services – a discussion document. Department of Health, London

Department of Health 1998f Modernising social services: promoting independence, improving protection, raising standards. Cm 4169. The Stationery Office, London

Department of Health 1999a Health Action Zones are the front-line in the war on health inequalities. Press release 1999/0182. Department of Health, London

Department of Health 1999b Saving lives: our healthier nation. Cm 4386. The Stationery Office, London

Department of Health 1999c New single body announced to regulate nurses, midwives and health visitors. Press release 1999/0070. Department of Health, London

Department of Health 1999d Fit for the future? National required standards for residential and nursing homes for older people: consultation document. Department of Health, London

Department of Health 1999e Making a difference: strengthening the nursing, midwifery and health visiting contribution to health and healthcare. Department of Health, London

Department of Health 2000a The NHS plan – a plan for investment; a plan for reform, Cm 4818. The Stationery Office, London

Department of Health 2000b A health service of all the talents: developing the NHS workforce, a consultation document. Department of Health, London

Department of Health 2000c A quality strategy for social care, a consultation document. Department of Health, London

Department of Health 2000d Meeting the challenge: a strategy for the allied health professions. Department of Health, London

Department of Health 2000e Minister outlines plans for learning disability strategy. Press Release 2000/0597. Department of Health, London

Department of Health 2000f Radical reform will put patients at centre of NHS. Press Release 2000/0717. Department of Health, London

Department of Health and Social Security 1972 Report of the Committee of Nursing (the Briggs Report). Cm 5115. HMSO, London

Department of Health and Social Security 1978 Services for the mentally handicapped in Northern Ireland – policy and objectives 1978. HMSO, Belfast

Department of Health and Social Security 1979 Report of the Committee of Enquiry into Mental Handicap Nursing and Care (the Jay Report). Cm 7648. HMSO, London

Department of Health and Social Services 1995 Review of policy for people with a learning disability. DHSS, Belfast

Department of Health and Social Services 1997 Health and well-being: into the next millennium. Regional strategy for health and social well-being 1997–2002. HMSO, Belfast

Department of Health and Social Services 1999 Fit for the future – a new approach. DHSS, Belfast

Donnelly M, McGilloway S, Mays N et al 1994 Opening new doors: an evaluation of community care for people discharged from psychiatric and mental handicap hospitals. HMSO, London

Donovan T, Allen D 1986 The AWS from a parent's point of view. Part 1 – attitudes to integrated services. Mental Handicap 14:19–21

English National Board for Nursing, Midwifery and Health Visiting 1999 Key areas in learning disability nursing – a review of programmes. 1999\06\GMB. ENB, London

Espie C A 1998 Health needs and learning disabilities: an overview. Health Bulletin 56:603–611

Felce D, Grant G, Todd S et al 1998 Towards a fuller life: researching policy innovation for people with learning disabilities. Butterworth Heinemann, Oxford

Harrison S, Pollitt C 1994 Controlling health professions: the future of work and organisation in the NHS. Open University Press, Buckingham

Health Act 1999 Chapter 08. The Stationery Office, London

House of Commons 2000a Care Standards Bill, Part IV. The Stationery Office, London

House of Commons 2000b Health and Social Care Bill. The Stationery Office, London

House of Commons Health Select Committee 1999a The relationship between health and social care. First report, HC 74-1. The Stationery Office, London

House of Commons Health Select Committee 1999b Primary care groups. Second report, HC 153. The Stationery Office, London

House of Commons Health Select Committee 1999c Future NHS staffing requirements. Third report, HC 38-1. The Stationery Office, London

Humberside and Yorkshire Credit Award Scheme 1999 Final report. Unpublished. HYCAS, Leeds

Learning Disability Awards Framework 2000 Statement of aims. LDAF, Chesterfield

Lewisham, Southwark and Lewisham Health Authority/Lewisham Social Services 1998 Strategy for adults with a learning disability. Lewisham Partnership, London

Means R, Smith R 1999 Community care: policy and practice, 2nd edn. Macmillan, London

National Audit Office 1992 Implementing
Project 2000. HMSO, London
National Health Service Executive 1996
Education and training planning guidance
(96)46. Department of Health, London
National Health Service Executive 1997a
Signposts for success in commissioning and
providing health services for people with
learning disabilities. Department of Health,
London
National Health Service Executive 1997b
Devolution of responsibilities to education
consortia. EL(97)30. Department of Health,
London
National Health Service Executive 1999 Once
a day: one or more people with learning
disabilities are likely to be in contact with
your primary healthcare team. Department
of Health, London
National Health Service Executive 2000a
Modernising regulation – the new
Nursing and Midwifery Council, a
consultation document. Department of
Health, London
National Health Service Executive 2000b
Modernising regulation – the new Health
Professions Council, a consultation
document. Department of Health, London
Nocon A 1994 Collaboration in community
care in the 1990s. Business Education
Publishers, Tyne and Wear
Ovretveit J 1994 Co-ordination community
care services: multidisciplinary teams and
care management. Open University Press,
Buckingham
Ovretveit J, Mathias P, Thompson T (eds)
1997 Interprofessional relations in health
and social care. Baillière Tindall, London
Owens P, Glennerster H 1990 Nursing in
conflict. Macmillan, London
Ramcharan P, Roberts G, Grant G, Borland J
(eds) 1997 Empowerment in everyday life:
learning disability. Jessica Kingsley
Publishers, London
Royal College of Nursing 1964 First report of
a Special Committee for Nurse Education: a
reform of nursing (the Platt Report). RCN,
London
Scottish Home and Health Department/
National Medical Advisory Committee 1993
The future of mental handicap hospitals in
Scotland. HMSO, Edinburgh

Scottish Office 1988 Scottish health authorities
review of priorities for the eighties and
nineties. HMSO, Edinburgh
Scottish Office 1998a Review of services for
people with a learning disability.
Department of Health, Edinburgh
Scottish Office 1998b Designed to care:
renewing the National Health Service in
Scotland. The Stationery Office, Edinburgh
Scottish Office 1999 Learning disabilities
nursing in Scotland – a position paper.
National Nursing, Midwifery and Health
Visiting Advisory Committee, Department
of Health, Edinburgh
Smith L 1999 The multi-skilled worker –
solution or problem? CAIPE Bulletin
16:12–15
Smither A 1994 All our futures. Channel 4
Publications, London
Towell D, Beardshaw V 1991 Enabling
community integration: the role of public
authorities in promoting an ordinary life for
people with learning disabilities in the
1990s. King's Fund, London
Training Organization for Personal Social
Services (England) 1999a Modernising the
social care workforce – the first national
strategy for England. TOPSS, London
Training Organization for Personal Social
Services (England) 1999b Modernising the
social care workforce – the first national
strategy for England: supplementary report
on learning disabilities. TOPSS, London
Trecare NHS Trust 1998 Needs-led staff
reprofiling in the NHS. Trecare NHS Trust,
Truro
United Kingdom Central Council for Nursing,
Midwifery and Health Visiting 1999 Fitness
for practice (the Peach Report). UKCC,
London
Weinstein J 1995 Sewing the seams of the
seamless services. CCETSW, London
Welsh Office 1983 The All-Wales strategy for
mental handicap. Department of Health,
Cardiff
Welsh Office 1994 The Welsh mental handicap
strategy – guidance. Department of Health,
Cardiff
Welsh Office 1996 Welsh health survey.
HMSO, Cardiff
Welsh Office 1998 Putting patients first. The
Stationery Office, Cardiff

2 Concepts of health and disability

Marc Saunders

KEY ISSUES

- Definitions of health
- Health as an evolutionary concept
- Pluralist perspectives of health
- Influences on health education and health promotion
- Attitudes to disability

INTRODUCTION

Health: at the end of the 20th century and the beginning of the 21st, what other word has enjoyed such attention and longevity of interest? Our collective fascination is all the more extraordinary as we contemplate a concept which is so difficult to define in a way that reflects our individual views, perceptions and circumstances. Yet the popular media, professional organizations and their publications as well as advertisers and product manufacturers are all increasingly happy to hang their messages on a health issue despite the risks associated with any lack of conceptual clarity. Like the constant ticking of a clock on the wall, the word 'health' has almost achieved the paradoxical status of momentous importance and complete insignificance at the same time.

This book aims very clearly to associate the real actions and activities of people working in services for people who have a learning disability with one or more conceptualizations of health. More specifically, it is anticipated that service users will experience tangible benefits from professionals' greater level of knowledge and understanding about health and related issues. This can only be achieved if the reader is first permitted the opportunity to consider health from many of its perspectives. This chapter aims to guide the reader through some of the principal issues, questions and debates as well as providing a basis for exploring and contemplating a range of related issues. Definitions of health are addressed as well as illness as a deviation from any particular definition. There is a historical view on the evolution of our understanding of health and a brief view of health and cultural influences on health, illness and health behaviour. In conclusion, the chapter will draw some of these themes together in terms of services provided to people who have a learning disability.

DEFINING HEALTH

Everyone has a view on what health is and what health means to themselves and those who are close to them. For the most part this does not facilitate a broad understanding of health which could be applied in any other context. Neither does it clarify its range of meanings so that service professionals might support people who have a learning disability to benefit from these insights. There are many questions: is health a continuum from ill health to good health? Should health be pursued as some kind of utopian ideal? Should disability be perceived as health which has been compromised? What special importance should health, perceptions of health and healthcare have for people who have a learning disability and how does this impact on service delivery?

For those who hope to find the perfect answer in their search for that apparently elusive definition of health, there is a danger of disappointment. There is little prospect of finding or developing a definition which reflects everyone's views on health, on what health means to us as individuals and what health means to us collectively. It is possible to identify definitions we might be comfortable with in any given context. However, the concept of health does not travel well and its application to different settings eventually leaves most definitions wanting. This has not prevented people from attempting to define health. Despite this, it seems the more we know about health and ill health, the more we realize there is further work to do.

ACTIVITY 2.1	Is 'complete health' possible for any person within society? What would this mean for people who have a learning disability?

Before looking further at definitions of health and ill health there is a final and perhaps somewhat controversial and challenging addition to this debate.

First, if we suppose that complete or ultimate health was an attainable goal for significant parts of our society, would we find this acceptable? At first it would seem that this would be a desirable state of affairs. However, brief reflection suggests that to some extent the ingenuity implicit in our humanity and our drive to solve problems are the product of there being problems to solve in the first place. If health is the ultimate goal, what else ought we to strive for?

Second, the issue of disability is an important part of this particular debate. Striving for health in its highest form focuses on the notion which has consistently been discredited, i.e. that people who have any type of disability are an unnecessary deviation from what is (usually) acceptable in Western society. This does not support the assertion that people who have a disability are in any way experiencing ill health. It does draw attention to the fact that society is already collectively intolerant towards people who have a disability and access to complete or ultimate health may only serve to emphasize or exacerbate any differences which exist. In such circumstances there is a basis for even greater intolerance.

There is plenty of evidence that this is already the case. People often think someone is *suffering* from Down's syndrome, that people who have a disability are dependent on charity and they are unable to contribute to our communities. On a more extreme level, people who have a disability are known to be victimized or bullied in their own homes.

Health, even if it is broadly considered to be concerned with the internal quality of a person's physical, mental, spiritual and social condition, cannot divorce itself from the context in which we all operate: the world around us. In an important text Dubos suggests:

Health and disease cannot be defined merely in terms of anatomical, physiological or mental attributes. Their real measure is in the ability of the individual to function in a manner acceptable to himself and to the group of which he is a part.

(Dubos 1959, p 206)

Many years on there seems to be an even greater need to focus on not only the internal qualities and attributes of each of us but also on how all the factors (internal and external) combine and interact to offer us the possibility of experiencing what we would call health. Or how they compromise our health.

The Black Report (Black et al 1982) examined the differences in health experiences between groups from differing social classes. It also suggested how public policy and planning could be redesigned to address some of this imbalance. Sir Douglas' committee needed a clear foundation upon which to undertake its work and so Chapter 1 of the Black Report explores concepts of health and inequality and states clearly that the variety of meanings which can be assigned to the term 'health' was not given due consideration at a public policy level. If this were accurate at the time of the report, it seems even more relevant in an era where the speed of developments and the expectations of service users have increased significantly. This is important because the very definition we attach to the term 'health' will affect how healthcare services and society respond in order to overcome a particular health issue or to maintain and promote the health of society as a whole.

The Black committee explored the ever-adapting nature of health and how changes in the many influencing factors such as medical knowledge, research, public anxiety and demands for services are reflected in any conceptualization of health. They comment on the increasing inclusiveness of definitions of health and ill health which have seen '... debility and different forms of incapacity ... come to play a more prominent part in social and medical conceptions' (Black et al 1982, p 35).

At the time this reflected society's notion that disability, and therefore learning disability, was a deviation from any number of definitions of health. There was, and still is, a possibility that financial incentives also reinforce this view. In the UK financial systems which are designed to support people who have a disability often require proof of incapacity as a deviation from health in order to gain access to state benefits. This is in no way intended as a criticism of people who have a disability who are required to cooperate with a system which is found to be inherently devaluing.

Over half a century ago when the World Health Organization (WHO) first assembled there was an attempt to define health as part of its constitution. Since then, the following definition of health has been frequently referred to.

Health is a state of complete physical, mental and social well-being, and not merely the absence of disease or infirmity. The enjoyment of the highest attainable standard of health is one of the fundamental rights of every human being without distinction of race, religion, political belief, economic or social condition.

(WHO 1946, p 29)

It is interesting to consider whether or not WHO would have attempted to define health were it set the task in the year 2000 and, moreover, would it have developed something similar? It is unlikely to have done so and the cynical amongst us might suggest that given what is now known about health, it would be easier to avoid the issue altogether than make any attempt at all. Certainly, subsequent publications have tended to quietly retreat from the 1946 definition and focus on the more functional aspects of health:

> ... the main social target of governments and WHO in the coming decades should be the attainment by all citizens of the world by the year 2000 of a level of health that will permit them to lead a socially and economically productive life.
>
> (WHO 1985, p 1)

It is all too easy to be critical of something which dates back over 50 years. However, the 1946 WHO definition continues to contribute to the debate on health. It is often referred to in texts on health and continues to be referred to by healthcare professionals and academics. If nothing else, this challenges us to try to do better. There is also a somewhat paradoxical quality to this particular definition. Some consider this view to be utopian or idealistic. Yet it might also provide an inappropriate justification for healthcare services to continue to focus on addressing disease and illness. Most people would now agree that a strategy based on prevention of ill health and health promotion, in order to enable people to experience '... a state of complete physical, mental and social well-being ...', is more appropriate.

Black et al (1982) are clear that service development in response to current and predicted demand has to be addressed in light of our collectively acknowledged definition of health. Given that the WHO definition (1946) is often taken as the accepted view on health and illness, we ought not to wonder at the inclusive nature of our services. If continued and complete health is the accepted minimum standard, as the WHO definition might suggest, then there are significant implications in terms of the pressure on health resources and our willingness to accept that priority setting (i.e. health service rationing) is necessary.

A number of writers adopt the stance that apparently brief and all-inclusive attempts at defining health are bound to fail. Seedhouse (1986) goes to some length to illustrate the complexities of developing a definition for health not least because of the complex nuances as well as the ambiguities that exist in our use of language. In response to this, he bases his ideas on the notion that health is the foundation for human achievement.

> A person's optimum state of health is equivalent to the state of the set of conditions which fulfil or enable a person to work to fulfil his or her realistic chosen and biological potentials. Some of these conditions are of the highest importance for all people. Others are variable and dependent upon individual abilities and circumstance.
>
> (Seedhouse 1986, p 61)

In recent years, there has perhaps been a preoccupation with the expression of any issue or concern in a positive way. One does not have an 'illness' but a 'health problem'. This may on occasion prevent the proper examination of naturally occurring phenomena which may impact upon us in a way we perceive as negative. Illness might be one such phenomenon. Considerable effort could be spent on defining health with the assumption that the antithesis of health will duly serve to define illness. Yet even if health providers, health researchers and academics are less than happy with the term 'illness', as far as our society is concerned the concept of illness is all too real. In the event, the public at large make endless references to the term and increase its currency as they do so. If this is ignored, there is a risk that service users will not receive the service they require.

Wolff-Lewis & Kuhn-Timby (1993, pp 26–27) reinforce the above perception by suggesting that health is what the individual regards health to be and that health can be assessed with reference to its component parts:

- physical health
- emotional health
- social health
- spiritual health.

In the final analysis health and illness are abstract concepts and only gather meaning from the context in which they are set. One might make a comparison with a work of art inasmuch as the view of the observer is critical.

HEALTH AS AN EVOLUTIONARY CONCEPT

The term 'health' is not a uniquely 20th century concept. Its derivation lies deep in history, in the work of Hippocrates, reputed to be the founder of Greek medicine, and philosophers such as Empedocles. Inevitably this section has a particular emphasis on the 20th century and how health is affected by the pressures and challenges of modern life.

One of the great challenges concerning our conceptualization of health and illness is our inability even to be clear whether or not we are talking about health as we see it, as we feel it and as we perceive it in our real worlds. Or whether we are talking about health, the word we use to describe what we see, what we feel and what we perceive. Seedhouse (1986) is familiar with this problem and argues that because we do not fully understand the world in which we live, we might be justified in feeling that at least the words we use to describe that world ought not to be quite so ambiguous. However, he recognizes that this clearly is not the case and that our lack of understanding about the world is reflected in the lack of clarity and focus in the words we use to describe it.

For many years there was remarkably little development in the conceptualization of health although there was considerable progress in addressing issues relating to health and illness through medical advancement in terms of treatment, research and health maintenance. Nevertheless, in the 18th century there were those who contradicted what was becoming a significant and continually developing body of knowledge.

The 19th and 20th centuries saw the overall understanding of the body reach new levels of sophistication and the crystallizing of human physiology as we understand it today. This has permitted us the luxury of further considering the notions of health and disease as concepts to be applied in 21st century settings. And in a sense the circle has been completed: the definition provided by WHO and others is the result of thousands of years of research, discussion, experiment and debate.

Health as a 21st century construct and its impact on people who have a learning disability

The discussion on health has led us to consider how contemporary cultures have impacted on perceptions of health. There is clearly an acknowledgement of the WHO (1946) definition; however, the overall construct has evolved so significantly that a view of health and 20th century life is critical to our understanding. There are a number of elements that have to be considered: changes in people's views on health in general and specifically on their own health, the structure and role of health services, the demands and pressures of 21st century life, the freedoms and challenges of modern communication, commercial considerations and technology, to name but a few.

Arguably the popular media have distorted the notion of health to fit their own agenda, often to the detriment of people who have a learning disability. Newspaper and broadcast journalists often confuse disability and learning disability with illness, either out of ignorance or for editorial convenience. Advertisers constantly throw up ideas of acceptability and human beauty which will consistently exclude people who deviate from these ideas and where any type of disability will almost inevitably represent a deviation.

The above observations notwithstanding, it is arguable that in the 21st century people virtually insist on being healthy without reference to any definition of health. This is because nearly all of us have tasted our own definitive view on health – the health associated with our youth. Our views often seem based on a Cartesian view of the human body, in this case perceived as a complex machine which receives instructions from the brain. Like a machine, we expect to be maintained, to receive healthcare like a car receives a service or repair. Yet it is not only our internal notion of health and the expectations which surround this notion which are an issue for us. There are other external influences which have both a positive and a negative impact on people's health status: lifestyle, the environment, technological developments and the consumer culture are all briefly considered. The whole conceptualization of health is influenced by our complex and continually shifting lifestyle. First, we need to be fitter and healthier for longer in order to aspire to achieve what others demand of us and what we demand of ourselves. Second, the way people work and live their lives actually places increased pressure on internal systems and resources in order to maintain an acceptable level of health. There is a clear dichotomy in that people are expected to work for longer and under more pressure than ever before, yet the costs are apparent in terms of the health of individuals which in turn impact on people's ability to operate in such a competitive environment.

ACTIVITY 2.3   What are the environmental and technological factors that influence the health status of people who have a learning disability?

There is an increasing awareness of the effects the environment can have on the individual and collective health status of society. Today there is more evidence than ever to suggest that the way the macro-environment is maintained or abused can have an impact upon people's health; for example, pollution, waste disposal, transport policy and so on.

Some of these environmental factors have already led healthcare professionals to revise their views on health and healthcare provision because of the increased health consequences associated with these issues. In essence, environmental determinants of health status are, at least in part, caused by the collective lifestyle of society in the 21st century.

Technological developments have impacted on both our lifestyle and the environment. These developments have also contributed to people's reassessment of their own health status, of healthcare and how the healthcare system should respond to their needs. In many ways they have given people expectations of their health status that go beyond their own ability to achieve and beyond the ability of the system to deliver for them.

The development of increasingly sophisticated technology in healthcare services has coincided with an increase in our expectations about what healthcare can achieve. Healthcare and health interventions have become a victim of their own success, leading to the possibility that people might be less conscientious about protecting their own health because they feel the technology is there to retrospectively 're-charge' them with good health.

Over the last few years a belief has developed that the market can deliver to us most of the things we would like, providing we are prepared to work to achieve this. In addition, most people feel they contribute in some way to the healthcare system that they hope to make use of should this become necessary. But the commercial and market-led world of the 21st century has moved these expectations by a significant degree. The ever-increasing display of healthy people eating apparently healthy products on the television or in magazines might lead us to believe that it is perfectly possible to achieve that image of health merely by buying that particular product, irrespective of how we live our lives.

How all of this impacts upon people who have a learning disability and how they are supported (or not) in order to function, in a society which virtually proclaims its competitiveness as one of its redeeming features, is a complex question. We have the understanding, the technology and quite possibly the resources to ensure that people who have a learning disability are fully subsumed into the fabric of society in such a way that they feel valued and that society benefits from this inclusion. Unfortunately the potential and the reality are barely comparable and whilst this is merely an observation without reference to any empirical evidence, there is a case to be made that people who have a learning disability are continuously and severely disadvantaged by this quiet but significant cultural evolution to the extent that there might arguably be a direct health cost to people who have a learning disability.

PLURALIST PERSPECTIVES OF HEALTH

It seems there is no end to the arrogance of the Western world which often looks critically down on the medical and physiological belief systems of other cultures irrespective of the fact that our own belief systems have continually been found to be wanting in many respects. Even today, healthcare professionals are still only able to rely completely upon a relatively small number of interventions to consistently deliver the outcomes they were designed to deliver. In contrast, Ramesh & Hyma (1984) reported on a WHO meeting on the promotion and development of traditional medicines where it was noted that, despite an increasingly sceptical view of 'traditional' systems of medicine, these systems continued to be used in both rural and urban settings and continued to meet the health needs of the populations in question.

Across the globe there are many different approaches to the conceptualization of health and how health needs are met within the populations in question. These may not look technologically advanced when compared with Western cultures, but in terms of how they represent health, address health issues and deliver outcomes to their respective populations, they should not be viewed with such scepticism.

For example, the Ethiopian Amhara tribe's concept of the physiological construction of a person behaves almost as a conceptual model of human physiology. They believe the stomach contains a colony of worms which turn food and drink into waste. In turn, this can explain the symptoms they experience when they are in pain or feel nauseous (Young 1991).

The Gnau of Papua New Guinea have developed a concept of health which presumes a growing ability to resist illness during the early years of life which then decreases in later years. Thus the deaths of older members or very young members of their society are looked upon as unremarkable compared with the death of someone in early adulthood (Lewis 1991).

ACTIVITY 2.4 How do you ensure that the health needs of people from different ethnic backgrounds are met within your service?

When considering pluralistic perspectives of health there are two specific foci: first, the issue of ethnicity and patterns of health and ill health within particular ethnic groups and second, how ethnicity affects health beliefs and health behaviour. There is some need for caution. Smaje (1995) points out that 'culture' is often given as a means of explaining diversity in patterns of health and health experience, particularly where other explanations do not come immediately to hand (p 85). He also suggests that culture in its broadest sense is often identified as a variable in its own right. Indeed, Murray & Zentner (1989) confirm that it is possible to find a whole range of illnesses which are only present in certain groups and absent in others. However, it is probably acceptable to note different patterns of health and ill health on the basis of culture and ethnicity but to suggest that these are the only determining factors is to hugely oversimplify the complexity of other cultures and is probably indicative of an overall lack of understanding.

For the most part it is likely that a behaviour or belief system within a given culture actually influences health and health experience. In short, it seems a little condescending to acknowledge countless variables which influence health in our own cultures and yet make the assumption that 'culture' in its own right is a sufficient explanation for health experiences in other groups which may vary from our own.

Whilst there may be many behaviours and beliefs that distinguish one culture from another, including medical belief systems, most cultures hold in common the conceptualization of health and illness. There is also likely to be some method for maintaining health and eradicating illness and disease (effectiveness notwithstanding across all cultures and societies) and the bases upon which health and (especially) illness will occur.

MODERN CONSTRUCTS OF HEALTH AND THEIR INFLUENCE ON HEALTH EDUCATION AND HEALTH PROMOTION

It is a little ironic that, despite the developments in health promotion and health education, particularly in an effort to support people who have a learning disability, the debate on the conceptualization of health has not progressed to a similar degree. As this book focuses on health and health issues relating to people who have a learning disability, the methods and motivations of health education and health promotion are explored in much greater detail, particularly in Chapter 7. Therefore, this section briefly touches on health education and health promotion in the context of the definitions of health and ill health.

Often, those involved with health education and health promotion find their work is undermined by society's collective attitudes to the messages designed to enable people to make healthier choices. On a more individual level, people who receive health education messages decide whether or not they will heed the message given. It is their right to make that choice. There is an increasingly large body of knowledge on factors which promote health or which can contribute to poor health and, critically, Ewles & Simnett (1985) suggest that this is knowledge which '... has the potential to affect the health of *every* human being' (p 10) (italics added).

Earlier the observation was made that people appear disinclined to actively acknowledge health promotion messages, possibly because of the perception that healthcare services can resolve most deviations from their internalized definition of health. The interplay between health definitions and concepts of health education and promotion is not at first obvious. However, each individual's internalized definition of health will impact on how that individual interacts with their environment and this includes the responses they make to health education and promotion messages.

In addition, health commissioners and providers will also have views on health, albeit shifting over time dependent on information and circumstance. This view will affect strategy on the development of healthcare services and their delivery. It might be considered an argument for the explicit definition of health which would guide commissioners and providers in the delivery of healthcare services. Over time policy has, to some extent, attempted to galvanize our view on health; for example, *Health of the nation* (DoH 1992) and *Saving lives: our healthier nation* (DoH 1999). However, even these have not been able to focus on any one single definition of health.

With regard to people who have a learning disability, some very real questions and concerns can be raised about how these messages are communicated. Arguably, the non-learning disabled population are being engaged in an almost individualized debate on how they view health, their own particular conceptualization of health and the implications for current and future health services. In short, many of us may not be conscious of the debate about definitions of health but each of us will have implicitly defined health for our own purposes and will in some way be able to engage in the debate about health and health services. People who have a learning disability also ought to be engaged in this debate. Unfortunately, this is clearly easier said than done.

ACTIVITY 2.5   How do you engage people who have a learning disability in discussions about their health?

Over recent years steps have been taken to engage people who have a learning disability in understanding their health; for example, the publication of *The healthy way* (DoH 1998) as well as documents aimed at supporting those who care for people who have a learning disability (DoH 1995). Many people whose jobs depend upon a comprehensive understanding of health cannot be relied upon to agree with each other on a definition of health or even deliver the debate in such a way that non-learning disabled lay people could engage in this important discussion. On this basis, the possibility of people who have a learning disability becoming actively involved in this discussion is perhaps somewhat remote. We need to be much more sophisticated in our approaches if people who have a learning disability are to become more involved.

The literature powerfully supports the idea of health education providing a sound base for health promotion (see Chapter 5, p 93 for clarification of definitions). Health education for people who have a learning disability has to have a springboard from which developments can occur. Defining health in a way which is meaningful to people who have a learning disability, i.e. not reflecting the notion that health and disability are in some way mutually exclusive, has to be at least one of the starting points.

Illness as a deviation/deficit from current constructs of health

It seems questionable only to address the issue of health from the perspective that it might be a consistently achievable state without addressing the possibility that ill health is in any way linked to the reality we all understand. Somewhat pragmatically, the notion of ill health is explored in this section along with factors that may contribute to the occurrence of ill health in individuals and in groups. In addition, there is a view on disability and how this is sometimes confused with concepts of ill health.

Cassell (1978) has a perspective on illness which might be described as amusing or even a little dry.

> Illness is what the patient feels when he goes to the doctor; disease is what he has on the way home from the doctor's surgery. Disease is something an organ has; illness is something man has.
>
> (Cassell 1978, p 23)

The real experience of ill health is different for every individual. And therein lies the challenge for those who aspire to define ill health. It is also an error to assume all individuals find ill health unwelcome. Some are reported to almost enjoy the process of being ill. Herzlich & Pierret (1991) describe the views of someone who almost wishes they could be excused their involvement in the everyday events of their life. They note the parallels which exist in psychoanalysis where the individual will avoid situations by 'escaping into illness'.

Whitehead (1988) defines illness as '... the subjective experience of symptoms of ill health'. She goes on to note the paradox of people who can '... be diseased without feeling ill and feel ill without having a medically recognisable disease' (Whitehead 1988, p 224).

Herzlich (1973) identified three ways of conceptualizing ill health: as a destructive event, as a liberating event or as an occupation. Active people who felt that ill health had had a desocializing effect on them saw ill health as a predominantly destructive event. Ill health as a liberating event also has a desocializing element but on this occasion this element is welcomed. Finally, ill health as an occupation requires the individual to acknowledge their state of ill health and to see themselves as one person in a population of many who are sharing their experiences of a particular condition.

Ill health behaviour cannot always be associated with appropriate behaviour. Asher (1984) comments on his time as a physician during the war in a paper he wrote on malingering. It is evidence of a further problem facing people who have a disability. If the argument is that people who have a disability are in some way suffering ill health then there is the chance that this may not be genuine and that they have made a deliberate decision to opt out of their role in society by using their disability. Before long a further devaluing label is attached to people who have a disability.

Second, the complex social roles associated with ill health are not easily absorbed and therefore complied with by people who have a learning disability. This is an additional hurdle for people who have a learning disability. The socially acceptable behaviours associated with being ill are many and varied. However, there is inevitably a range of what might be considered appropriate in any particular illness. People who have a learning disability often do not comply with these unwritten rules because they have not had the opportunity to develop the necessary insights. Therefore, not only do they have to contend with a general view that their disability is some kind of illness but when they are genuinely ill, their behaviours are not always within the range of socially recognizable responses.

ATTITUDES TO DISABILITY, LEARNING DISABILITY AND THE SUPERIMPOSITION OF HEALTH AND ILL HEALTH CONSTRUCTS

Much of this discussion concerns evidence on how society as a whole and in part (for example, the media) responds to disability and in particular learning disability, as if it was synonymous with illness or evidence of some kind of health deficit. However, accepted definitions of health and ill health have to be reviewed in the light of such concerns. The WHO (1946) definition which proposes that health is a kind of ideal state and not just an absence of disease or infirmity is most concerning. It has a double impact on people who have a learning disability. First, it describes health as not only the 'absence of infirmity' but 'a state of complete physical, social and mental well-being'. All of which means that, to those not directly involved, people who have a learning disability could quite possibly be perceived as failing to 'achieve' health. They cannot claim to have an absence of infirmity nor can they aspire to the state of complete physical, social and mental well-being, if indeed anyone could.

Of course, the criticisms directed at the WHO definition might also be directed at other definitions and other apparently disadvantaged groups or groups devalued by society. People who have a disability, not necessarily a learning disability, might also feel aggrieved at the various definitions of health and their implications in terms of society's attitudes towards them. One of the problems is that the health/ill health label is too convenient for society and its representatives in the media. It also provides a basis for people to feel sympathy and sorrow. After all, it might be acceptable to feel sorry for someone if they are ill so these feelings are legitimized if we are allowed to perceive people who have a disability as having some kind of illness.

There was a temptation at this point to stray from what is currently acceptable terminology and to use the term 'disabled people', because there is a growing feeling among people who have a disability that their disability is not something they should be ashamed of or wish to deemphasize. If we wish to lose the idea that disability is associated with lesser value and that comparisons with ill health are inappropriate, then perhaps we should be less focused on playing with words in order to shift emphases. Particularly if by implication we are suggesting the 'disability' is an inappropriate state. In short, is the term 'disabled people' inappropriate?

Evidence of the superimposition of ill health concepts on to people who have a disability and in particular people who have a learning disability is all about us. Quite often, the choice of words is a good indication. Even in the 21st century it is still accepted to assume that someone *suffers* with a learning disability. It is something of a cliché but most people who use a wheelchair will have found that the wheelchair seems to indicate to others that they are also deaf. But the issue is broader than this and there is a possibility (not proven, but interesting to debate) that people from other groups which at times might be considered as disadvantaged may find this ill health label inappropriately applied to them. For example, people from minority ethnic groups (particularly people from the Afro-Caribbean population) experience increased levels of diagnoses of mental ill health, older people are automatically associated with infirmity and homosexual people, particularly as a historical experience, are treated for their sexual orientation as if it were a genuine physical or mental illness that would be amenable to treatment.

Some readers may not appreciate the topic being raised in this way but people who have a learning disability are often supported or looked after by nurses. Historically, hospitals were considered the service base of choice for many people who have a learning disability in some form of colonizing process, once again providing a degree of legitimacy to the notion that people who have a learning disability are suffering from some level of ill health.

HEALTH AND QUALITY OF LIFE

Like the term 'health', the concept of quality of life is not always easy to define in terms of what it might mean for individuals. This has not prevented many writers attempting to establish a conceptual base for quality of life, how it can be articulated and how it can be measured (e.g. Cragg & Look 1992, King's Fund 1980, O'Brien 1987).

ACTIVITY 2.6	Identify the ways in which you think health and health status influence the quality of life a person is able to experience. What does this mean for people who have a learning disability? How do you and the service you work in help to mediate some of these issues?

Conceptually there are a number of similarities. For example, how health as a 'commodity' can be delivered to people who have a learning disability might be considered a similarity, as is the influence of the external environment on health as well as quality of life. There is clearly a relationship between both although defining or specifying this is challenging. At a very basic level a high quality of life appears partly dependent upon the idea that people generally experience a degree of good health on a consistent basis. Equally, much of the available research suggests good health is to some degree dependent upon the quality of life that people experience.

There is an interesting subtext to this debate in that there is a danger that people who have a learning disability experience less than ideal services on the basis that most members of the population also experience less than ideal services. This is one of the dangers of using norm referencing as a way of establishing or measuring quality of life. In essence, such a system would implicitly accept that a poor service is acceptable providing it is poor for everyone and not just for people who have a learning disability. However, there is another argument; that if a service is generally inadequate then it is often especially inadequate for people who have a learning disability.

From an ordinary living perspective (King's Fund 1980), which argues that people who have a learning disability have the same human value as any other member of society and therefore the same human rights, the argument for equity between people who have a learning disability and non-disabled people is a powerful one. An exponent of social role valorization (e.g. Wolfensberger 1972) might argue that value is imparted only if the very best support for people who have a learning disability is provided. This has to be seen in terms of health as well as other aspects of their life. If this is conceptually relevant to other aspects of life for people who have a learning disability then the issue of health-care ought to be seen as another component of this and be treated no differently.

Seedhouse (1986) described a perspective of health which is briefly touched upon earlier in this chapter. He argued that many definitions of health were inadequate because they missed the reasons why good health is so valued and that health should therefore be viewed in terms of its context for each individual, almost as a means to an end. He termed this the *foundation for achievement*. Whether or not this particular view of health is acceptable to a majority is not relevant but it is worth considering that health could conceivably be a foundation for a life of acceptable or valued quality. In other words, people who have a learning disability ought to receive all the necessary support to ensure that variations in their health do not become a barrier to all these potential opportunities or become another opportunity to devalue individuals who have a learning disability.

Health screening and primary care

Screening of people who have a learning disability has the potential to become one of the contentious issues of the new millennium. The rule of thumb applied to most commercial and service developments is one of cost and benefit and health screening is no exception to this. However, the issues are complex and difficult to untangle, especially for people who have a learning disability. It may seem to an enlightened readership that the cost of focused screening for particular conditions in people who have a severe learning disability is a necessary and therefore justifiable expense.

There are many pressures facing commissioners and politicians which mean that a continued focus on the health needs of people who have a learning disability will remain important for some time to come. However, the broader agenda of the effectiveness of healthcare interventions and screening is as important to people who have a learning disability as it is to any other group and at times more important. In short, if screening can be shown to offer health and quality of life benefits to people who have a learning disability, particularly to those whose disability is of a complex nature, then resources might appropriately be directed to achieve this.

The policy context of primary healthcare services possibly has not helped: GPs find their practices almost discriminated against if they have more than the average number of people who have a learning disability on their list because it is possible this group of service users may need a larger share of healthcare interventions and monitoring than the non-disabled population. Having made these points, the publication of *Once a day* (NHSE 1998) has perhaps started to redress the balance in favour of people who have a learning disability.

Complex healthcare interventions

People who have a learning disability also need access to the more complex spectrum of healthcare interventions. Currently in the USA radical surgery is being used to correct the visible characteristics associated with disability, notably surgery to reduce the impact of features of Down's syndrome. Whilst there are bound to be defenders of this use of healthcare services, this seems to provide a drastic illustration of a disable-ist and disabling society at work. Worse still is the possibility that you might only be able to access this type of healthcare if you can pay for it. There will be many people for whom sophisticated secondary interventions would genuinely contribute something to their quality of life but who are unable to access them because the cost is prohibitive.

In the UK the picture is currently less disturbing although the cynical could suggest this has more to do with the passage of time than any ethical purity. That said, if the issue around primary healthcare is about resources to support people who have a learning disability then access to secondary level healthcare is the same only more so. Periodically there is media interest in service shortfalls which seem applicable only to people who have a learning disability; for example, stories where parents have to make strong cases for their child who has a learning disability to receive the same treatment as non-learning disabled people. One major difference is the arguments that can be levelled in order to prevent action being taken. Consent to treatment is the double-edged sword often working both for and against people who have a learning disability. This issue is sometimes overcome by strength of will but often it is not overcome and it is a suitably convenient barrier to prevent people accessing services that most other members of the population would have little problem in demanding for themselves.

CONCLUSION

This chapter has considered a whole range of issues, debates and insights into concepts of health, ill health and their importance to people who have a learning disability and those who work to support them. It is clear that simple definitions of health and ill health which suit all people in all contexts are not achievable. It is also clear that a deeper understanding of health and ill health will help service providers to more effectively support service users to take more inclusive roles in society. This will only happen if the sustained efforts to achieve this include further public education and involve service users in the process.

There are some powerful debates about health and illness and how the concept can be applied to people who have a learning disability without once again contributing to the catalogue of issues that moves such a vulnerable group of individuals to where they are almost silently discriminated against. If the issue of health (conceptually) and what all of this means can be reengineered to effectively support people who have a learning disability to begin to understand and engage in the discussion then other groups might also be engaged more successfully.

Paradoxically, the engagement of people who have a learning disability in the debate about health, health education and ill health has not really happened to any meaningful degree. At the moment there remains so much indecision on health and ill health at all levels from the popular media to academia that it is difficult to see how people who have a learning disability will ever be effectively engaged in such a debate.

Only when the whole debate moves away from the idea that health is some kind of utopian dream and that it is conceptually very dependent upon the state and circumstances of the person concerned as well as their beliefs and behaviours will those who have a learning disability feel that the pursuit of a positive personal health state is the key to accessing improvements in quality of life. The infrastructure which will help people make that journey is in health education, health promotion, a better understanding of the views of people who have a learning disability and responsive, not discriminating, services. It is not in the arguments about resources, nor is it in the debate on human quality as if it were some kind of continuum from acceptable to unacceptable. If all human life is of equal value then access to healthcare (and the rationing of healthcare) has to be on an equitable basis. It seems that people who have a learning disability are not really demanding new conceptualizations of health or even healthcare services which are remarkably different; they just wish to access what the non-disabled population demands in order to maintain an equitable quality of life.

FURTHER READING

Seedhouse D 1986 Health: the foundations for achievement. John Wiley, Chichester
This is a significant text explaining the definitions of health from a variety of perspectives.

Department of Health 1998 The healthy way. DoH, London
This is one of the first documents about health that is aimed at peope who have a learning disability. It can be a useful tool to aid in increasing a person's understanding about their own health.

REFERENCES

Asher R 1984 Malingering. In: Black N, Boswell D, Gray A, Murphey S, Popay J (eds) Health and disease: a reader. Open University Press, Milton Keynes

Black D, Morris J N, Smith C, Townsend P 1982 Inequalities in health: the Black report. Penguin Books, London

Cassell J E 1978 The healer's art: a new approach to the doctor–patient relationship. Penguin, Harmondsworth

Cragg R, Look R 1992 Compass: a multi-perspective evaluation of quality in home life. Cragg and Look, Birmingham

DoH 1992 Health of the nation: a strategy for health in England. HMSO, London

DoH 1995 The health of the nation: a strategy for people with learning disabilities. DoH, Wetherby

DoH 1998 The healthy way. DoH, London

DoH 1999 Saving lives: our healthier nation. The Stationery Office, London

Dubos R 1959 Mirage of health: utopias, progress and biological change. George Allen and Unwin, London

Ewles L, Simnett I 1985 Promoting health: a practical guide to health education. John Wiley, Chichester

Herzlich C 1973 Health and illness: a social psychological analysis. Academic Press, London

Herzlich C, Pierret J 1991 Illness: from causes to meaning. In: Currer C, Stacey M (eds) Concepts of health, illness and disease. Berg, New York

King's Fund 1980 An ordinary life: comprehensive locally-based services for mentally handicapped people. King's Fund, London

Lewis G 1991 Concepts of health and illness in a Sepik society. In: Currer C, Stacey M (eds) Concepts of health, illness and disease. Berg, New York

Murray R B, Zentner J P 1989 Nursing concepts for health and health promotion. Prentice Hall, New York

NHSE 1998 Once a day. DoH, London

O'Brien J 1987 A guide to personal futures planning. In: Bellamy G T, Wilcox B (eds) A comprehensive guide to the activities catalog. Paul H Brookes, Baltimore

Ramesh A, Hyma B 1984 Traditional Indian medicine in practice in an Indian metropolitan city. In: Black N, Boswell D, Gray A, Murphey S, Popay J (eds) Health and disease: a reader. Open University Press, Milton Keynes

Seedhouse D 1986 Health: the foundations for achievement. John Wiley, Chichester

Smaje C 1995 Health, race and ethnicity: making sense of the evidence. King's Fund Institute, London

Whitehead M 1988 The health divide. Pelican Books, London

Wolfensberger W 1972 The principle of normalization in human services. National Institute on Mental Retardation, Toronto

Wolff-Lewis L V, Kuhn-Timby B 1993 Fundamental skills and concepts in patient care. Chapman and Hall, London

World Health Organization 1946 Constitution.
World Health Organization, Geneva

World Health Organization 1985 Target for
health for all: targets in support of the
European regional strategy for health for all.
World Health Organization, Copenhagen

Young A 1991 Internalising and externalising
medical belief systems: an Ethiopian
example. In: Currer C, Stacey M (eds)
Concepts of health, illness and disease. Berg,
New York

3 Influences on health

Mavis Arevalo

KEY ISSUES

- Health as a multifactorial phenomenon
- The role of genetic inheritance and biology in health
- The impact of age and generation on health experience
- Sex, gender and health inequalities
- Socialization, lifestyle and health behaviour
- Race, ethnicity and culture in healthcare
- Social class and health inequalities
- The role of the education system in relation to health behaviour
- Health-diminishing effects of occupation, work environment and unemployment
- Health and social exclusion

INTRODUCTION

Health is influenced by a range of factors from the individual's genetic structure and biology to the physical and sociocultural environment in which they live. Hart (1985, p 50) suggests that recent improvements in human health have been 'embedded in the general rise in living standards which began in the 19th century and which continued at an accelerating pace in the 20th'. This rise is still evident today as we begin the 21st century; however, the existence of inequalities relating to economic and social position demonstrate that the rise in living standards has not been the same for everyone and for many people who have a learning disability, this is a particular issue. This is specifically relevant in the context of models of aggregate living. Hart (1985) adds, therefore, that 'health is a product of society'.

It is essential to consider, however, that the pathway to health/ill health is multifactorial with interaction between different factors being a key feature. As O'Brien (1995, p 193) states, there has been 'a widening of the meaning of health from an absence of disease or physical functioning to include social issues'. He adds: 'The extended concept places health at the intersection of key life experiences and conditions and implies a multidimensional agenda for health policy and practice'.

This chapter aims to explore these features of society in order to develop an understanding of their impact, particularly their negative impact, on individual health. Whilst much of this chapter will focus upon generic information this is pertinent, as such data are equally relevant to people who have a learning disability. Where additional influences exist that are specific to this group of people, this information will also be included.

FIGURE 3.1   *Factors influencing health.*

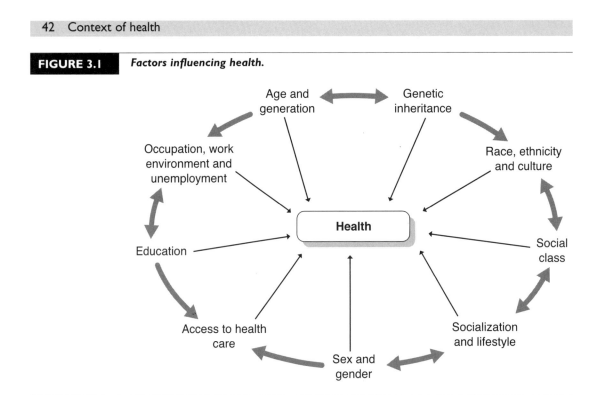

To explore the factors that impact on human health, these need to be considered individually but in the real world interaction between the elements must always be at the forefront of practitioner assessment. To enable appropriate assessment, this chapter will initially consider the factors influencing the health of all people. These factors will then be considered in relation to the specific issues relating to individuals who have a learning disability. There is no specific relevance attached to the order in which these factors are discussed.

GENETIC INHERITANCE AND BIOLOGY

For an individual to aspire to health, each organ of their body needs to operate efficiently and appropriately within the overall organization of the body. These basic features of structure and functioning are dependent on the genetic information contained in each cell. Errors in the sequencing of the genetic information can lead to alterations of form and functioning, often with disastrous consequences for long-term survival. As more of the human genome is 'decoded', there is a greater awareness of the role of genes in disease processes.

However, to suggest that genes alone are the key to understanding disease is to misunderstand the impact of the physical and social environment on genetic processes. In reality, although many diseases are known to have a genetic base, an environmental trigger is usually required for those genes to be expressed in the form of a disease. Very recent evidence is also beginning to suggest that other features in the cell may control the ways in which genes are activated. According to Knight (1999, p 16) 'As well as genes, cells have a set of instructions that tell genes when to be active'. He adds: 'This "epigenetic" instruction manual means different cells can use the same set of genes to develop distinctive identities ... there have also been hints that epigenetic instructions can be inherited'. The expression of genetic information would therefore appear to be far more complex than genetic determinism would suggest.

The occurrence of disease is therefore more appropriately conceived as an amalgam of genetic, stress-related, behavioural and socioeconomic features. The tendency to cite a single cause is based on the doctrine of specific aetiology as it arises within the medical model, but this is detrimental to our understanding of the processes involved. It also leads research into 'laboratory medicine' rather than epidemiology, further weakening our understanding of the relationship between genetic structure and disease.

In relation to individuals who have a learning disability, Down's syndrome is perhaps one of the better understood genetic conditions. Trisomy 21, the presence of three strands of chromosome 21, produces the characteristic features of the syndrome. Research in this area has enhanced our understanding of genetic expression but it also reinforces the view that, even with an identical genetic anomaly, the physical manifestations vary enormously between individuals.

Craft et al (1985) identified approximately 26.5% of people who have a learning disability as being associated with genetic causes. For those individuals with Downs syndrome, their genetic make-up has the potential to influence their health status. This can include, for example, increased likelihood of cardiovascular disease, musculoskeletal difficulties, epilepsy, increased prevalence of leukaemia and dementia. Information such as this is therefore essential when considering the health needs of this group of people.

AGE AND GENERATION

There is a tendency in modern society to use chronological age as a marker for function and competency, with little regard for biological development. This particular trend can make achievement and acceptance difficult for people who have a learning disability. Socially constructed features have also compounded this confusion. These features are evident in life events such as retirement, which occurs at a particular chronological age, supported by social norms regarding the behaviour of those who are retired. However, the functional level of the individual may well be at variance with these features with some individuals remaining well and active for many further years but with others needing to retire earlier.

In terms of age and health, the very young and the very old are deemed to be more vulnerable to ill health. However, there are also important cohort features that need to be borne in mind. As Jones (1994, p 344) suggests, the concept of generation refers to 'the commonalities, public events and patterns of social change which bind the cohort together'. Each cohort shares a particular life experience that may have an impact on their subsequent individual health. This is supported by O'Donnell (1997, p 446) who suggests that the experience of each age group is constructed by 'the state of the economy, the availability of work ... how individuals make sense of the situations which confront them'.

The use of the drug thalidomide, for example, had a very serious physical impact on children who were conceived during a particular time frame, as well as an emotional impact on that generation of parents. Evidence from studies conducted on individuals who underwent starvation whilst pregnant (during

World War II) has demonstrated that although the babies from these pregnancies were apparently well and grew normally once normal food intake was restored, as adults the females have had significantly higher levels of small babies. The suggestion therefore is that the impact of the starvation was on the germ cells of the babies, not the babies themselves. The effect on this particular cohort was to influence the health of the grandchildren of the affected women, not their children. As Jones (1994, p 344) states in relation to pre- and postwar children, 'The experiences of these different generations will be quite distinctive'. The life experience of each cohort or generation is therefore important for their overall health.

The fact that age and generation are important elements to consider in relation to health and well-being is particularly true for individuals who have a learning disability where the ageing process may be accelerated, with possible early onset of degenerative conditions. One common feature for this group of people, therefore, is the differential mortality rates with comparatively fewer people surviving into old age. In a society which uses chronological age to determine service provision, e.g. retirement, early onset of the ageing process can be a problem. It can also be viewed negatively by others if an individual is unable to perform the social role of an adult because of physical deterioration. From the perspective of people who have a learning disability, increasing numbers of individuals have been born during the last 20 years who may not have survived in earlier decades. This is giving rise to an increasing number of people who have extremely complex health needs and whose health status may follow a very different pattern from those with which we are familiar.

Generation is important in relation to the cohort experience of individuals with a learning disability, as this may include a history of institutional care and the effects of the transfer into community living. These lived experiences are likely to have had and will continue to have an influence on individual health. The memories, the joys and fears of life in institutional care have been clearly articulated by individuals who have physical disabilities in a BBC2 series (BBC 1999) and it is reasonable to assume that similar effects have been felt by individuals who have a learning disability. The long-term impact on physical health, self-esteem and mental health must be taken into consideration when exploring the factors influencing the health of people who have a learning disability, particularly those born before moves to community care became widespread.

SEX AND GENDER

The links between gender and health have been explored quite widely and several anomalies have been discussed. Evidence suggests that women see their GP more often than men (Naidoo & Wills 1994, p 33) and have higher morbidity (Townsend et al 1992, p 243). They are also more likely to be on psychotropic drugs and more likely to be admitted to a psychiatric unit (Naidoo & Wills 1994, p 32). Despite this, men are more likely to commit suicide than women (Acheson 1998, p 107) and they die younger (Townsend et al 1992, p 243). As Hart (1985, p 55) states, 'Male death rates are almost double those of females in every class'. She also adds: 'The sex differential tends to increase with age'. However, although never equal, these differences are less in societies or communities where gender roles converge, for example in kibbutzim (Jones

1994, p 251). The question to be addressed, therefore, is why is it that although women are apparently sicker than men, they actually live longer.

Biological factors

The first response to the question relates to the genetic and therefore biological differences between the sexes. Male fetuses are more likely to miscarry or be stillborn (Jones 1994, p 252), possibly due to weakness associated with the single X chromosome. Similar problems are also evident in a range of other diseases and health issues such as colour blindness and haemophilia, which are expressed predominantly in males. As Acheson (1998, p 24) states, 'At each age in childhood and on into adulthood, the age-specific mortality rates for boys is higher than for girls'.

Another biological feature that explains some of the surplus deaths of men in late middle age is the hormonal protection available to women until the onset of the menopause (Jones 1994, p 252). Nevertheless, the lack of protection for men should be balanced by the serious problems that may occur in pregnancy and in other areas related to fertility, particularly where absolute poverty exists. This can be an issue for women who have a learning disability, particularly as they are likely to fall into the 'poverty trap' and may also experience the difficulties associated with different class status when accessing healthcare. However, as Turner (1995, p 108) suggests, 'These differences persist even when problems relating specifically to reproduction are removed from the statistical calculations of male/female differences'. It is apparent, therefore, that biology can only account for a small proportion of the gender inequalities in health.

Masculine/feminine behaviour

The second feature of gender inequalities in health relates to the issue of masculine and feminine behaviour. Sociobiologists argue that behaviour differences derive from biology (Jones 1994, p 249) and the need to survive. Within this context differences in male and female behaviour may be seen as 'natural' and enhancing the survival of the species. Behaviours often cited as masculine/feminine include aggression/passivity, expression of emotion and risk taking. These are deemed to be important in the male/female divide between hunting and child rearing. Whilst sociobiologists suggest that these are innate, feminists argue that they are learned through socialization. Whatever their origins, they impact on health inequalities mainly through their influence on lifestyle and leisure activities. As Jones (1994, p 253) suggests, 'Tobacco, alcohol and illegal substances are more frequently used by men'. Leisure activities involving risk, speed and height, for example, are more frequently pursued by men. It is also apparent that male suicide attempts tend to use irreversible methods.

Female/male work roles

The third area of gender inequalities in health relates to the more common types of employment. When looking at the nature of work undertaken and its impact on health, it becomes apparent that male occupations tend to involve more physical danger, whilst female occupations tend to be more repetitive. This has a definite impact on mortality, with industrial accidents resulting in higher mortality in men but chronic disease such as tenosynovitis (repetitive strain injury or RSI) causing significant morbidity in women.

The importance of employment to a person's feelings of self-worth and mental health and well-being is well documented. Equally well noted is the dearth of employment opportunities for people who have a learning disability. Many places continue to operate on traditional models of adult training centres and day centres which, whilst providing some aspects of value to service users, typically do not provide meaningful occupation with an accompanying living wage. York People First 2000 noted the inequity in financial remuneration that many of them had experienced with no increase in 'salary' between 1981 and September 1999. Whilst in September 1999 they received a 50% increase, this still only took those people in 'day occupation' to an income level of £1.50 per day.

Gender stereotypes and labelling

The final feature of health inequality relates to stereotypes of gender, particularly those relating to sexuality. According to Turner (1995, p 90), 'Women's bodies and female sexuality have often been seen as threatening to the moral and social fabric of human societies'. He adds (citing Roussell 1988), 'In both classical and Christian times, man's sexual desire for woman has been regarded as a threat to personal reason and to the social order'. This social anxiety about female sexuality has been expressed historically through religious and medical discourse, the latter focusing on the notion of hysteria. This was a disease that was believed to occur in the absence of normal sexual activity (occurring within marriage and designed to bring about reproduction). It underpinned the stereotype of women as 'the weaker sex, given to fits of weeping, fainting and uncontrollable laughter' (Turner 1995, p 91). The implication was that women could only lead healthy lives if they were sexually connected to a man in a lawful marriage, which had the aim of reproduction. Sexual relations outside marriage were associated with another sexual disorder – nymphomania. Sexual freedom in men could be tolerated but not in women.

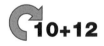

It could be argued that people who have a learning disability fall into an additional category created by society, that is asexual. In essence, people who have a learning disability have in the past been seen as eternal children and the concept that they are sexual beings is one that society continues to find uncomfortable. This relates not only to the prescribed role in society of reproduction but also to the physical act of sexual intercourse. It terms of the concept of 'person-hood', this has implications for the health of the individual, particularly in light of the impact an asexual label can have on a person's self-value and self-worth.

Within the medical literature both menstruation and pregnancy are regarded as medical problems; there is a basic logic to the medical view that 'constitutes women as patients' (Turner 1995, p 109). The impact of these beliefs has led medical ideology to constitute women as psychologically and socially vulnerable and therefore in need of close medical (male) surveillance, advice and guidance. It has also permitted the development of patriarchal control of caring, much of which is carried out by females. Many people who have a learning disability are placed within this patriarchal caring structure for much of their lives, either in the context of formal service provision or in the context of their family home.

When all these elements are drawn together, it is possible to argue that gender inequalities in health, although having a limited biological base, occur predominantly because of sociocultural features of gender and gender role. The challenge for service providers is to be aware of the influence of gender on how services are structured and also on staff–client relationships in order to genuinely move towards a system which supports the empowerment of the service user.

SOCIALIZATION AND LIFESTYLE

Learning a designated gender role forms part of the process known as socialization, through which the individual learns the culture of their society. As Taylor et al (1995, p 7) state, 'This is a lifelong process ... but the most important part probably takes place during a person's early years'. They also add: 'Socialization is closely linked to social control' to maintain the standardized and predictable behaviour without which society could not operate. This is supported by Fulcher & Scott (1999, p 124) who state: 'Human beings are social animals and the process through which someone learns to be a member of a particular society is termed socialization'. They add: 'It is through socialization that a person acquires a sense of social identity and an image of his or herself'.

Having acknowledged the importance of being a member of society in order to acquire a social identity, it must also be noted that historically large numbers of people who have a learning disability have spent their formative years in institutions where this learning experience was not available. Even in the context of care in the community, people may find themselves segregated from such experiences. This may be as a consequence of something as simple as access to appropriate transport systems or may be about the individual's lack of a social network or the non-inclusive nature of the community in which they live. Irrespective of the cause, the effect on the health of a person who has a learning disability is the same.

Socialization is influential in relation to health because of its impact on identity (and therefore mental well-being) and on lifestyle (physical well-being). As Hart (1985, p 68) states: 'Part of the culture of any social group is concerned with ideas and practices about health'. The 'regulation of bodies' inherent in the biomedical model (Turner 1995, p 205) is, in part, implemented through socialization. Individuals may be actively encouraged, particularly through secondary socialization from education and the mass media, to adopt a 'healthy lifestyle', to look after their bodies. As Hart (1985, p 69) states: 'The major causes of death today are increasingly thought of as the outcome of degenerative processes, of human bodies literally wearing out ... people should be capable of regulating the life of bodies in some degree by looking after them properly'. Individuals are therefore expected to take responsibility for their bodies, the reward offered being a longer, healthier life. However, some are socialized into health-diminishing behaviours through peer group pressure and family influence. The outcomes can be quite different and it is suggested that this may widen the health gap as those who have knowledge of and access to the healthier lifestyle become healthier than the rest, whereas peer group pressure may be hard to resist for those who have a poor sense of self, thereby compounding an existing problem.

Hart (1985, p 69) also suggests that 'The culture of an advanced industrialized society is heavily influenced by science and technology and by universal literacy'. This has further implications for health as most health information and, indeed, access is dependent on an expected level of literacy and numeracy (see below). This has implications for individuals who have a learning disability, who may not be able to interpret the available health information in order to make informed choices and decisions regarding their health. Health is about making choices, often related to cultural norms and beliefs, but also sometimes in defiance of these. Enabling individuals who have a learning disability to become involved in all decisions relating to their health is an important practitioner intervention.

RACE, ETHNICITY AND CULTURE

A further aspect of living that influences health and life chances relates to membership of minority racial/ethnic groups. Health may be affected by a diverse range of issues relating to these features, particularly cultural elements of both host and migrant settler. However, social class is also an important feature of ethnic/racial health difference.

According to Taylor et al (1995, p 6), 'Culture is a social blueprint, the way of life of a society'. It comprises the collection of ideas and habits which they learn, share and transmit from generation to generation through the process of socialization. Without a shared culture, members of society would be unable to communicate and cooperate and confusion and disorder would result. Culture, therefore, has two essential qualities: it is learned and it is shared.

Cultural development is influenced by a range of natural features such as climate, natural resources, geography and biological/genetic factors, some of which have a specific impact upon the incidence of learning disability. It also has an impact on a range of behaviours and activities including language, food preference, exchange of goods and services, sexual and family patterns, artistic expression, recreational and leisure activities and religious ideas and practices. Members of the same cultural group also share a history or ancestry although this may be more imagined than real (Anderson 1991). However, little attention has been paid to whether people who have a learning disability have a cultural identity. This appears to be in contrast to the clear identity associated with disabled people which is illustrated through the work of disabled action groups. Groups such as People First are beginning to address this imbalance. In doing so, they are starting to challenge many of the cultural stereotypes people experience and subsequently contributing to changes in the overall group identity. This in turn can only influence each individual's health positively.

'Cultural' tends to be used to identify the way of life of the dominant group; however, migration of populations has created the feature known as the ethnic group or, more recently, the ethnie. According to Jary & Jary (1991, p 202),

'Ethnicity can incorporate several forms of collective identity'. Members see themselves as culturally distinct and are seen to be so by others. According to Cashmore (1984, p 98), an ethnic group is the creative response of a people who feel somehow 'marginal to the mainstream society'. He argues that it reflects the positive tendencies of 'identification and inclusion'. As Taylor et al (1995) suggest, members have a 'shared culture and regular social interaction'. They participate in shared activities built around their common origin or culture. Ethnicities are never singular, they exist in systems and one ethnicity implies at least one other. Distinctions between ethnicities are also rarely neutral; there tend to be marked inequalities of wealth and power and antagonism between groups. The ethnie may be sociologically and psychologically important to its members or its role may be administrative or classificatory. A nation may be defined as an ethnie with statehood (Oomen 1997, p 20).

The word 'race', on the other hand, entered the English language at the beginning of the 16th century and was used primarily to indicate common features present because of shared descent. From the 19th century, however, 'race' has come to indicate a sense of 'type' designating species of humans, distinct both in physical constitution and mental capacities: caucasoid, negroid and mongoloid. Unfortunately, this approach was founded on the need to justify New World slavery (Miles 1989, pp 31–32) and forms the basis of the 'scientific racism' which has troubled society over the last century, leading to the creation of 'social races' (see below). However, although there is some medical significance of race, it is impossible to draw genetic boundaries between human groups.

The final meaning defines a 'race' as a group of people who are socially defined in a given society as belonging together because of physical markers such as skin pigmentation, hair texture, facial features, stature and the like. Where these *social races* exist, there is invariably an attribution of social and behavioural importance to physical markers, usually related to intellectual, moral and behavioural characteristics (Oomen 1997, p 63). As Taylor et al (1995) suggest, 'People construct racial categories which they then impose on their own and other groups'. They add that people 'use physical appearance to mark out the social boundaries between groups and they draw the false conclusion that the moral and intellectual achievements of groups are a result of their physical features'. 'Race' therefore reflects the negative tendencies of dissociation and exclusion.

Racism is the attribution of social significance to particular patterns of phenotypical and/or genetic difference, which leads to discrimination, and ideas of superiority. As mentioned above, modern forms of racism emerged from the 'scientific racism' of last century. Once colonization began, the idea of European innate superiority evolved slowly. Racism grew out of the need to control slaves and to justify slavery (Fenton 1999, p 44). At the same time there was a need to create a racial identity that would unify diverse Europeans and obscure the real motive for slavery and white superiority – the maintenance of wealth and privilege for a small elite. Racism therefore describes the dynamic relationship between racial prejudice, institutional discrimination, economic inequality and culture. This is sometimes described as individual racism, cultural racism and institutional racism. However, it must be stressed that people are oppressed and the ruling hierarchy is maintained by a number of other bases besides race: sex, social class, ethnicity and sexual orientation form other distinct but interrelated social cleavages.

Ethnocentrism is distinguished from racism and comprises the belief that one's own culture is superior to other cultural forms. It is typified by an attitude of prejudice or mistrust towards outsiders and also involves an incapacity to acknowledge that cultural differentiation does not imply the inferiority of those groups who are ethnically distinct from one's own (Jary & Jary 1991, pp 203–204).

A wide range of theories from psychology, social psychology and sociology have been put forward to explain the origins of racist beliefs and the nature of racism. These have in turn influenced the strategies adopted to address the problem. In the earlier part of the 20th century, drawing on the work of Freud, Allport and Adorno, racism was conceptualized as being based on an individual pathology. Ideas concerning attitude formation, prejudice, stereotyping and the authoritarian personality were very influential in constructing the view that racism occurs because of individual problems (Gross 1996, p 459). This generated the belief that not all people are racist and promoted assimilation as the optimum race relations strategy. In this approach the racial/ethnic group is absorbed into the host culture, adopting its cultural norms and ways of behaving (Jary & Jary 1991, p 32). This has been the case for many Eastern European groups who have abandoned their national identity and become 'British'. This often involves changing customs and language and even anglicizing their names. Also prophesied was the emergence of 'the brown Englishman', but phenotype cannot be altered in the way that learned behaviour can and racism has persisted even in the face of long-term residence in this country. The assimilation approach is criticized because of the resulting loss of identity, loss of 'roots'.

During the 1970s, the work of Tajfel (cited in Banton 1997, p 50) in the area of intergroup relations provided a useful explanation for some of the issues relating to the relationship between minority groups and the host culture. The understanding of the role of social categorization, social comparison and social identity and the tendency to be favourable to self has gone some way to identifying how group polarization can lead to in-group/out-group conflict and the amplification of difference. Important evidence was also provided to demonstrate that group polarization is exaggerated when there is competition for scarce resources (Banton 1997, p 50). Prejudice can be seen to occur as part of this process and is therefore always more evident in times of societal problems such as high unemployment, when competition increases. As such, during times of economic crisis people who have a learning disability and other disadvantaged groups are often further marginalized.

Ideas of multicultural approaches to race relations developed from these theories of intergroup relations, where it was believed that understanding of difference would reduce conflict between groups. Learning about 'other cultures' whilst in school was heralded as a way forward. Believed by some as having been very effective in reducing racism in school, the approach has been discredited because it may inadvertently reinforce the very stereotype that it is trying to combat (saris, samosas and steel bands approach).

Structural theories consider racism as a feature of the way society is organized. Myrdal, for example, writing in 1944, suggested that white racism was dysfunctional, a relic from the past. He argued that there was conflict between the American ideal of egalitarianism and racial stratification and he believed that racism would slowly disappear over time (cited in Solomos 1993, p 16).

Liberal reformist views from the 1960s, however, felt that this 'relic' would not disappear on its own and they argued for legislation to correct injustices from the past. Their position supported the view that individuals needed an equal opportunity to participate in society and compete, otherwise the balance would never be redressed. Marxist and neo-Marxist views, on the other hand, in criticizing the capitalist mode of production, stress the potential benefits to capitalism of the 'reserve army of labour' which may be created by the presence of migrant workers. Migrant settlers, they argue, may also be used as scapegoats when capitalism is in recession, when they are blamed for the problems that occur (Miles 1989, p 81). Gramsci (1971) also adopted a Marxist perspective but he viewed racism as part of the cultural domination exerted by the power bloc. For Gramsci, racism is deeply embedded in culture and transmitted through socialization, encouraged by capitalism as part of a 'divide and rule strategy'. These ideas have underpinned the development of theories of institutionalized racism, the active and pervasive operation of racist attitudes and practices at societal level.

The approach to racism known as antiracism has arisen from the study of institutionalized racism, where it has been found that discrimination often occurs because of inadvertent or sometimes deliberate policies that create problems for some racial/ethnic groups (Solomos 1993, p 80). For example, jobs may be advertised in magazines that are only read by the dominant group or the uniform may be unacceptable to certain groups. The approach of antiracism describes a process of monitoring and dealing with issues of inequality. Positive action is one way of addressing inequalities but in the USA, stricter affirmative action is used. Criticisms of this approach cite the unfairness of positive discrimination and the problems of a white backlash. Social work has been one area where antiracism has been influential.

In the 1990s there was an increasing move towards ethnic and racial separatism, with powerful speakers arguing that incompatible groups should not attempt to live together but that separate homelands should be created. This approach is also heavily criticized because of the escalation of conflict that often results from separation.

As can be interpreted from the discussion above, membership of minority racial and/or ethnic groups has an impact on both physical and mental health and well-being. This arises both directly from overt racism and indirectly through discriminatory processes occurring at a societal level. Amongst the problems that may be faced by families from minority ethnic/racial groups, the presence of an individual who has a learning disability may compound their difficulties. In addition, the individual themselves may also experience double discrimination. They may face issues of institutionalized racism in relation to service provision or anglocentric practitioner views, which may condemn cultural practices. In addition, the current goal of independent living may be in conflict with the ethnic group's cultural norms and values.

SOCIAL CLASS

Whilst traditional societies tended to be based on rigid social hierarchies with little movement between the layers, modern industrial societies are deemed to be much more meritocratic, still hierarchical but based on occupational achievement. Social mobility is suggested as offering equal chances to all, with those who work hard or have greater intelligence rising to the top. For those who are less able, the welfare state is deemed to provide a financial safety net and healthcare that is free at the point of use. Based on these beliefs, it came as a shock to many when the Black Report (1980, in Townsend et al 1992) demonstrated the extent to which life expectancy and morbidity show social class gradients, with social class I experiencing significantly less sickness and much greater life expectancy than class V. When these findings were replicated in *The health divide* (1988, in Townsend et al 1992), with evidence that the gap had grown wider, significant debate was initiated as to the features of social class that may be responsible for the inequalities. More recently, the *Independent Inquiry into Inequalities in Health* (Acheson 1998) has attempted to utilize the major findings to suggest government policy but debate continues to rage regarding the causative factors. In addition to social class differentials, Singh (1997) noted the higher level of health needs experienced by people who have a learning disability combined with a reduced rate of access to general practitioner services.

For Turner (1995, p 216) one of the major difficulties is 'the contradictory pull between the political process of democracy with respect to citizenship rights and the continuity of economic inequality which is closely related to the character of a capitalist society, namely the existence of social class'. He argues: 'While there have been rising expectations of healthcare, there has also been a persistent demand for equal access to healthcare services ... in other words, expectations have been rising, but they have also been within the context of a broader demand for social equality'. For Graham (1985, pp 35–36), 'Disentangling social class from personal health is a complex process' yet, she argues, 'It is crucial for this model that we can distinguish "natural health" from the cumulative impact of inequality on those at the bottom of the occupational hierarchy'.

Evidence from the reports mentioned above identifies four potential explanations for social class inequalities that need to be considered. However, it is often the dominant political perspective that is as influential in accepting and/or rejecting these explanations as the explanations themselves. Perhaps the most powerful variable relates to personal and cultural explanations regarding whether individuals are primarily responsible for their position in the social order or whether the structures of society place individuals in particular positions. The reality is a mixture of the two. Whilst society may limit the choices available to individuals based on their position in the hierarchy, it is nevertheless true that some choices are made at an individual level based on locally operating norms and values and therefore explanations should encompass a mixture of the two approaches.

The first explanation considered and predominantly discounted is that the figures constitute an artefact. 'This approach suggests that both health and class are artificial variables thrown up by attempts to measure social phenomena and that the relationship between them may itself be an artefact of little causal significance' (Townsend et al 1992, p 105). The argument here hinges on issues such as shrinkage of poorer classes and associated relative upward mobility of the healthier members of the class, leaving smaller numbers of less healthy individuals in the lowest social grouping. This approach continues to be used by individuals wishing to discount the findings although Townsend et al (1992, pp 209–210) clearly demonstrate that the phenomenon of social inequalities in health is not an artefact.

The second explanation considered is that of natural and social selection. Briefly, the argument here suggests that the strong rise to the top whereas the weak sink to lower levels of society. As Townsend et al (1992, p 105) suggest, 'The occupational class structure is seen as a filter or sorter of human beings and one of the major bases of selection is health'. They add: 'It is postulated that affected people *drift* to the bottom rung of the Registrar General's occupational scale'. In reality, however, there is little evidence to suggest that this occurs. In fact, it would be difficult for an individual to undertake most manual jobs unless they were in good health and relatively strong.

The third explanation, which relates to material and structural features of individuals' lives, locates the problem of health inequalities within the socio-economic structure of society. The argument here suggests that economic and material deprivation are key elements in the issue of health, even in the early 21st century. As Townsend et al (1992, p 110) suggest, even in advanced industrialized societies 'Profit is realized through hazardous, punishing and physically stressful work'. When this is added to poor living conditions and a nutritionally inadequate diet the vicious circle of poverty becomes evident.

The final explanation considers cultural and behavioural features of social class groups as being important in the development of health inequalities. This approach views individual lifestyle as the key element, but links this with behaviour in social groups. As Townsend et al (1992, p 110) state, 'Such explanations, when applied to modern industrial societies, often focus on the individual as the unit of analysis emphasizing unthinking, reckless or irresponsible behaviour or incautious lifestyle as the moving determinant of poor health status'. They add: 'What is implied is that people harm themselves or their children by the excessive consumption of harmful commodities ... or by their under-utilization of preventive healthcare'.

However, it can also be argued that choices in consumption of goods and services may be limited by social position. Recent evidence suggests that the poor pay more for food and goods than people in higher social classes. This has arisen because the purchase of cheaper commodities tends to require bulk purchase from 'out-of-town' facilities leading to the need for transport and storage facilities. Day-to-day purchasing at the local shop, where goods are more expensive, is often the only option. It is also important to consider that so-called 'healthy foods' tend to be sold at higher prices because of their appeal to the health-conscious middle classes. Similar arguments can be applied to leisure pursuits where, although the activities may be subsidized for the poor, cost and transport remain important issues. As well as relating to different activities, these arguments also illustrate what people who have a learning disability may experience.

The cultural explanation, therefore, although a powerful argument, on its own is unable to provide a full explanation for the development of inequalities in health. It is also important to consider that the ways in which people think and feel about themselves and others are profoundly influenced by their position in society. It can be suggested that such 'world views' shape the ways in which people act and hence their future lives. Explanations for health inequalities need to take account of both material inequalities and cultural differences.

Gender and social class

Women have traditionally been classified by husband's occupation though many work in their own right. However, class gradients in health change if women are studied based on their own occupation. Cancers of the reproductive system, for example, are more common among professional women than female manual workers (Jones 1994, p 256). Nevertheless professional women experience lower levels of sickness overall than female manual workers.

In relation to people who have a learning disability, the factors influencing the general social group will also have an effect. Added to this, parents and carers in social classes IV and V may be dependent on state provision whilst those in higher social classes will be in a position to seek extra help and to purchase services. In effect, people who have a learning disability in the lower classes will be doubly disadvantaged relative to their peers in the higher social classes.

THE EDUCATION SYSTEM

Following from the discussion of social class, it is important to consider the impact of the education system in the development of inequalities in health. However, it cannot be ignored that many of the issues arising from schooling are closely linked to those of social class. The importance of education, as Fulcher & Scott (1999, p 231) state, is that it 'plays a crucial part in the process of socialization'. Because of this, Acheson (1998, p 36) argues, 'Education plays a number of roles in influencing inequalities in health'. The report goes on to identify the education system as: directly affecting socio-economic position; influencing practical, social and emotional knowledge and skills; preparing children to participate in society; and influencing health directly through the environment it provides and the culture it espouses.

In the context of people who have a learning disability, the impact of segregated schooling upon social and emotional development as well as integration into society must be considered. For many children experiencing the special school system, their opportunity to mix with their peers and form lasting relationships is limited to the school day. Whilst most people enter adolescence with a peer group with whom they can develop their own ideas and formulate their personal identity, many adolescents who have a learning disability do not have the same peer support structures. The lack of access to such support structures can be detrimental to both social and emotional health and well-being.

Despite the repeated attempts to ensure equity in the education system, there continues to be evidence of inequalities in access and in individual educational achievement based on class, gender and race/ethnicity. The first such attempt comprised the 1944 Education Act, which was based on meritocratic principles (Fulcher & Scott 1999, p 242). The aim of the Act was to give every pupil an equal chance to develop their talents and abilities to the full within a free system of state education. This Act did not, however, cover the needs of people who have a learning disability. It was not until the 1970 Education Act that this group of people were classed as 'educable'. Over time, it became apparent that intelligence testing (the 11+ exam) was an inadequate base for the division of children into different types of school. It also became evident that the supposed 'parity of esteem' (Taylor et al 1995, p 275) of the schools was not seen in that light by pupils and their parents. The more common view was that a pass would lead to a superior school, whereas a fail indicated a poor student fit only for an inferior school. It is argued that the resulting low self-esteem created a self-fulfilling prophecy (Taylor et al 1995, p 276) and the system continued to reflect the divisions in society, particularly social class. As a result of these criticisms, comprehensive schooling was developed and 'By the end of 1978 just over 80% of state secondary education was organized along comprehensive lines' (O'Donnell 1997, p 102). The system of schooling for people who have a learning disability, however, stayed clearly outside these developments.

The debate regarding schooling and equality of opportunity escalated with the passing of the 1988 Education Reform Act which allowed schools to opt out of local authority control and, if they wished, return to a degree of selection in allocating places to pupils. A further major change in this Act was the introduction of the National Curriculum. This had 'the aim of developing a shared national culture and identity ... however, while it reflects a strong concern with national culture, the substantial increase in non-national curriculum time brought about by the Dearing review (1994–95) allowed more scope' (O'Donnell 1997, p 130). It also attempted to ensure that the content of teaching was very similar in all schools through the introduction of a series of key stages with associated abilities. This also permitted comparative testing of children against age-related standards and, more recently, the introduction of 'league tables'.

Despite changes and attempts to ensure equality of opportunity for all children, statistics and exam results continue to reveal major differences between lower and higher social classes (Macionis & Plummer 1998, p 539). The introduction of league tables and other performance measures can be seen to militate against the inclusion of people who have a learning disability in mainstream schools.

The higher the social class of the parents, the more successful the child will be in education. Inequality begins in primary school and higher education is dominated by the professional and semiprofessional classes. Many reasons have been given to explain working-class underachievement. Perhaps one of the foremost is the issue of intelligence and how it is measured. The use of tests and exams may introduce a bias against the lower classes and also people who have a learning disability because they are reliant on particular levels of literacy and numeracy. They are also biased because they are located within a particular culture framework, reflecting the beliefs and values of the testers (Taylor et al 1995, p 294). Material and cultural factors are also important as poverty and low wages can affect school performance and concentration at school (Fulcher & Scott 1999, p 233), through factors such as poor diet and money problems. Low wages/unemployment leading to a lack of educational toys and books can affect educational development before and during school education. Lack of money can mean going without sports equipment and clothing, school trips, calculators and music lessons.

Poor housing conditions such as overcrowding, poor heating and damp can lead to homework difficulties and higher levels of sickness may affect school attendance, where the child misses lessons and falls behind. Financial support can be a problem and it may be difficult to support and maintain children in post-16 education, despite their abilities (Taylor et al 1995, p 295). Pupils may be encouraged to leave school and get a job or join a job-training scheme to support themselves or to bring money into the home as the benefit system doesn't encourage or enable further education.

Encouragement is also held to be a factor as studies show that higher social class parents are more likely to encourage and take interest in their child's progress (Fulcher & Scott 1999, p 233). They are more likely to visit school, to discuss exam options and career choices and they encourage their child to stay on beyond 16. They can afford further education and they place higher value on getting educational qualifications. Working-class parents may see education as having little relevance to their own jobs which may lead to poor motivation in children and lower levels of achievement and expectations regardless of ability. On the other hand, it is argued that working-class parents do encourage their children but are not evident in school because their own experience of the education system was so negative. Parents may be adversely influenced by their own low self-esteem and may therefore find it difficult to encourage and support their child's development. When the child has a learning disability this may be further compounded by low expectations of the child's abilities and an inability or unwillingness on the part of the parents to challenge 'authority figures' to ensure their child is given the optimum support.

Another feature of the education system that is deemed to be relevant to the problems experienced by lower social class children is that of language use. According to Bernstein (1971, cited in Meighan & Siraj-Blatchford 1997), 'School is necessarily concerned with the transmission and development of universalistic orders of meaning'. He suggests a relationship between social class and language use (speech patterns) and described two types of speech pattern: restricted code and elaborated code.

Restricted code is used by all groups, particularly between people who have so much in common that there is no need to make meanings explicit in speech, such as friends, married couples and family members. Since they have a shared experience(s) and understanding, it is unnecessary to spell out their meanings and intentions in detail; these are conveyed more by gesture, voice intonations, and the context within which the communication occurs (Taylor et al 1995, p 297). Thus meanings are limited to a particular social group and not readily available to outsiders. As Meighan & Siraj-Blatchford (1997, p 149) state, 'The social relations of a particular group ... will generate a *system of communication* specific to that group and their conditions of life'.

Restricted code is a kind of shorthand speech, characterized by short, grammatically simple, often unfinished sentences with a limited use of adjectives and adverbs. Elaborated code, on the other hand, explicitly verbalizes many of the meanings used in the restricted code. It fills in the details, spells out the relationships and provides explanations (Fulcher & Scott 1999, p 234). The listener need not share the experience and understanding of the speaker. In principle, it is available to all as the meanings have been made explicit. There is a tendency in the higher social classes to encourage children to develop their elaborated code, thereby enabling them to communicate more effectively with a wider range of people. However, as a consequence of different experiences and opportunities, it is possible that some people who have a learning disability will not have developed their understanding of the elaborated code sufficiently to make appropriate use of it.

The elaborated code is also used in school (Fulcher & Scott 1999, p 234), as it is more suited to understanding textbooks, writing essays and exam answers. Given that children from the higher social classes use it at home they find the transition to school much easier and learn more than a working-class child using a restricted code (Meighan & Siraj-Blatchford 1997, p 150). The teacher may also mistake the working-class child's restricted use of language as a lack of ability and therefore expect less. Children who are capable of understanding within their restricted code may view themselves as lacking intelligence if they are unable to respond when elaborated code is used. Thus a self-fulfilling prophecy may come into effect (Taylor et al 1995, p 299).

A further feature relating to educational inequalities is that of culture clash. Schools are mainly middle-class institutions and stress the middle-class way of life (Taylor et al 1995, p 299). This includes the importance of hard work and study and the idea of making sacrifices now for future rewards, also known as deferred gratification (Fulcher & Scott 1999, p 233). Therefore middle-class children are more tuned in to the atmosphere of school, of doing homework, of foregoing TV, of good behaviour and cooperative attitudes to teacher. Working-class children may find the atmosphere and values of school to be unfamiliar and different from home, therefore resulting in a culture clash (Meighan & Siraj-Blatchford 1997, p 150). Teachers, who are also middle-class, may compound the problem by their tendency to view middle-class children as more intelligent and lower class pupils as 'troublemakers'.

Given the already acknowledged links between success in the education system and improved health behaviour, it is not difficult to see that children with difficulties in school are more likely to experience health problems. At its most basic level this arises from lack of knowledge and understanding. However, the picture is complicated by the impact of poor communication and interpersonal skills on the individual's ability to access health information and the influence of low self-esteem on self-concept and overall mental well-being.

In relation to pupils who have a learning disability, an additional problem that may occur is that the child's needs may not be fully apparent prior to school entry and he or she may experience problems in coping with the learning environment. This could include hostility from other pupils and may lead to the child being labelled as a low achiever by the teaching staff. Since the implementation of the 1981 Education Act it is expected that all children with special needs will have the opportunity to be statemented prior to entering the education system. This is intended to be a positive experience that ensures that schools are prepared to receive the children prior to their arrival. Unfortunately, the system does not always work as it should and not all children are identified as having a learning disability before entering school. The impact this may have on the child's self-esteem and mental health should not be underestimated. In addition, not all children or their parents wish their child to be statemented as this can confine the child to the segregated education system rather than allowing appropriate and supported access to mainstream education.

The issue of placing children who have a learning disability in mainstream education continues to be debated as advantages and disadvantages are explored. The gains for all children of contact with all abilities and the long-term benefit in understanding and appreciation of each other's needs that can accrue have to be offset against the possibility of the detrimental effects of out-group membership. Concern amongst parents obviously remains when some parents opt for cosmetic correction of the features of Down's syndrome. As Legge (1998) states, 'The parents say they are doing the best they can for a child they hope will be able to enter mainstream education without their classmates bullying and jeering them'. However, correction of features does not alter the ability of the child to perform and the underlying issue of enabling participation is not addressed.

It is important to consider that without appropriate schooling, the child with a learning disability may be less articulate and may not acquire the necessary interpersonal skills to deal effectively with their own health needs. In this situation, parents or carers may have to provide support. The ability of these individuals to provide that support will also be influenced by their own educational experience.

OCCUPATION, WORK ENVIRONMENT AND UNEMPLOYMENT

In a society which has been heavily influenced by the 'Protestant work ethic', much emphasis is placed on the importance of work in relation to status and social class. It also has a powerful influence on our view of work, making us reluctant to see it as a cause of ill health. As Taylor et al (1995, p 317) state, 'Work has a major influence on people's lives ... it can affect their income, standing in the community, leisure activities and political views'. According to Fulcher & Scott (1999, p 504), the creation of separate workplaces has meant that the experience of work has become 'a distinct part of life'. They add that 'Those in paid work were spending a considerable proportion of their daily lives in the workplace' and that 'This experience was shaped by aspects of the work that were largely outside their control'. As Acheson (1998, p 44) states, 'Employment plays a fundamental role in our society ... people are often defined, and define themselves, through what they do for a living'.

However, it is important to acknowledge that 'the technology, the pace of work, and the work environment' are 'controlled by the worker's employer' (Fulcher & Scott 1999, p 504). This is not without its problems as there is evidence to suggest that 'An imbalance between psychological demands and control, and lack of control at work are associated with increased risk of coronary heart disease, musculoskeletal disorders, mental illness and sickness absence' (Acheson 1998, p 48). As Hart (1985, p 54) states, there are also 'inequalities within occupational groups'. She further suggests (p 66) 'In their contribution to the *social division of labour*, manual workers must systematically expose their health to greater risk'.

The emphasis on the importance of work, however, has an adverse effect on those individuals who, for whatever reason, are not employed. The personal and social effects of unemployment are extensive and usually detrimental to health, although release from a stressful work environment may have some benefits. Also important in relation to work and non-work is the issue of poverty. As Graham (1985, p 32) states, 'Poverty can only be understood in the context of wealth; in the context of a society organized around economic differences between people'. Poverty is therefore closely linked to social class and has a direct influence on where and how people lead their lives. It influences the area where they are able to live and the quality and type of housing to which they have access. Because of this, Jones (1994, p 178) states, 'Poverty shapes health in a number of ways'. The difficulties experienced by people who have a learning disability in accessing valued and meaningful employment immediately place many of them in the category of unemployed, with all the associated health risk factors.

5

ACCESS TO HEALTHCARE

All the issues addressed thus far link together under the banner of 'access to healthcare'. All influence an individual's access to services in different ways and it is this combination of effects that is so problematic. According to Tudor-Hart (cited in Hart 1985, p 59), there is widespread evidence of an 'inverse care law' where those whose needs are greatest get the least. This is reinforced by the work of Singh (1997), Band (1998) and Lindsay (1998), all of whom clearly acknowledge the increased health risks and health needs of people who have a learning disability. This increased need is also balanced with the apparent decrease in accessibility to many generic healthcare services such as screening and GP clinics (Shaughnessy 1999, Singh 1997).

Care services may be implicated in this through the operation of three features. The first of these involves the physical placement of facilities and services. Primary care facilities (GP, dentist, optician and pharmacy) are, for example, far less evident in poorer/deprived areas. Arguments against their placement in these areas are very powerful, ranging from the risk of vandalism and theft to the unwillingness of people to access the facilities, thereby leading to underuse. Whether the validity of these arguments has been really tested is debatable but these are accepted truths and the need for transport to access more distant facilities therefore becomes an issue. In addition, physical access may be an issue from the perspective of people who have a learning disability, as well as other practical issues such as appointment times (Lawrie 1995, p 32), which are often too short for people who have communication difficulties. Also unhelpful waiting times can cause problems for people who have a learning disability who are unable to understand the system in place.

The second feature relates to the relationship between the individual and the professional services. GPs, for example, were found to spend far less time with their patients from lower social classes during research carried out in 1976 by Cartwright & O'Brien (cited in Hart 1985, p 59). This situation may be further compounded for service users who have little or no verbal communication (Lawrie 1995, p 32). Without skilled support GPs will often find this group of people difficult to work with. People from the lower social classes and those who have a learning disability may also fail to get the necessary services because of general lack of knowledge about health issues and problems in articulating their needs based on their poor experience of the education system (Matthews 1996, p 36). Practitioner stereotypes based on class, gender and race/ethnicity may also be problematic. A particular issue in this area is that of informed consent, especially in the context of invasive procedures. Evidence suggests that some people are being excluded from screening afforded to the rest of the female population as a consequence of this issue (Shaughnessy 1999). As Taylor et al (1998, p 60) suggest, a failure to identify specialist needs can 'devalue people with a learning disability by failing to meet their health requirements'.

The third feature that can increase inequalities between groups is the issue of health promotion, an activity based on middle-class values of deferred gratification and individual success. For the general public, access to health-enhancing behaviours may be limited by poverty and availability, whilst indulgence in health-diminishing behaviours is often a result of strategies to cope with stress. In relation to people who have a learning disability, these may be compounded by poor access to services as discussed above. As Lawrie (1995, p 32) states, 'It is clear that many services are not providing the basic aspects of healthcare, and that the current emphasis on health promotion may not be filtering through to the services delivered to people with learning disabilities'.

CONCLUSION

Overall, these problems in access to healthcare appear to be widening the health gap between rich and poor. For Wilkinson (1996, p 215), however, this widening gap in health is more about the destruction of social cohesion that is occurring as a result of the widening wealth gap between rich and poor. He states: 'The material environment is merely the indelible mark and constant reminder of the oppressive fact of one's failure, of the atrophy of any sense of having a place in a community, and of one's social exclusion and devaluation as a human being'. He further adds: 'To feel depressed, cheated, bitter, desperate, vulnerable, frightened, angry, worried about debts or job and housing insecurity; to feel devalued, useless, helpless, uncared for, hopeless, isolated, anxious and a failure: these feelings can dominate people's whole experience of life, colouring their experience of everything else'. 'It is the chronic stress arising from feelings like these which does the damage', he argues.

For people who have a learning disability, whose role is already generally undervalued, the stress and anxiety associated with failure to succeed are great. Social exclusion continues to be evident for this group in society to the probable detriment of their health and well-being. According to Rodger (1996), for example, 'People with learning disability are known to experience a greater number of health problems than other people but use health services less than the general population'. This is made even worse by the inadequate provision of appropriate healthcare services. As Marwick (1998) states, 'Service providers must address the issue of inequalities in health care provision for people with learning disabilities and charge health care providers with the task of closing the divide between the experiences of the general public and those of this client group'.

This chapter has examined some of the factors that have an impact on the health of individuals. It has also briefly related these to the specific area of learning disability. The reality unfortunately remains that, whilst an individual can make some improvements in their own health, the bulk of health-related issues rests very firmly with the role of society in the provision of equal and accessible services to all citizens.

FURTHER READING

Fulcher J, Scott J 1999 Sociology. Oxford University Press, Oxford. Taylor P, Richardson J, Yeo A et al 1995 Sociology in focus. Causeway, Ormskirk
These two introductory sociology texts provide a useful exploration of the key concepts and ideas in sociology. They also provide background reading relevant to the study of the areas of social cleavage that impact on health – gender, social class and race/ethnicity.

Jones L 1994 The social context of health and health work. Macmillan, Basingstoke
This text applies the concepts of sociology directly to the issues of health and healthcare practice. It provides a good grounding in the subject area and is easy to read and understand.

Naidoo J, Wills J 1994 Health promotion: foundations for practice. Baillière Tindall, London
This is a well-written text, based in practice, which considers approaches to health promotion within a framework of the wider factors that impact on individual health.

Townsend P, Davidson N, Whitehead M 1992 Inequalities in health. Penguin, Harmondsworth. Acheson D 1998 Independent inquiry into inequalities in health. The Stationery Office, London
These are sequential reports exploring inequalities in health arising from social class. I would recommend them as essential reading for anyone working in healthcare.

Turner B S 1995 Medical power and social knowledge, 2nd edn. Sage, London
This is a more indepth critique of medical power, particularly in relation to issues of gender. It is an advanced text requiring a prior understanding of the sociological concepts under discussion but is nevertheless a very interesting read for individuals working in healthcare practice.

Wilkinson R 1996 Unhealthy societies. Routledge, London
This is a very interesting and thought-provoking account which takes a different stance on the ways in which social class may produce inequalities in health, particularly emphasizing the size of the gap between rich and poor as a factor. This is an important read for anyone interested in the study of inequalities in health.

REFERENCES

Acheson D 1998 Independent inquiry into inequalities in health. The Stationery Office, London
Anderson B 1991 Imagined communities. Verso, London
Band R 1998 Health for all. Mencap, London
Banton M 1997 Ethnic and racial consciousness. Longman, London
BBC 1999 Disabled century. BBC, London
Cashmore E E 1984 Dictionary of race and ethnic relations, 2nd edn. Routledge, London
Craft A, Bicknell J, Hollins S 1985 Mental handicap. Baillière Tindall, London
Fenton S 1999 Ethnicity: racism, class and culture. Macmillan, Basingstoke

Fulcher J, Scott J 1999 Sociology. Oxford University Press, Oxford

Graham H 1985 Health and welfare. Nelson, Walton-on-Thames

Gramsci A 1971 Selections from the prison notebooks. Lawrence and Wishart, London

Gross R 1996 Psychology: the science of mind and behaviour, 3rd edn. Hodder and Stoughton, London

Hart N 1985 The sociology of health and medicine. Causeway, Ormskirk

Jary D, Jary J 1991 Dictionary of sociology. HarperCollins, London

Jones L 1994 The social context of health and health work. Macmillan, Basingstoke

Knight J 1999 Hidden legacy. New Scientist 164:2212

Lawrie K 1995 Better healthcare for people with learning disability. Nursing Times 91(19):32–33

Legge A 1998 Face values. Nursing Times 94(40):36

Lindsay M 1998 Signposts for success. DoH, London

Macionis J, Plummer K 1998 Sociology: a global introduction. Prentice Hall, New Jersey

Marwick A 1998 Healthcare for people with learning disability. Nursing Times 94(36):64–65

Matthews D 1996 Learning disability: the challenge for nursing. Nursing Times 92(27):36–38

Meighan R, Siraj-Blatchford I 1997 A sociology of educating, 3rd edn. Cassell, London

Miles R 1989 Racism. Routledge, London

Naidoo J, Wills J 1994 Health promotion: foundations for practice. Baillière Tindall, London

O'Brien M 1995 Health and lifestyle: a critical mess? In: Bunton R, Nettleton S, Burrows R (eds) The sociology of health promotion. Routledge, London

O'Donnell M 1997 Introduction to sociology. Thomas Nelson, Walton-on-Thames

Oomen T K 1997 Citizenship, nationality and ethnicity. Polity Press, Cambridge

Rodger D 1996 Strengthening primary care. Nursing Times 92(33):61–62

Shaughnessy P 1999 Better cervical screening for women with learning disabilities. Nursing Times 95:44–45

Singh P 1997 Prescription for change. Mencap, London

Solomos J 1993 Race and racism in Britain. Macmillan, Basingstoke

Taylor G, Pearson J, Cook H 1998 Family planning for women with learning disability. Nursing Times 94(40):60–61

Taylor P, Richardson J, Yeo A et al 1995 Sociology in focus. Causeway, Ormskirk

Townsend P, Davidson N, Whitehead M 1992 Inequalities in health. Penguin, Harmondsworth

Turner B S 1995 Medical power and social knowledge, 2nd edn. Sage, London

Wilkinson R 1996 Unhealthy societies. Routledge, London

Health needs of people who have a learning disability

Steve Turner

KEY ISSUES

- A wide range of chronic and acute health problems are more common among people who have learning disabilities than among the general population
- Some health problems are associated with the cause of the learning disability
- Lifestyle plays an important role in the health of people who have learning disabilities
- Nevertheless, many people who have learning disabilities enjoy good health

INTRODUCTION

Earlier chapters of this book have made it clear that people who have learning disabilities are an extremely diverse group. A wide range of causes are responsible for learning disability and these causes have an even wider range of direct and indirect consequences for the health and well-being of the individuals affected. This chapter will detail what is known about the diseases, conditions and susceptibilities that seem to be particularly prevalent among people who have learning disabilities. Many of these problems may severely restrict and even shorten their life. People with particular syndromes like Down's syndrome and fragile X syndrome have a high risk of certain physical and neurological conditions but many health problems are indirect consequences, resulting from the social, economic and employment restrictions that intellectual disability often brings (Pitetti & Campbell 1991, Rimmer et al 1994). It is therefore important to recognize that many people who have learning disabilities are capable of enjoying a long-term level of health which is as good as their non-disabled peers. For example, a study of 500 people living in three types of residential care (village communities, residential campuses and dispersed housing) in England and Scotland found that between 14% and 20% had no reported health problems (Emerson et al 1999).

Establishing an accurate and comprehensive picture of the physical health of people who have learning disabilities is a complex task. There are several reasons for this. First, information relating to the health of people who have learning disabilities in practice often refers only to those known to agencies providing services to them; that is, the population base for any conclusions about disease prevalence is defined administratively.

This definition is likely to overrepresent those who have severe learning disabilities and those living in hospital, hostel or other staffed accommodation. Their dependence on services, especially residential services, may mean that their health is more often monitored, recorded and researched. In contrast, the large group of people who have mild or moderate learning disabilities – up to 10 times as many as those who have severe disabilities – are often not in contact with services, particularly once they have left school. As a result, the health status of this group is also largely unknown. There is also evidence that people from ethnic minorities are underrepresented among those known to learning disability services and there is little evidence to say whether their health needs differ from other groups of people who have learning disabilities (Chaplin et al 1996).

Second, much research evidence on health and learning disability has in the past come from studies of long-stay institutional populations. Even though this group has declined dramatically in number in recent years, the research base has tended to lag behind. Some health problems reported in the literature may be at least partly the result of long-term institutional living, rather than the person's learning disability, especially when healthcare has been less than optimal. When interpreting such research evidence, it is worth asking the question: are these findings just as likely to apply in a community setting?

A third difficulty is that administrative definitions of learning disability vary from country to country. In the US, where much information on health and learning disability originates, the administrative label of 'mental retardation' gives eligibility to welfare payments and so people who have mild or moderate disabilities are more visible. Information on health status which is based on this broader definition of learning disability may not be helpful when considering the risks to health of adults in contact with services in the UK. It is particularly difficult to judge the relevance of disease prevalence studies when they fail to report the range of severity of learning disability found in the study population or to examine whether prevalence rates vary across the profound, severe, moderate and mild subcategories.

Fourth, the picture may be distorted by the fact that one condition, Down's syndrome, has been given more attention in epidemiological studies than others. This is partly due to it being the most commonly diagnosed cause of learning disability, accounting for 40% of all those identified as learning disabled, and partly because until quite recently, the remaining 60% was composed of people with rare conditions or those for whom no cause had been ascertained. Fragile X syndrome, which may be more common than Down's syndrome (but does not always lead to identifiable learning disability), was not recognized until 1977 and many people with fragile X remain undiagnosed. Many studies which report the incidence or prevalence of morbidity distinguish simply between two groups of people who have learning disabilities – those with Down's syndrome and those identified as being learning disabled as a result of a number of disparate or undiagnosed causes. Thus, there is no doubt that many associations between aspects of physical ill health and particular causes of learning disability are as yet unidentified.

Finally, there is the difficult problem of interpreting studies of morbidity which use different comparison groups and different statistical criteria for their conclusions. In recent years, studies of disease prevalence have followed the fashion in reports of clinical trials by using odds ratios as a kind of statistical shorthand to compare risks or treatment effects. Thus, an odds ratio of 2 means that morbidity or mortality is twice as high in one group compared with another. However, studies involving small numbers of people are less likely to achieve reliable results than larger studies and reported odds ratios which appear to demonstrate a higher prevalence or incidence of disease may be misleading, being due to some unidentified bias or chance factors. Larger studies are less likely to suffer from this problem. Unfortunately larger studies are also more expensive and therefore less common. Where they do occur, they may be more likely to use institutional populations and may therefore be a poor guide to health problems and risks which may occur in community settings.

In order to reflect this situation, this chapter is organized in the following way. First, a review is made of the evidence linking the two most common causes of learning disability – Down's syndrome and fragile X syndrome – with a higher risk of mortality and ill health. Then, findings about ill health and learning disability which are not tied to a particular syndrome or condition are presented. Finally, the importance of risk factors and lifestyle is discussed. Wherever possible, research findings are reported with reference to the setting (i.e. institutional or home based) and the comparison group used (people who have other forms of learning disability or the general population). Because of the need to concentrate on conditions and risks which non-specialist staff are more likely to encounter during their practice, this chapter does not review the evidence on health problems related to less common conditions such as Rett's syndrome or Prader–Willi syndrome.

DOWN'S SYNDROME

Infections and immune deficiencies

For many years the biggest threat to the lives of people with Down's syndrome was respiratory infection, which may have been responsible for at least half of all deaths (Carter & Jancar 1983), representing a 62-fold increase in mortality compared with the general population. Increased susceptibility to infection may be due to institutional living, the combined effect of heart disease and general debilitation, the presence of pulmonary vascular abnormalities and pulmonary hypertension and immunological deficiencies (Thase 1982).

In the last few decades, the risk of death from respiratory infection has retreated. McGrother & Marshall (1990) report that such deaths among a Down's syndrome cohort born in Leicestershire between 1980 and 1985 represented 5% of all deaths, compared with 50% in Carter's 1958 study. The decline in mortality has been attributed to improved treatment, including the use of antibiotic therapy, and better institutional care (Nelson & Crocker 1978). While the risk has decreased, death rates due to infection remain high compared with the general population (Table 4.1).

Historically, deaths from other infectious diseases have also been significantly higher among people with Down's syndrome than among the age-matched general population (Oster & Van Den Temple 1975). Hepatitis virus infection has been reported as having a high prevalence among people with Down's syndrome living in institutions in the US, Spain and Belgium (Devuyst & Maesen-Collard 1991, Garcia Bengoechea et al 1989, Hershow et al 1989). While the danger of infection may be declining as fewer people live

TABLE 4.1	*Down's syndrome, mortality and prevalence of disease*	
People with Down's syndrome, compared with	**(a) the general population**	**(b) others who have learning disabilities**
are *more* likely to die from …	Congenital heart conditions (×30–74)	Congenital heart conditions (×10)
	Respiratory infection (×62)	
are *more* likely to suffer from …	Hypothyroidism	Hypothyroidism (×3–5)
	Leukaemia (×10–20)	Leukaemia (×?)
	Hepatitis B (×28)	Hepatitis B (×5)
	Alzheimer's	Alzheimer's (×4)
	Epilepsy	
	Alzheimer's with epilepsy (×8)	Alzheimer's with epilepsy
	Atlantoaxial instability (×7)	
	Degenerative spinal disorders (×4)	
	Gastrointestinal tract abnormality	
	Hearing impairment	Hearing impairment (×2–18)
	Visual impairment (×4 for functional blindness)	
	Muscular weakness	Muscular weakness
are *less* likely to suffer from…	Hepatitis A	Epilepsy (if dementia free)

long term in institutions, there is evidence that hepatitis B is also common among people with Down's syndrome living at home. Renner et al (1985) estimated that the prevalence of hepatitis B in this group was five times higher than among people with other forms of learning disability also living at home and 28 times higher than among the general population. The same authors concluded that hepatitis A, which has a different route of infection, may be *less* common among people with Down's syndrome than in the general population.

The high risk of respiratory and hepatitis B infections may be at least partly due to the weakened autoimmunological status of this group. Immunological deficiencies in people with Down's syndrome relating to T cell abnormalities have been identified, which could result in a higher susceptibility to infections (Pueschel 1987). It is also possible that these abnormalities may account for the increased prevalence of age-related disorders among people with Down's syndrome. As normal individuals age, they express an increased number of a type of lymphocyte identified as 3G5+ T cells. Children with Down's syndrome have been found to have the same proportion of these age-related (3G5+) T cells as normal 50–70-year-old persons (Rabinowe et al 1989).

Autoimmune disorder related to immune deficiency of the T-lymphocyte system may also be the reason for the observed high prevalence of thyroid disorders among people with Down's syndrome (Levin et al 1975, Mani 1988, Whittingham et al 1977). Compared with people who have other causes of learning disability, the risk of hypothyroidism may be between three and five times higher (Hughes et al 1982, Kinnell et al 1987).

Heart and other congenital disorders

There is evidence that congenital heart disease is now the biggest single cause of death among people who have Down's syndrome. Estimates range from 35% (Deaton 1973), through 50% (Hurst & Logue 1970) to 65% (McGrother & Marshall 1990). Murdoch (1984), in a study of 134 children with Down's syndrome aged 0–10 living at home, found that the risk of congenital heart disease was 74 times that of non-disabled children of the same age. By adulthood, the increase over expected occurrence has been estimated to be 30-fold (Greenwood & Nadas 1976, Katlic et al 1977). Chaney et al (1985) found that the death rate from congenital heart disease was 10 times higher among people with Down's syndrome aged 0–30 than among people who have other kinds of learning disabilities. There is also evidence that heart problems may manifest themselves in later years. Goldhaber et al (1987) found valvular heart abnormalities in 25 out of 35 asymptomatic young adults (mean age 26 years). The most frequent problems were mitral valve prolapse and aortic regurgitation. Geggel et al (1993) also studied 35 patients with Down's syndrome with no known congenital heart disease and found heart valve dysfunction in 16. They suggest that screening for the development of valve dysfunction should be continued during the teenage and young adult period.

CASE STUDY 4.1

The health of young people with Down's syndrome

For most people, early adulthood is a period free from worries about health. While many young people with Down's syndrome enjoy good health, for some it can be a time when chronic childhood problems have an increasingly restricting effect on life opportunities and these problems may be compounded by new problems like weight gain or loss of fitness once they leave school. Such problems can affect the whole family. Here are four examples.

Gill is 20 and lives with her parents. Her heart condition was diagnosed before she started school and has worsened in recent years, preventing her from walking far. She also has a long-standing hearing problem. Her health problems have recently been compounded by the discovery that she has a chronic skin condition. This condition is related to immune deficiency, which may lie behind a lot of health problems suffered by people with Down's syndrome. Gill is less fit than she was while at school and has put on weight. All these health problems seriously affect her college, home and social life. Her mother is concerned about her future health and angry that she has not received optimal treatment in the past. She also regrets the effect that all these problems have had on Gill's younger sister.

Anthea is 23 and also lives at home. Throughout her childhood she has had chronic problems with her hearing, although this has improved recently, and skeletal problems in her hip and neck. She has a pin in her hip and one leg is several inches shorter than the other. Her mother has been told by the consultant that a hip replacement operation is not yet advisable because she does not meet his criterion of being in severe pain. However, Anthea's mother believes there is reluctance to operate because Anthea has Down's syndrome. Her hip seriously restricts her social life and daytime activities.

CASE STUDY 4.1 *(Cont'd)*

Frank is a polite and well-liked young man. Unfortunately, he has a serious heart complaint which damaged his lungs when he was quite young. His parents were told not to expect him to live beyond adolescence. He is now 22. He has oxygen for 16 hours each day to help ease his condition, as well as taking other medication. His mother says she has to build him up before any event so that he does not become exhausted. If he does too much he may feel unwell for up to 2 days afterwards. There are no centres appropriate to Frank's needs and given his health, she is quite happy to have him at home. His parents have no idea how long he will live and treat every day as a bonus.

Billy is now 20 and left school at 19. His health is a major concern. His father says Billy needs a triple transplant and believes that he hasn't had it because he has Down's syndrome. His heart has been a major restriction on activities at school and since, and he has a wheelchair which he sometimes uses when he goes out. He has always slept poorly, but does not take his prescribed sleeping tablets because they made him too tired during the day. Now his parents don't think too much about the future, but there remains some defiant hope: 'They said he'd never walk and talk; he did. They said he'd never live past the age of 5; he did. Now he's 21 in March, we're thinking of inviting everyone who said he wouldn't do things to his party. I don't know if they'd come, like.'

Other congenital conditions have been described in the literature which are likely to have implications for the physical health of adults with Down's syndrome. MacLachlan et al (1993) found that atlantoaxial instability, a condition affecting the strength of the neck joints, was seven times more likely among people who have Down's syndrome than among normal controls. This study reports that 13% of adults with Down's syndrome were at risk of dislocation of the neck, while Cremers et al (1993) found a prevalence of 32% among children aged 6–17. The high prevalence of atlantoaxial instability among children with Down's syndrome is usually asymptomatic (Pueschel 1987) and may not necessarily preclude physical activity (Cremers et al 1993). However, a high incidence of degenerative cervical arthritis may be associated with such skeletal abnormalities (Howells 1989). MacLachlan et al (1993) also found that degenerative spinal disorders were nearly four times as common as in normal controls. Hresko et al (1993) report a high prevalence of hip abnormalities, not all of which were manifest during childhood. The 28% of patients with such abnormalities had significantly inferior walking ability, which worsened with age. Levy (1992) found high prevalence of gastrointestinal tract abnormalities, including oesophageal atresia, duodenal stenosis, imperforate anus and Hirschsprung's disease. A possible association with coeliac disease (intolerance to gluten) has also been found (Simila & Kokkonen 1990).

Neurological disorders

Evidence of premature ageing has been well documented in persons with Down's syndrome. Early onset of clinically apparent dementia of the Alzheimer type develops in approximately 40% of people with Down's syndrome by the sixth decade of life, while neuropathological evidence of Alzheimer's disease can be seen in many (if not all) people with Down's syndrome by the fourth decade (Ball & Nuttall 1980, Burger & Vogel 1973, Crapper et al 1975, Ellis et al 1974, Wisniewski et al 1985). According to Schupf et al (1989), people with Down's syndrome aged over 50 were 3–4 times more likely to regress than those under 50 or matched controls. In a large-scale study, Collacott et al (1992) compared 371 people with Down's syndrome aged 16–78 with people who have other forms of learning disabilities and found the risk of dementia was nearly 17 times higher in the Down's syndrome group. The incidence of deaths from dementia may be expected to increase as longevity increases among people with Down's syndrome (Thase 1982).

It is important to bear in mind that the relationship between clinical symptoms and brain pathology is not at all clear. Frequently Alzheimer's disease is diagnosed only at postmortem, with no previous observable clinical symptoms (Dalton 1992, Dalton et al 1993, Karlinsky 1986, Mann 1988). In an early study, Olson & Shaw (1969) reviewed the cases of 26 Down's syndrome individuals who had subsequently died and found that the three people who had lived longer than 35 years all showed the distinct pathological signs of Alzheimer's disease. However, only one of these had a history of dementing behaviour. Obviously the sample size is very small but it highlights the need for caution in assuming a link between this kind of functional degeneration and Down's syndrome. One possible explanation is that symptoms of depression or other disorders may mask the signs of dementia (Burt et al 1992). The issues relating to the diagnosis of dementia have been examined in detail by Aylward et al (1997).

Epilepsy is known to be more common in people of all ages with Down's syndrome than in the general population (Strafstrom 1993). For younger age groups there appears to be no difference between those with Down's syndrome and people who have other conditions (Van Schrojenstein Lantman-de Valk et al 1997). However, this study found that for those aged over 50, the risk of epilepsy was nearly three times higher in the Down's syndrome group. Among people with Down's syndrome and dementia of the Alzheimer type, the incidence of epileptic seizures has been noted to be up to eight times higher (i.e. up to 84%) compared to people with dementia of the Alzheimer type who do not have Down's syndrome (Evenhuis 1990, Lai & Williams 1989). While it has been argued that Down's syndrome, Alzheimer's disease and Parkinson's disease may be linked to a common pathogenic mechanism underlying observed neuronal degeneration (Lai & Williams 1989, Raghaven et al 1993), it does not necessarily follow that the high prevalence (vis-a-vis the general population) of epilepsy among the over-50s is due entirely to the elevated incidence of Alzheimer's. Collacott (1993) suggests that only late-onset epilepsy may be associated with Alzheimer's disease.

Cancers

It has been noted that people of all ages with Down's syndrome have a far higher risk of death from leukaemia than do members of the general population. This association has been documented for over 50 years and incidence is estimated at between 10 and 20 times that in the general population (Fong &

Brodeur 1987). Although peaking in the childhood years, the increased risk may also extend into adulthood (Fong & Brodeur 1987, Scholl et al 1982). Buckley et al (1994) found that the risk of acute lymphocytic leukaemia was three times higher among children with Down's syndrome compared with normal controls. An association with testicular cancer (Braun et al 1985) has also been reported.

Obesity

Compared with people who have other forms of learning disability, Down's syndrome appears to increase the risk of being overweight (BMI >25). The increased risk has been estimated as 2.5 times for men and 13.5 for women (Bell & Bhate 1992). Prasher (1995), in a study of 201 hospital and community residents in the West Midlands, did not confirm this gender difference, reporting 52% of men and 47% of women as obese and 84% of men and 80% of women as overweight/obese. This gives an odd ratio vis-a-vis the general population of 8.7 for male obesity and 5.9 for female obesity and 2.1 for male overweight/obesity and 2.5 for female overweight/obesity.

It would be wrong to assume that obesity is related to Down's syndrome in a simple causal manner. Both Prasher (1995) and Rimmer et al (1992) found higher levels of obesity among those living in the community. One possible explanation for such differences is that institutional life (school or residential care) may impose some influence on diet and physical activity which is absent for adults living in the community. There may also be familial influences at work: Sharav & Bowman (1992) found no difference in body mass between children with Down's syndrome and their siblings. Prasher (1995) also found that BMI tended to decline with age (the opposite trend to that in the general population). It is possible that higher mortality among younger people who have learning disabilities and who are obese may partly explain this. It is also worth pointing out that the tendency for people with Down's syndrome to be short and stocky in build may suggest that BMI norms are inappropriate for this population.

Obesity is recognized to have serious implications for health, including cardiovascular disease. However, Rimmer et al (1994) report no difference in risk of coronary heart disease due to abnormal blood lipid levels and obesity between people with Down's syndrome and other people who have mental disabilities.

Vision and hearing problems

Milder forms of vision and hearing loss may be difficult to diagnose among people who have learning disabilities, as investigation often requires a degree of active cooperation (Van Schrojenstein Lantman-de Valk et al 1997). Studies therefore tend to concentrate on conditions which have clear physiological symptoms and it is likely that prevalence of sensory problems is underestimated.

In addition to the high incidence of vision and hearing problems which manifest themselves during childhood among people with Down's syndrome (Pueschel & Gieswein 1993), deterioration of vision and hearing during adulthood is likely. A high frequency (30–60%) of acquired cataracts have been reported (Pueschel 1987) and estimations of the increased risk from two studies of institutional populations vary from 2.5 to 8 times that for the general population (Van Schrojenstein Lantman-de Valk et al 1994, Walsh 1981). Keratoconus (thinning and bulging of the central cornea), sometimes associated with cataract and glaucoma, may appear at puberty and prevalence has been estimated at 5% (Catalano 1992). The increased risk may be 4–30-fold that of the general population, again based on studies of institutional populations (Van Schrojenstein Lantman-de Valk et al 1994, Walsh 1981). The risk of functional blindness (visual capacity <0.1) has been estimated to be 3.7 times that of normal controls (Walsh 1981).

Hearing impairment has been estimated at between 2 and 18 times more likely among people with Down's syndrome than among people who have other learning disabilities (Squires et al 1986, Van Schrojenstein-Lantman-de Valk et al 1994). This higher risk applies to both adults and children (Dahle & McCollister 1986). Presbyacusis or hearing loss due to ageing has also been noted in individuals with Down's syndrome at an earlier age than in both the general population and adults who have learning disability without Down's syndrome (Buchanan 1990). Presbyacusis is evident by the second decade of life among people with Down's syndrome.

FRAGILE X SYNDROME

Fragile X syndrome is now recognized to be the most common cause of hereditary learning disability in all populations and ethnic groups (Sherman 1991). It is the most common of 100 or more X-linked syndromes currently recognized, which together account for 20–30% of all learning disability (Feldman 1996). The syndrome has been characterized as presenting with mild to severe mental impairment, elongated face with large ears and megalo-testes in males. However, none of these indicators is conclusive and all three are present in only 60% of fragile X males (Jacobs et al 1983, Mattei et al 1981). Most significantly, not all males and only one-third of females with a fragile X chromosome show intellectual impairment. Unlike with Down's syndrome, therefore, there is a considerable problem of underdiagnosis, which has implications for the detection of associated health problems and consequently for health screening and health maintenance programmes.

Males with fragile X do not appear to have a lower life expectancy than the general population (Hagerman 1991). The main conditions which appear to be associated with males with fragile X syndrome are abnormalities of palate, skeleton, endocrine system and connective tissue (Vieregge & Froster-Iskenius 1989). Skeletal and connective tissue problems include scoliosis (lateral spinal curvature), flat feet and laxity of the joints (Davids et al 1990). A high prevalence of cardiac defects has also been reported, the most frequent being mitral valve prolapse (Loehr et al 1986, Sreeram et al 1989). Vision problems are common (Maino et al 1990), specifically strabismus (squint) (Storm et al 1987). Conductive hearing loss due to prolonged otitis media is likely to exacerbate the underlying language dysfunction associated with the syndrome (Hagerman et al 1987).

Unlike Down's syndrome, where a link with Alzheimer's disease has been established, no neurological, electroencephalographic or neuroradiological

TABLE 4.2	Fragile X syndrome, mortality and disease prevalence

Men with fragile X syndrome, compared with the general population

are *more* likely to die from ...	Congenital heart abnormalities
and *more* likely to suffer from ...	Middle ear infections
	Epileptic seizures, especially in childhood
	Skeletal problems
	Abnormalities of the endocrine system
	Vision problems

abnormalities have been consistently shown to be specifically associated with fragile X syndrome. While increased levels of hyperactivity and poor attention span have been found, it has been argued that affected individuals are no more susceptible to autism, psychiatric disorders, hyperactivity, attention deficit or seizures than other males who have mental disability (Fisch 1993, Vieregge & Froster-Iskenius 1989). However, Hagerman (1991) cites an overall prevalence rate of clinical seizures among males of 17%. Unlike in Down's syndrome, where epilepsy is more common among older people, epilepsy in fragile X males is most common in childhood (Hagerman 1991).

ACTIVITY 4.1	Identify a group of people who have learning disability using the service in which you work. By checking records and talking to staff and carers, try to establish the causes of the disability for as many of the group as possible. Using the information in this chapter and others in this book, what health problems could these individuals be at risk of, taking into account the aetiology of their disability, their age, level of disability and lifestyle (e.g. living alone)? What evidence is there that they have been screened for these health risks?

HEALTH PROBLEMS NOT RELATED TO CAUSE OF LEARNING DISABILITY

Many studies report health issues relating to people who have mental disability as a whole, without necessarily establishing a link with any particular condition. Here we shall review these other health concerns described in the literature as having elevated incidence or prevalence among this population, omitting those, like Alzeimer's, which are clearly related to a particular syndrome.

Infections

Evidence on mortality due to respiratory and other infections tends to relate predominantly to institutional populations and therefore may not necessarily reflect the level or pattern of risk for those living in the community. From the evidence available, infections continue to play a disproportionate role in the mortality of people who have learning disabilities. The risk of death from respiratory infection appears to be about 8–10 times higher for people who have learning disabilities, at least among those living in an institutional setting. This cause accounts for about half of all deaths among people who have learning disability in institutions (Carter & Jancar 1983) compared with 5–7% of deaths in the general population. People who have a profound level of learning disability are considerably more at risk from respiratory disease than are individuals in the mild or severe categories. Thus, Chaney et al (1979) found that 75% of people who have profound learning disability die from this cause, compared with 58% of those who have a lesser degree of learning disability. Similarly, in a US study O'Brien et al (1991) report that respiratory diseases caused 52% of all deaths among institutionalized residents who have profound learning disabilities and 23% and 28% respectively among those who have severe and mild/moderate learning disabilities.

It has been suggested by Fryers (1984) that there are two reasons for this pattern of respiratory mortality. First, people who have profound learning disability tend to suffer from a variety of additional medical problems which shorten life and specifically render them susceptible to respiratory infection. Second, they are likely to suffer from an inadequate level of self-care, which will also increase the possibility of infection.

However, a large-scale study in Denmark (Dupont et al 1987) confirmed that excess mortality due to respiratory infection was not confined to institutional populations or to those who have severe or profound disabilities. Analysis of causes of death among 7134 people diagnosed as having a mild learning disability (71% of whom lived in the community) found an excess mortality from respiratory disease among males aged 15–64. Hepatitis virus infection also has had a high prevalence among institutional populations, particularly, as we have seen, among those with Down's syndrome (Devuyst & Maesen-Collard 1991, Garcia Bengoechea et al 1989, Hershow et al 1989). A study of tuberculosis in a UK mental handicap hospital population of 400 people found a prevalence of 27 per 10 000, substantially higher than in the general population (Wiggins et al 1989).

Cancer

Cancer appears to remain a less common cause of death among people who have learning disabilities than it is in the general population. The death rate from cancer in an institutional population in England between 1986 and 1995 was 13.6%, compared with 26% in the general population (Cooke 1997). Despite this comparatively low level of cancer-related deaths, there is evidence that these cases may be on the increase among people who have learning disability. Jancar (1990) found the death rate from cancer in an institutional population increased markedly from 10% of all deaths in the period 1931–80 to 17% in the period 1976–85 and concludes that this was due mainly to the increasing longevity of clients.

Cooke (1997) reports a high rate of cancer of the gastrointestinal tract, which supports findings from Jancar's earlier studies at the same institution (Jancar 1990) and those of O'Brien et al (1991) in the US. Cooke suggests that high rates of chronic constipation and of gastrooesophageal reflux may indicate

TABLE 4.3	*Non-syndrome specific mortality and disease prevalence*

People who have learning disabilities, compared with the general population

are *more* likely
to die from ...   Gastrointestinal cancer
                                    Respiratory infections

are *more* likely
to suffer from ...   Hepatitis
                                    Vision and hearing problems
                                    Dental problems

are *less* likely
to die or suffer
from ...   Hypertension
                                    Road traffic accidents
                                    Pulmonary cancer

abnormalities which increase the risk of cancer. Such problems may also be more directly fatal. In a UK study, Roy & Simon (1987) report that deaths from non-malignant intestinal obstruction are particularly high compared with the general population.

The possibility that death from cancer may also be becoming more common in populations living in non-institutional settings is suggested by Dupont et al (1987), who report an excess mortality from cancer among males aged 15–64. For females the pattern was closer to that of the general population. One reason for this may be the reported gender difference in prevalence of cancer of the reproductive organs. Dexeus et al (1988) and Thornhill et al (1988) report an increased prevalence of cancer of the reproductive organs among men who have learning disabilities, while the rate among women appears to be lower than in the general population, possibly because of a lower level of sexual activity (Huovinen 1993).

Cardiovascular disease

In a UK study, Cole et al (1994) reported that cardiovascular disease was the second most common cause of death among 60 patients who had learning disability studied at autopsy. A study in Norway, on the other hand, found 4% of deaths from this cause (Haugeberg & Kris 1991). These discrepant figures may represent differences in selection of the population under consideration. In the UK general population this condition accounts for about 26% of all deaths and is the largest single cause of death.

Evidence of the prevalence of cardiovascular disorders among older people comes from a study in Holland (Evenhuis 1997). Of 70 people who have learning disabilities aged 60 and over living in residential settings, 34% were found by their general practitioner to have symptoms of cardio- and cerebrovascular disease, including 13% with coronary heart disease. The author reports that this compares with a figure of 14% with coronary heart disease in an ageing UK general population.

Vision and hearing

Vision problems in the Down's syndrome and fragile X syndrome populations have been reviewed above and the high prevalence of problems in these groups is reflected in studies of the learning disabilities population as a whole. Aitchison et al (1990) found that 59% of 367 patients in two mental handicap hospitals in Bristol, England, had one or more eye abnormalities and this figure only reduced to 54% when the Down's syndrome group were excluded. Jaworski (1993) reports that exposure corneal disease (keratopathy) due to incomplete blinking was a significant problem among people who have learning disabilities, affecting 18% of 210 patients.

In a Danish study, Parving & Christensen (1990) report a prevalence of 33–40% of defective hearing among people who have learning disabilities living at home. Of the 17% judged to require a hearing aid, none was using one. Two US studies report a high level of conductive hearing loss due to impacted earwax among adolescents and adults who have learning disabilities (Brister et al 1986, Crandell & Roeser 1993). In the latter study, prevalence of conductive hearing loss due to this cause was 28%, compared with 2–6% in the general population.

Dental health

The dental health of people who have learning disabilities has attracted a considerable amount of research interest. Kendall (1992a,b), in a study of 350 people who have learning disability attending day centres, found great variation in dental health. Those who were less learning disabled had better oral hygiene, less gingival inflammation, more fillings and fewer teeth extracted because of caries. However, a Swedish study reports contradictory findings, with those who have milder learning disabilities living in the community having a higher caries incidence and prevalence than those who have moderate or severe learning disabilities (Gabre & Gahnberg 1997).

There is some evidence that dental care and dental health begin to decline after leaving school. A study of the dental health of children who have learning disabilities in South Glamorgan (Evans et al 1991) suggests that special schools were making efforts to ensure their children were regularly monitored. The majority were receiving regular dental care and results showed that 12- and 14-year-olds in special schools had a better history of caries than children of the same age in other state schools. But in a study of dental care among adults in Birmingham, Shaw et al (1989) found far less restorative care than among members of the general population.

Age-related trends in health

Age-related ill health among people who have learning disabilities is a subject of some imprecision. Evidence from the US, where a number of studies have been completed since the 1980s (Jacobson et al 1985, Janicki & Jacobson 1982, Janicki & MacEachron 1984), points to age-related increases in chronic disease conditions involving the cardiovascular, digestive, musculoskeletal, sensory and respiratory systems and increases in neoplastic diseases. Major deterioration in hearing, vision and mobility have also been reported.

Comparing a group of 55–64-year-olds with a group aged 65 and over, Janicki & Jacobson (1982) found a 25% increase in these problems for the older group. Aitchison et al (1990) found that vision problems among people who have learning disabilities living in hospitals were significantly more prevalent among those over 40. Twenty nine per cent of this group had two or more ocular defects: 17% suffered from a combination of strabismus (squint), refractive error and cataract. Stone et al (1989) found that movement disorders (dyskinesia and Parkinsonism) were more common among the US learning disabled population than in the general population, although dyskinesia prevalence was comparable with that among psychiatric and institutionalized geriatric populations. Parkinsonism was found to increase with age for men, while dyskinesia increased with age for women.

Such considerations can only increase in importance. Janicki et al (1999) report that many people who have learning disabilities in the US now live as long as adults in the general population. The mean age of death of 2752 adults over 40 who had intellectual disability who died over a 10-year period was 66.1 years and the most common causes of death – cardiovascular disease, cancers and respiratory disease – were similar in both groups.

This evidence from US studies of generally poor health in older people who have learning disability may, however, be misleading. Because of the eligibility for welfare factor mentioned at the beginning of this chapter, such studies tend to include many more people who have mild learning disability than would normally be eligible for, and therefore known to, services in the UK. As a result, research on the physical health status of older people in the UK has been at odds with the US evidence. For example, Moss et al (1993a), in a study of 105 moderate to severely disabled people aged over 50, found relatively low levels of morbidity, particularly that which could be classed as 'severe'. The authors suggest that among a more tightly defined and therefore more severely disabled population, those with poor physical health would tend to die relatively young, leaving the older age groups composed of the fitter individuals. This 'differential mortality' effect would be less marked in US service populations, while the effects of ageing would be correspondingly greater.

Moss et al (1993b) nevertheless report that among those aged 65 or more, both those who have learning disability and people of similar age without learning disability had high prevalence of gastrointestinal disorders (28% prevalence among those who have learning disabilities, 23% in the general population), foot disorders (23% and 26% respectively) and arthropathy (55% and 47% respectively). Incontinence was much more prevalent in the group with learning disability (51% versus 12%), as were obesity (17% versus 4%) and visual disorders (64% versus 43%, although the authors warn that the detection methods differed somewhat in the two groups). A Dutch study (Van Schrojenstein Lantman-de Valk et al 1997) found that increasing age was associated with higher prevalence of dementia, vision and hearing impairment for both people with Down's syndrome and those who have other forms of learning disability and also report that the non-Down's syndrome group had increasing levels of hypertension with age, but decreasing prevalence of epilepsy. For those with Down's syndrome, epilepsy became more prevalent with age. Cooper (1997), in a study of over-65s living in Leicestershire, found that in this age

group the effect of ageing on morbidity outweighed any differential morta[ ]
effect. In a related study, Cooper (1999) found that physical health was sign[ ]
cantly associated with dementia among people who have learning disabilities
aged 65 and over and recommended that psychiatric assessments should be
accompanied by physical assessments.

RISK FACTORS AND LIFESTYLE

Although studies both in the UK and elsewhere have examined aspects of the
lifestyles of people who have learning disabilities, they have tended to be rather
limited in scope; for example, covering individuals from one particular institution, one age group or with a specific condition. None has covered the full range
of risk factors listed in *The Health of the Nation* (DoH 1992) and none has
attempted to look in detail at the influences and determinants of lifestyles and risk
factors. However, evidence from the UK literature in regard to diet, obesity and
physical activity indicates some substantial problems within this population. At
the same time, there appears to be increasing recognition of these issues by service
purchasers and providers. Turner et al (1995) found that a number of community
care plans developed by health and local authorities in England and Wales made
specific reference to health promotion policies for people who have learning
disabilities. Initiatives reported include a series of health fairs held in day centres,
the appointment of specialist dieticians, routine health checks by specially trained
GPs and training of residential and day care staff in the preparation of healthy
diets, including the use of supplements and vitamin tablets.

Obesity

Obesity has been cited as a risk factor for cardiovascular and renal disease,
some forms of cancer, hypertension, diabetes, respiratory problems and other
conditions, both in the general population (Royal College of Physicians 1983)
and among people who have learning disabilities (Burkhart et al 1985).
Prevalence in the general UK population is reported to be 13% (OPCS 1995),
and in a three-country comparative study of over 5000 subjects aged 16–50,
Laurier et al (1992) found the prevalence of obesity to be 15% in the US,
9% in the UK and 7% in France.

Studies in both the US and the UK suggest that obesity is higher among
people who have learning disabilities than among the general population. In the
UK Wood (1994) found a obesity prevalence of 14% among 35 people living in
staffed hostels or houses. Bell & Bhate (1992) studied 183 day centre attenders,
most of whom lived in the family home. They report prevalence rates of 19%
for men and 35% for women. Rates were particularly high for the 58 people
who have Down's syndrome (men 32%, women 42%). The Welsh Health and
Community Care Survey (Welsh Office 1996) found more obese and more
underweight people and a particularly high obesity rate for women, compared
with the general population. Moss et al (1993b), in a study of people over 50,
found 17% of the study population to be obese compared with 6% of the
control group of individuals without learning disability. Rimmer et al (1993)
found obesity levels in the US of 27.5% for men and 58% for women. The rate
for women was twice that estimated for the general US population. Studies of

TABLE 4.4	Obesity in the general and learning-disabled populations			

Body Mass Index category	General population		Learning-disabled population	
	Health Survey for England 1993[1] n = 15 284		Welsh Health Survey[2] n = 1553	
	Men (%)	Women (%)	Men (%)	Women(%)
Underweight	5	7	14	13
Normal	38	44	39	30
Overweight	44	32	29	28
Obese	13	16	18	30

[1]OPCS 1995 [2]Welsh Office 1996. Only the Health Survey for England used direct measurements

obesity among children who have learning disabilities are rarer and are restricted to US studies. One study reports a prevalence of 22% among 337 5–15-year-olds (Fox et al 1985).

There is some evidence from US studies that in the learning-disabled population, obesity may be more prevalent among people who have mild or moderate developmental delay and those living in non-institutional settings (Burkhart et al 1985, Emery et al 1985). However, these two factors may be confounded. Rimmer et al (1993) compared rates for different living arrangements while controlling for severity of disability. They conclude that those who have severe or profound disability living with carers in the family home were much more likely to be obese than those of a comparable level of disability living in an institution.

The limited evidence from UK studies suggests that this finding may also apply in the UK. Wood (1994) cites evidence from an unpublished study of 733 institutionalized patients indicating an 8% prevalence of obesity. This compares with 14% of 35 adults living in a staffed home in the same area of North East England (Wood 1994) and 26% in a study of 183 people who have learning disabilities predominantly living in the family home (Bell & Bhate 1992). Overall, results from UK and US studies indicate a high prevalence of obesity, which is higher among women and those living in the community. It is widely accepted that weight control, together with maintenance of physical fitness, is an important component in the maintenance of good health, particularly in respect to congenital heart disease and stroke. Apart from the direct health benefits, however, there is also evidence that appropriate interventions could have a wider impact for people who have learning disabilities. For example, it has been reported that self-injurious and other challenging behaviour may be positively related to obesity (Gabler-Halle et al 1993, Neri & Sandman 1992). It has also been argued that acceptance by, and integration into, the wider community may be furthered by weight loss (Rimmer et al 1993).

While some specific syndromes have implications for obesity, it is clear that lifestyle is also highly relevant. Treatment therapies specifically designed for this population have been developed in the US but results have been mixed, with considerable problems regarding variations in response and relapse following the end of interventions. US research suggests that changes in both diet and exercise are essential for sustained effectiveness.

ACTIVITY 4.2

Devising a weight loss and fitness gain intervention

Working with dietician and physiotherapist support, investigate the level of interest among people who have learning disabilities in losing weight and getting fitter. The following principles reflect research findings reviewed in this chapter regarding weight loss and fitness gain.

■ Self-monitoring of performance and results, which helps participants relate changed habits with outcomes. Examples of self-monitoring include self-weighing, recording of food consumed, self-timing in exercise regimes and internalization of the adverse effects of relapse.

■ Progressive replacement of staff supervision and external rewards by self-reinforcement. This may be made easier by the use of simple exercises and techniques which avoid the need for special equipment or close supervision and by aiming for integration in mainstream exercise or dieting programmes. Involvement of carers and parents in the motivation, monitoring and reinforcement process has been shown to be important.

■ Limiting the influence of external eating cues. Availability of food may be reduced by limiting eating to a few specific settings, reducing portion size, slowing down the eating process and substituting other pleasurable activities.

■ Generalization of behaviour change to a variety of situations and settings beyond the training setting. This can be made less challenging by making the training setting as close as possible to the natural environment; for example, by using actual foods and eating settings or non-specialized fitness equipment.

■ There appears to be a consensus that, because of metabolic changes in the body during dieting, relatively slow losses of half to one pound per week are more sustainable. The literature also suggests that neither exercise nor diet is effective alone for long-term maintenance of weight loss.

It is important to note that there are methodological problems in defining obesity and thus in estimating and comparing prevalence rates. Litchford (1987) compared various ways of calculating percentage body fat and concluded that Body Mass Index (BMI: weight in kg/height in m^2) is the most appropriate measure for the learning-disabled population. BMI of 30 or more is the most common measure of obesity for both the general population and people who have learning disability. However, Burkhart et al (1985) argue that differences in growth rate and physical make-up relating to particular clinical conditions (for example, Down's syndrome) may invalidate the use of the same standard cut-off as used in the general population. The comparison of weight with height alone does not take account of skeletal, muscle and body fluid weights, which for clinical reasons may be atypical in people who have learning disabilities. A more direct measure of obesity used in several studies entails the use of calipers to measure triceps skinfold thickness. However, Rimmer et al (1987) concluded that this measurement alone may result in large errors for some subjects. There is no accepted methodology which defines the number of sites to be used in skinfold measurements, how data are to be combined or whether these measures should be combined with height/weight ratio.

The implication of these methodological problems is that estimates of prevalence of obesity in the population of people who have learning disabilities must be treated with caution.

Physical fitness

Studies of physical fitness of people who have learning disabilities mainly reflect the view that cardiovascular capacity is the most important indicator of overall fitness (Lavay & McKenzie 1991, Pitetti et al 1993). Cardiovascular fitness is bound up with the lowering of risk factors for coronary heart disease and may be optimized by exercise, lowering of cholesterol through diet control and non-smoking (Rimmer et al 1994). Flynn & Hirst (1992) compared a UK sample of young people who have learning disabilities aged 14–22 to a matched sample of non-disabled young people and found that the proportion taking part in sports was considerably lower and that much of their time was spent in passive activities. In a large-scale US study, Rimmer et al (1994) reported that of 329 subjects living in hostels, the family home or group homes, 40% were found to have high cholesterol levels plus one or more background risk factors and thus were likely to benefit from cardiovascular fitness interventions. The authors conclude that cardiovascular health should be a major concern for people who have learning disabilities.

In addition to cardiovascular fitness, muscular strength and endurance have been shown to influence health and well-being. The relative lack of strength and endurance in people who have learning disabilities (Pitetti & Campbell 1991) may limit work performance and possibly increase the possibility of re-institutionalization on ageing (Fernhall 1993). Although poor levels of fitness among people who have learning disabilities have been linked with a sedentary lifestyle and lack of exercise (Fernhall et al 1988, Pitetti et al 1993), there may also be clinical causes. Pitetti et al (1992) report that the leg muscle strength of children and adults with Down's syndrome was significantly weaker than that of normal controls and of others with developmental delay from other causes. This suggests that people with Down's syndrome are a special group and should be treated separately in studies of fitness. Fernhall et al's study (1989) supports others in suggesting that people who have learning disabilities may have a lower maximal heart rate in addition to any lack of cardiovascular fitness and this may partly explain their relatively poor performance in fitness programmes.

Participation in exercise has been shown to have certain behavioural and other effects in the general population (e.g. Folkins & Sime 1981). Studies which seek to establish similar effects for people who have learning disabilities are reviewed by Gabler-Halle et al (1993). They conclude that participation in exercise programmes produces immediate but not durable benefits in intellectual functioning, behaviour, including stereotypic behaviour, and self-concept. However, there is a need for more investigation of the factors which may cause these changes. As with obesity, there are certain methodological problems in using definitions of fitness developed in the general population for people who have learning disabilities.

Smoking and alcohol consumption

The smoking and alcohol consumption habits of adults who have learning disabilities have received relatively little attention. The Welsh Health and Community Care Survey (Welsh Office 1996) found that 13% of people who have learning disabilities living at home were current smokers, 7% ex-smokers and 81% had never smoked. Two of these rates are lower than those found in the general population by The Health Survey for England (OPCS 1995), which gives figures of 27% current smokers, 25% ex-smokers and 44% who had never smoked. In the US, O'Brien et al (1991) report that tobacco use was positively correlated with IQ level among adults in a large institution. It was also positively correlated with presence of cancer at death.

Alcohol consumption appears to be low among people who have learning disabilities. Using the Department of Health's 1995 definition of sensible and harmful levels of alcohol consumption, the Welsh Health and Community Care Survey (Welsh Office 1996) identified 1% as harmful level drinkers, 39% as sensible level drinkers and 60% as non-drinkers. The figures in the general population are 30%, 64% and 7% respectively. Both surveys report that men drank significantly more than women. A US study (Krishef & DiNitto 1981) linked alcohol abuse among people who have learning disability to a high rate of alcohol-related arrests.

IMPLICATIONS FOR PRACTICE

The challenge of responding to the health needs of people who have learning disabilities has proved to be a difficult one for health services, which have been criticized for inadequacies in the detection and treatment of established conditions (particularly mental illness) and in the preventive care aimed at reducing risk factors. Part of the problem stems from the reliance on the self-report of symptoms and health concerns in order to trigger healthcare. People who have learning disabilities acting unaided may be unable to fulfil this expectation and healthcare professionals may lack the communication skills necessary to compensate. For example, failure to report or detect visual or hearing defects is likely to compound learning difficulty and cause communication difficulties and isolation. In the same way, not reporting side-effects of medication may encourage poor prescribing practices. Practitioners should be aware of the dangers of repeat prescribing, particularly of antiepileptic and other neuroleptic drugs, and of polypharmacy, where a range of medications are prescribed and not necessarily adequately monitored.

Training programmes for GPs and other primary care team members, service users and carers, as separate groups, may be one way to overcome such problems. A number of authors, including Greenhagh (1994), Howells & Barker (1990) and Martin et al (1997), have suggested that primary care and community learning disability teams should adopt a common healthcare protocol to identify opportunities for health gain in such areas as vision, hearing, communication, mobility, epilepsy and other specific conditions. The targets outlined could be translated to a clinical level as a basis for individual teams' standards. This would mirror and broaden the national strategic approach of *Our healthier nation* (DoH 1998).

CONCLUSION

This chapter has examined what is known about patterns of morbidity and mortality among people who have learning disabilities. The range of health problems which they face require continued surveillance and monitoring to optimize detection, treatment and management. Problems such as sensory impairments and dental health represent major causes of avoidable ill health which are clearly open to effective intervention and consequent improvement in health. While mortality from the biggest killers in the general population is still relatively low, people who have learning disability increasingly share the same risk factors relating to cardiovascular disease, cancers, mental illness, sexual health and accidents. The evidence from US research suggests that, at least among those who have mild to moderate learning disability, such risks will increasingly influence the pattern of mortality. In particular, the risk factors of obesity and physical inactivity, much more common among people who have learning disability than in the general population, are likely to impact on rates of cardiovascular disease and cancer. In consequence, government strategies aimed at reducing the impact of major causes of mortality and morbidity in the general population are also recognized as having relevance to people who have learning disabilities (DoH 1995).

FURTHER READING

Department of Health 1995 The health of the nation: a strategy for people with learning disabilities. HMSO, London
This booklet aimed to direct health service purchaser and provider organizations to the special considerations involved in planning and providing services for people who have learning disabilities. It discusses the particular contributions of different professionals and has proved influential in recent service developments for this group. The document concludes that the objectives of all five key areas are equally relevant to people who have learning disabilities and that their health needs are best met by promoting access to sensitive and responsive mainstream services and the strengthening of specialist healthcare, surveillance and health promotion programmes.

Van Schrojenstein Lantman-de Valk H M J, Haveman M J, Crebolder H F J M 1997 Comorbidity in people with Down's syndrome: a criteria-based analysis. J Intellect Disability Res 40:385–399
This paper attempts to discriminate between studies which reach a certain level of reliability through careful methodology, size of populations studied and the attainment of significant odds ratios to identify high risk and those which do not. This approach results in the clear identification of hearing and vision problems, congenital heart disease, hypothyroidism and hepatitis B (among those in residential facilities) as 'clustering' with Down's syndrome. This does not necessarily imply that these problems are caused by Down's syndrome, only that they are more common in its presence.

Cooper S A 1999 Clinical study of the effects of age on the physical health of adults with mental retardation. Am J Mental Retard 102:582–589

A useful and up-to-date picture of the health problems encountered by the increasing numbers of people who have learning disability living beyond 65 years of age. The study is based on a survey in the UK and compares morbidity patterns between older and younger groups.

Barr O, Gilgunn J, Kane T, Moore G 1999 Health screening for people with learning disabilities by a community learning disability nursing service in Northern Ireland. J Adv Nurs 29:1482–1491
This paper reviews the literature regarding the changing health profile of people who have learning disabilities, and suggests ways in which health screening in the community can inform service provision to this group.

Martin D M, Roy A, Wells M 1997 Health gain through health checks: improving access to primary care for people with intellectual disability. J Intellect Disability Res 41:401–408
This study is unusual in that it goes beyond the identification of morbidity by offering an intervention based on primary care which is then evaluated by analysing case notes. Health gains were demonstrated in physical disorders but not in mental health problems. The study offers a model for the improvement of health through primary care teams.
*   This paper appears in a special issue of the Journal of Intellectual Disability Research containing a number of papers covering aspects of primary healthcare for people who have learning disabilities.*

REFERENCES

Aitchison C, Easty D L, Jancar J 1990 Eye abnormalities in the mentally handicapped. J Mental Defic Res 34:41–48

Aylward E H, Burt D B, Thorpe L U, Lai F, Dalton A 1997 Diagnosis of dementia in individuals with intellectual disability. J Intellect Disability Res 41:152–164

Ball M J, Nuttall K 1980 Neurofibrillary tangles, granulovascular degeneration and neuron loss in Down's syndrome: qualitative comparison with Alzheimer dementia. Ann Neurol 7:462–465

Bell A, Bhate M 1992 Prevalence of overweight and obesity in Down's syndrome and other mentally handicapped adults living in the community. J Intellect Disability Res 36:359–364

Braun D, Green M, Rausen A et al 1985 Down's syndrome and testicular cancer: a possible association. Am J Pediatr Hematol Oncol 7:208–211

Brister F, Fullwood H L, Ripp T, Blodgett C 1986 Incidence of occlusion due to impacted cerumen among mentally retarded adolescents. Am J Mental Defic 91:302–304

Buchanan L 1990 Early onset of presbyacusis in Down syndrome. Scand Audiol 19:103–110

Buckley J D, Buckley C M, Ruccione K et al for the Children's Cancer Group 1994 Epidemiological characteristics of childhood acute lymphocytic leukemia. Analysis by immunophenotype. Leukemia 8:856–864

Burger P C, Vogel F S 1973 The development of pathologic changes of Alzheimer's disease and senile dementia in patients with Down's syndrome. Am J Pathol 73:457–468

Burkhart J, Fox R, Rotatori A 1985 Obesity of mentally retarded individuals: prevalence, characteristics and intervention. Am J Mental Defic 90:303–312

Burt D B, Loveland K A, Lewis K R 1992 Depression and the onset of dementia in adults with mental retardation. Am J Mental Retard 96:502–511

Carter C 1958 A life-table for mongols with the cause of death. J Mental Defic Res 2:64–74

Carter G, Jancar J 1983 Mortality in the mentally handicapped: a 50-year survey at the Stoke Park group of hospitals 1930–1980. J Mental Defic Res 27:143–156

Catalano R A 1992 Ophthalmologic concerns. In: Pueschel S, Pueschel J (eds) Biomedical concerns in persons with Down syndrome. Paul H Brookes, Baltimore

Chaney R, Eyman R, Miller C 1979 Comparison of respiratory mortality in the profoundly mentally retarded and in the less retarded. J Mental Defic Res 23:1–7

Chaney R, Eyman R, Miller C 1985 The relationship of congenital heart disease and respiratory infection mortality in patients with Down's syndrome. J Mental Defic Res 29:23–27

Chaplin R H, Thorp I A, Collacott R A et al 1996 Psychiatric disorder in Asian adults with learning disabilities: patterns of service use. J Intellect Disability Res 40:298–304

Cole G, Neal J W, Fraser W I, Cowie V A 1994 Autopsy findings in patients with mental handicap. J Intellect Disability Res 38:9–26

Collacott R 1993 Epilepsy, dementia and adaptive behaviour in Down's syndrome. J Intellect Disability Res 37:153–160

Collacott R, Cooper S A, McGrother C 1992 Differential rates of psychiatric disorders in adults with Down's syndrome compared with other mentally handicapped adults. Br J Psychiatr 161:671–674

Cooke L B 1997 Cancer and learning disability. J Intellect Disability Res 41:312–316

Cooper S A 1997 Clinical study of the effects of age on the physical health of adults with mental retardation. Am J Mental Retard 102:582–589

Cooper S A 1999 The relationship between psychiatric and physical health in elderly people with intellectual disability. J Intellect Disability Res 43:54–60

Crandell C C, Roeser R J 1993 Incidence of excessive/impacted cerumen in individuals with mental retardation: a longitudinal investigation. Am J Mental Retard 97:568–574

Crapper D R, Dalton A J, Skopitz P, Scott J W, Hachinski V C 1975 Alzheimer degeneration in Down's syndrome. Arch Neurol 32:618–623

Cremers M J G, Bol E, De Roos F, Van Gijn J 1993 Risk of sports injuries in children with Down syndrome and atlantoaxial instability. Lancet 342:511–514

Dahle A J, McCollister F P 1986 Hearing and otological disorders in children with Down syndrome. Am J Mental Defic 90:636–642

Dalton A J 1992 Dementia in Down syndrome: methods of evaluation. In: Nadel L, Epstein C J (eds) Down syndrome and Alzheimer disease. Wiley Liss Inc, New York, pp 51–76

Dalton A J, Selzer G B, Adlin M S, Wisniewski H M 1993 Association between Alzheimer

disease and Down syndrome; clinical observations. In: Berg J M, Karlinsky H, Holland A J (eds) Alzheimer disease, Down syndrome and their relationship. Oxford University Press, Oxford, pp 54–69

Davids J, Hagerman R, Eilert R 1990 Orthopaedic aspects of fragile X syndrome. J Bone Joint Surg 72:889–896

Deaton J G 1973 The mortality rate and causes of death among institutionalized Mongols in Texas. J Mental Defic Res 17:117–122

Devuyst O, Maesen-Collard Y 1991 Hepatitis B in a Belgian institution for mentally retarded patients: an epidemiological study. Acta Gastroenterol 54:12–18

Dexeus F, Logothetis C, Chong C, Sella A, Ogden S 1988 Genetic abnormalities in men with germ cell tumors. J Urol 140:80–84

DoH 1992 The health of the nation. Cm 1986. HMSO, London

DoH 1995 The health of the nation: a strategy for people with learning disabilities. HMSO, London

DoH 1998 Our healthier nation. The Stationery Office, London

Dupont A, Vaeth M, Videbech P 1987 Mortality, life expectancy and causes of death of mildly mentally retarded in Denmark. Upsala J Med Sci 4(Suppl): 76–82

Ellis W G, McCulloch J R, Corley C L 1974 Presenile dementia in Down's syndrome. Neurology 24:101–106

Emerson E, Robertson J, Gregory N et al 1999 A comparative analysis of quality and costs in village communities, residential campuses and dispersed housing schemes. Hester Adrian Research Centre, University of Manchester, Manchester

Emery C L, Watson J L, Watson P J, Thompson D M, Biderman M D 1985 Variables related to body-weight status of mentally retarded adults. Am J Mental Defic 90:34–39

Evans D J, Greening S, French A D 1991 A study of the dental health of children and young adults attending special schools in South Glamorgan. Int J Paediatr Dentist 1:17–24

Evenhuis H M 1990 The natural history of dementia in Down's syndrome. Arch Neurol 47:263–267

Evenhuis H M 1997 Medical aspects of ageing in a population with intellectual disability. III. Mobility, internal conditions and cancer. J Intellect Disability Res 41:8–18

Feldman E J 1996 The recognition and investigation of X-linked learning disability syndromes. J Intellect Disability Res 40:400–411

Fernhall B 1993 Physical fitness and exercise training of individuals with mental retardation. Med Sci Sports Exercise 25:442–450

Fernhall B, Tymeson G, Webster G 1988 Cardiovascular fitness of mentally retarded individuals. Adapted Physical Activity Quart 5:12–28

Fernhall B, Tymeson G, Millar L, Burkett L 1989 Cardiovascular fitness testing and fitness levels of adolescents and adults with mental retardation including Down syndrome. Educ Training Mentally Retard 24:133–138

Fisch G 1993 What is associated with the fragile X syndrome? Am J Med Genet 48:112–121

Flynn M, Hirst M 1992 This year, next year, sometime …? Learning disability and adulthood. National Development Team/Social Policy Research Unit, London

Folkins C, Sime W 1981 Physical fitness training and mental health. Am Psychol 36:373–389

Fong C, Brodeur G 1987 Down's syndrome and leukemia: epidemiology, genetics, cytogenetics and mechanisms of leukemogenesis. Cancer Genet Cytogenet 28:55–76

Fox R, Hartney C, Rotatori A, Kurpiers E 1985 Determined incidence of obesity among retarded children. Educ Training Mentally Retard 20:175–181

Fryers T 1984 The epidemiology of severe intellectual impairment: the dynamics of prevalence. Academic Press, London

Gabler-Halle D, Halle J, Chung Y 1993 The effects of aerobic exercise on psychological and behavioral variables of individuals with developmental delay: a critical review. Res Dev Disabilities 14:359–386

Gabre P, Gahnberg L 1997 Inter-relationship among degree of mental retardation, living arrangements, and dental health in adults with mental retardation. Special Care Dentist 17:7–12

Garcia Bengoechea M, Legarda J J, Cortes A, Enriquez I, Arriola J A, Arenas J I 1989 Mentally deficient patients and infection caused by hepatitis B virus. Prevalence in our area. Medicina Clinica Barcelona 93:10–13

Geggel R, O'Brien J, Feingold M 1993 Development of valve dysfunction in adolescents and young adults with Down syndrome and no known congenital heart disease. J Pediatr 122:821–823

Goldhaber S, Brown W, Sutton M 1987 High frequency of mitral valve prolapse and aortic regurgitation among asymptomatic adults with Down's syndrome. JAMA 258:1793–1795

Greenhalgh L 1994 Well aware: improving access to health information for people who have learning difficulties. NHS Executive, Anglia and Oxford Regional Health Authority

Greenwood R, Nadas A 1976 The clinical course of cardiac disease in Down's syndrome. Pediatrics 58:893–897

Hagerman R J 1991 Physical and behavioral phenotype. In: Hagerman R J, Siverman A C (eds) Fragile X syndrome: diagnosis, treatment and research. Johns Hopkins University Press, Baltimore

Hagerman R, Altshul-Stark D, McBogg P 1987 Recurrent otitis media in boys with the fragile X syndrome. Am J Dis Child 141:184–187

Haugeberg G, Kris S 1991 Causes of death among mentally retarded. Naerlandheimen Central Institution for the Mentally Retarded. Tidsskr Mor Laegeforen Norway 111:2255–2257

Hershow R, Chomel B, Graham D et al 1989 Hepatitis D virus in Illinois state facilities for the developmentally disabled. Epidemiology and clinical manifestations. Ann Int Med 110:779–785

Howells G 1989 Down's syndrome and the general practitioner. J Roy Coll Gen Pract 39:470–475

Howells G, Barker M 1990 A protocol for primary healthcare. Occasional papers. Royal College of General Practitioners, London

Hresko M, McCarthy J, Goldberg M 1993 Hip disease in adults with Down syndrome. J Bone Joint Surg 75:604–607

Hughes V C, Cameron J, Goonetilleke A S 1982 The prevalence of thyroid dysfunction in mentally handicapped in-patients. J Mental Defic Res 26:115–120

Huovinen K J 1993 Gynecological problems of mentally retarded women. A case-control study from southern Finland. Acta Obstet Gynecol Scand 72:475–480

Hurst J W, Logue R B 1970 The heart. McGraw-Hill, New York

Jacobs P, Mayer M, Matsuura J, Rhoads F, Yee S 1983 A cytogenetic study of a population of mentally retarded males with special reference to the marker X syndrome. Human Genet 7:471–489

Jacobson J W, Sutton M S, Janicki M P 1985 Demography and characteristics of aging and aged mentally retarded persons. In: Janicki M P, Wisniewski H M (eds) Aging and developmental disabilities: issues and approaches. Paul H Brookes, Baltimore

Jancar J 1990 Cancer and mental handicap: a further study. Br J Psychiatr 156:531–533

Janicki M P, Jacobson J W 1982 The character of developmental disabilities in New York State: preliminary observations. Int J Rehabil Res 5:191–202

Janicki M P, MacEachron A E 1984 Residential, health, and social service needs of elderly developmentally disabled persons. Gerontologist 24:128–137

Janicki M P, Dalton A J, Henderson C M, Davidson P W 1999 Disability. Rehabilitation 21:284–294

Jaworski C N 1993 Exposure keratopathy in a mentally retarded adult population. J Am Optomol Assoc 64:723–725

Karlinsky H 1986 Alzheimer's disease in Down's syndrome. A review. J Am Geriatr Soc 34:728–734

Katlic M, Clark E, Neill C, Hall J 1977 Surgical management of congenital heart disease in Down's syndrome. J Thorac Cardiovasc Surg 74:204–209

Kendall N P 1992a Differences in dental health observed within a group of non-institutionalised mentally handicapped adults attending day centres. Commun Dental Health 9:31–38

Kendall N P 1992b Oral health of a group of non-institutionalised mentally handicapped adults in the UK. Commun Dent Oral Epidemiol 19:357–359

Kinnell H G, Gibbs N, Teale J D, Smith J 1987 Thyroid dysfunction in institutionised Down's syndrome adults. Psychol Med 17:387–392

Krishef C H, DiNitto D M 1981 Alcohol abuse among mentally retarded individuals. Mental Retard 19:151–155

Lai F, Williams R 1989 A prospective study of Alzheimer disease in Down syndrome. Arch Neurol 46:849–853

Laurier D, Guiguet M, Chau N P, Wells J A, Valleron A J 1992 Prevalence of obesity: a comparative study in France, the United Kingdom and the United States. Int J Obesity Related Metabol Disord 16:565–572

Lavay B, McKenzie T L 1991 Development and evaluation of a systematic run/walk program for men with mental retardation. Educ Training Mental Retard 26:333–341

Levin S, Nir E, Moglilner B 1975 T-system immune-deficiency in Down syndrome. Pediatrics 56:123–126

Levy J 1992 Gastrointestinal concerns. In: Pueschel S M, Pueschel J K (eds) Biomedical concerns in people with Down's syndrome. Paul H Brookes, Baltimore, pp 119–126

Litchford M D 1987 Estimation of energy stores of mentally retarded individuals. Am J Mental Defic 91:532–536

Loehr J, Synhorst D, Wolfe R, Hagerman R 1986 Aortic root dilation and mitral valve prolapse in the fragile X syndrome. Am J Med Genet 23:189–194

MacLachan R A, Fidler K E, Yeh H, Hodgetts P G, Pharand G, Chau M 1993 Cervical spine abnormalities in institutionalized adults with Down's syndrome. J Intellect Defic Res 37:277–285

Maino D, Schlange D, Maino J, Caden B 1990 Ocular abnormalities in fragile X syndrome. J Am Optometry Assoc 61:316–323

Mani C 1988 Hypothyroidism in Down's syndrome. Br J Psychiatr 153:102–104

Mann D 1988 Calcification of the basal ganglia in Down's syndrome and Alzheimer's disease. Acta Neuropathol 76:595–598

Martin D M, Roy A, Wells M B 1997 Health gain through health checks: improving access to primary healthcare for people who have intellectual disability. J Intellect Disability Res 41:401–408

Mattei J, Mattei M, Aumeras C, Auger M, Giraud F 1981 X-linked mental retardation with the fragile X syndrome: a study of 15 families. Human Genet 59:281–289

McGrother C, Marshall B 1990 Recent trends in incidence, morbidity, and survival in Down's syndrome. J Mental Defic Res 34:49–57

Moss S C, Patel P, Prosser H, Goldberg D P, Simpson N, Rowe S, Lucchino R 1993a Psychiatric morbidity in older people with moderate and severe learning disability mental retardation. Part I: Development and reliability of the patient interview: the PAS-ADD. Br J Psychiatr 163:471–480

Moss S C, Goldberg D P, Patel P, Wilkin D 1993b Physical morbidity in older people with moderate, severe and profound mental handicap, and its relation to psychiatric morbidity. Social Psychiatr Psychiatr Epidemiol 28:32–39

Murdoch J C 1984 Comparison of the care of children with Down's syndrome with the care of matched controls. J Roy Coll Gen Pract 34:205–209

Nelson R, Crocker A 1978 The medical care of mentally retarded persons in public residential facilities. N Engl J Med 299:1039

Neri C L, Sandman C A 1992 Relationship between diet and self-injurious behaviour: a survey. J Dev Physical Disabil 4:194–198

O'Brien K, Tate K, Zaharia E 1991 Mortality in a large Southeastern facility for persons with mental retardation. Am J Mental Retard 95:397–403

Olson M I, Shaw C M 1969 Presenile dementia and Alzheimer's disease in Mongolism. Brain 92:147–156

OPCS 1995 The health survey for England 1993. HMSO, London

Oster J, Van Den Temple A 1975 A 21-year psycho-social follow-up of 524 unselected cases of Down's syndrome and their families. Acta Pediatr Scand 64:505

Parving A, Christensen B 1990 Hearing of the mentally retarded living at home. Ugeskr Laeger 152:3161–3164

Pitetti K H, Campbell K D 1991 Mentally retarded individuals – a population at risk? Med Sci Sports Exercise 23:586–593

Pitetti K, Climstein M, Mays M, Barrett P 1992 Isokinetic arm and leg strength of adults with Down's syndrome: a comparative study. Arch Phys Med Rehabil 73:847–850

Pitetti K H, Rimmer J H, Fernhall B 1993 Physical fitness and adults with mental retardation. An overview of current research and future directions. Sports Med 16:23–56

Prasher V P 1995 Overweight and obesity amongst Down's syndrome adults. J Intellect Disability Res 39:437–441

Pueschel S 1987 Health concerns in persons with Down's syndrome. In: Pueschel S et al (eds) New perspectives on Down's syndrome. Paul H Brookes, Baltimore

Pueschel S, Gieswein S 1993 Ocular problems in children with Down syndrome. Down's Syndrome Res Pract 1:129–132

Rabinowe S, Rubin I, Adri M, Eisenbarth G 1989 Trisomy 21 Down's syndrome: autoimmunity, aging and monoclonal antibody-defined T-cell abnormalities. J Autoimmunol 2:25–30

Raghaven R, Khin-Nu C, Brown A et al 1993 Detection of Lewy bodies in trisomy 21 Down's syndrome. Can J Neurol Sci 20:48–51

Renner F, Andrie M, Horak W, Rett A 1985 Hepatitis A and B in non-institutionalized mentally retarded patients. Hepato-gastro-enterology 32:175–177

Rimmer J H, Kelly L, Rosentswieg J 1987 Accuracy of anthropometric equations for estimating body composition of mentally retarded adults. Am J Mental Defic 91:626–632

Rimmer J H, Braddock D, Fujiura G 1992 Blood lipid and percent body fat levels in Down's syndrome versus non-Down's syndrome persons with mental retardation. Adapted Phys Activity Quart 9:123–129

Rimmer J H, Braddock D, Fujiura G 1993 Prevalence of obesity in adults with mental retardation: implications for health promotion and disease prevention. Mental Retard 31:103–110

Rimmer J H, Braddock D, Fujiura G 1994 Cardiovascular risk factor levels in adults with mental retardation. Am J Mental Retard 98:510–518

Roy A, Simon G 1987 Intestinal obstruction as a cause of death in the mentally handicapped. J Mental Defic Res 31:193–197

Royal College of Physicians 1983 Obesity: a report of the Royal College of Physicians. J Roy Coll Physic London 17:1–65

Scholl T, Stein Z, Hansen H 1982 Leukaemia and other cancers, anomalies and infections as causes of death in Down's syndrome in the United States during 1976. Dev Med Child Neurol 24:817–829

Schupf N, Silverman W P, Sperling R C, Zigman W B 1989 Down syndrome, terminal illness and risk for dementia of the Alzheimer type. Brain Dysfunction 2:181–188

Sharav T, Bowman T 1992 Dietary practices, physical activity and body-mass-index in a selected population of Down syndrome children and their siblings. Clin Pediatr 1:341–344

Shaw L, Shaw M J, Foster T D 1989 Correlation of manual dexterity and comprehension with oral hygiene and periodontal status in mentally handicapped adults. Commun Dentistry Oral Epidemiol 17:187–189

Sherman S L 1991 Genetic epidemiology of the fragile X syndrome with special reference to genetic counseling. Program Clin Biol Res 368:79–99

Simila S, Kokkonen J 1990 Coexistence of celiac disease and Down syndrome. Am J Mental Retard 95:120–122

Squires N, Ollo C, Jordan R 1986 Auditory brain stem responses in the mentally retarded: audiometric correlates. Ear Hearing 7:83–92

Sreeram N, Wren C, Bhate M, Robertson P, Hunter S 1989 Cardiac abnormalities in the fragile X syndrome. Br Heart J 61:289–291

Stone R K, May J E, Alvarez W F, Ellman G 1989 Prevalence of dyskinesia and related movement disorders in a developmentally disabled population. J Mental Defic Res 33:41–53

Storm R, Pe Benito R, Ferretti C 1987 Ophthalmologic findings in the fragile X syndrome. Arch Ophthalmol 105:1099–1102

Strafstrom C 1993 Epilepsy in Down syndrome: clinical aspects and possible mechanisms. Am J Mental Retard 98(suppl):12–26

Thase M E 1982 Longevity and mortality in Down's syndrome. J Mental Defic Res 26:177–192

Thornhill J, Conroy R, Kelly D, Walsh A, Fennelly J, Fitzpatrick J 1988 An evaluation of predisposing factors for testis cancer in Ireland. Eur Urol 14:429–433

Turner S, Sweeney D, Hayes L 1995 Developments in community care for adults with learning disabilities. HMSO, London

Van Schrojenstein Lantman-de Valk H M J, Haveman M J, Maaskant M A, Kessels A G H, Urlings H F J, Sturmans F 1994 The need for assessment of sensory function in ageing people with mental handicap. J Intellect Disability Res 38:289–298

Van Schrojenstein Lantman-de Valk H M J, Haveman M J, Crebolder H F J M 1997 Comorbidity in people with Down's syndrome: a criteria-based analysis. J Intellect Disability Res 40:385–399

Vieregge P, Froster-Iskenius U 1989 Clinico-neurological investigations in the FraX form of mental retardation. J Neurol 236:85–92

Walsh S Z 1981 Keratoconus and blindness in 469 institutionised subjects with Down syndrome and other causes of mental retardation. J Mental Defic Res 25:243–251

Welsh Office 1996 Welsh Health and Community Care Survey. HMSO, Cardiff

Whittingham S, Pitt D, Sharma D, Mackay I 1977 Stress deficiency of the T-lymphocyte system exemplified by Down syndrome. Lancet i:163–166

Wiggins J, Hearn G, Skinner C 1989 Recent experience in the control and management of tuberculosis in a mental handicap hospital. Respir Med 83:315–319

Wisniewski K E, Wisniewski H M, Wen G Y 1985 Occurrence of neuropathological changes and dementia of Alzheimer's disease in Down's syndrome. Ann Neurol 17:278–282

Wood T 1994 Weight reduction of a group of adults with learning disabilities. Br J Learning Disabil 22:97–99

2 STRATEGIES FOR IDENTIFYING HEALTH NEEDS

Public health has once again become a very important aspect of the healthcare system. Not only has it become a central plank of government initiatives, it is also a crucial subject area for all health and social care practitioners to explore. When considered in its new guise, it is essentially the fundamental driver through which the health of individual health communities and subsequently the nation will be achieved. As such, the first chapter is one of the few pieces of work that attempts to consider the relevance of public health for people who have a learning disability and those agencies that provide services for this group of people. The similarities and relevance outlined in this chapter are important aspects for practitioners to consider. This section continues with further explorations into some of the central tenets of the public health agenda such as assessing health needs – a skill area in which many professionals need to become more competent. Also considered is the area of health promotion and crucially the area of accessing health information. This chapter is particularly important as it considers this issue from the perspective of people who have a learning disability, not just from that of the professionals.

SECTION CONTENTS

5 **The public health agenda**
   Jeanette Thompson and Sharon Pickering

6 **The assessment of health needs**
   Elizabeth Newbronner

7 **Health promotion with people who have a learning disability**
   Philomena Shaughnessy and Susan Cruse

8 **Accessing health information**
   Nicola Taylor with Susan Smithurst

5 The public health agenda

Jeanette Thompson and Sharon Pickering

KEY ISSUES

- What is public health?
- Inequalities in the health of people who have a learning disability
- Promoting positive health for people who have a learning disability
- Strategies for involving communities
- Developing skills in public health

INTRODUCTION

The health of the nation has gained a new level of relevance in relation to government policy, as a consequence of the acceptance of the link between socioeconomic experiences and poor health. Acknowledging this has resulted in a fundamental shift in approach to improving the health of the nation. Whilst historically, public health has been seen to focus upon public sanitation, epidemiology, communicable diseases and the identification of health risks within populations, more recent approaches have broadened its agenda to encompass the psychosocial aspects of health and healthcare. This has led to an understanding of the impact of unemployment, poverty, poor housing, social isolation, low self-esteem, crime and drug abuse upon a population's health (Billingham 1997). In addition, public health departments have begun to accept and develop more qualitative approaches to assessing the health needs of any given population. While public health has begun to focus upon these issues, learning disability services have begun to explore areas such as health and social inclusion in relation to the quality of life experienced by people who have a learning disability. The interface between these two areas is the focus of this chapter.

Billingham (1997) identifies that over the last decade there has been a culture shift in what is acknowledged as 'good practice' in promoting the health of individuals, from directive advice giving to non-directive participatory care. This is illustrated in public health by the move from a professionally led, philanthropic approach towards a more emancipatory model which can more effectively respond to community health needs (Twinn 1996). Within this the solutions to today's health problems are not necessarily seen entirely in individual terms but also in environmental health measures, collaboration across agencies (e.g. education and housing) and community participation. This aspect of public health emphasizes the involvement of the public in improving their health, building social support networks and strengthening community action. For practitioners, this means looking further than the ill health-focused, individually based, everyday health education work that they may currently be involved in, to the new public health roles that they need to be involved in.

In this context, it is crucial that practitioners working in the area of learning disabilities consider the public health agenda and the interface between this and the quality of life experienced by people who have a learning disability. Whilst it is acknowledged that public health utilizes many approaches, this chapter will consider issues relating to health inequalities, promoting positive health and inclusion for people who have a learning disability by building and developing

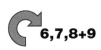

community participation. Other aspects of the public health function are addressed in Chapters 3, 4, 6, 7, 8 and 9, amongst others.

WHAT IS PUBLIC HEALTH?

Within the public health agenda, health is defined broadly in a way that encompasses both the health and social care needs that people have. This approach does not adhere to a strict medical definition of health such as the 'absence of disease or infirmity', as it operates from a much more holistic basis. As such, current definitions of public health acknowledge all the factors that can contribute to a person's overall health status. This approach to health is further underpinned by the belief that people's welfare is not only related to the individual and their medical conditions but also to the community and society's well-being. Therefore, public health is a way of looking at health which combines all factors that shape and influence the health of individuals and their communities. Public health can thus be defined as:

> a perspective which encompasses the roots and causes of ill health as well as its treatment … an approach which sees health within its overall social and political context, rather than an isolated medical event and looks for solutions in wider social action, individual empowerment and community development, as well as in clinical interventions.
>
> (DoH 2000)

In addition it is about:

- tackling the underlying causes of ill health and health inequalities
- building the capacity of those communities to promote positive health at the same time as preventing disease
- working with communities in order to assist them to improve their individual and collective health.

It achieves this through:

- exploring links between what is happening to an individual and their community
- identifying connections between the person and the social structures in which they operate
- extrapolating evidence in the context of epidemiological data
- exploring the influence of both medical and social models of health upon the community's overall well-being.

In essence, therefore, public health can be seen to be 'the science and art of preventing disease, prolonging life, promoting, protecting and improving health and well-being through organized efforts of society' (Lessof et al 1998). Improving the health of communities is therefore generally achieved by focusing upon needs assessment, epidemiology, influencing key stakeholders, influencing and implementing government policy, health education, promotion and screening and building communities. Many of these functions are the responsibility of public health departments across a variety of organizations and focus upon the population as a whole. However, public health is now being acknowledged as the business of all professionals, not just those operating at a strategic population level.

ACTIVITY 5.1   What public health roles are you involved in?

You may have considered your involvement in the following roles.

Public health role	Description
Health promotion/ education	Health promotion can be described as any deliberate or planned attempt to improve health or prevent or manage disease (Tones & Tilford 1994). Health education forms part of a health promotion activity and is about enablement by supporting people to set their own health agendas (French 1990).
Health screening/ protection	Health screening is the process of testing people for diseases or conditions in order to provide appropriate treatments. Health protection includes immunization and vaccination approaches. Both immunization and screening are targeted to groups at risk of particular conditions.
Health needs assessment	Identifying the health needs of a defined population. The population may be defined geographically, by care group or disease based.
Developing partnerships	This may include partnerships with service users, carers, other professionals, across organizations and across agencies.
Community building	Working to stimulate communities to express their needs and to support them in collective action aimed at meeting those needs (Ewles & Simnett 1995).
Acting as expert resource	Providing knowledge and expertise to whoever may need this information. This may be service users, carers, other professionals, non-professionally qualified workers, policy makers, managers, etc.
Developing services to meet local needs	This may mean identifying gaps in services and providing the impetus to establish these services or working with existing services to ensure they meet the needs of people who have a learning disability. This would include supporting generic services to more effectively meet the needs of service users.
Operationalizing local health strategy	Implementing the local health improvement programme and other health strategies. This includes the process of translating the strategies into a relevant and understandable format for local communities. A spin-off from this process should be the feeding back of relevant information to the policy makers.
Raising awareness	This is a two-way process and includes raising awareness of health issues within the local community, some of which may be difficult

ACTIVITY 5.1	*(Cont'd)*	
		issues for the community to deal with. It is also the process of raising awareness amongst professionals, service providers and policy makers about the needs of the local population.
	Influencing political agendas	This is the macro picture and involves the collation of all the soft and hard data accumulated about a given population in the process of undertaking any or all of the public health roles outlined above. This information should then be passed to the relevant authorities and organizations to influence the development of local and national policies.

Collating health assessment data

Public health has an exclusively population-based approach and public health specialists often focus upon particular tasks and provide an overview of the health status and needs of specific populations. The value of such information is to inform the strategic planning and delivery of healthcare services at all levels. The collation of this data set is important in effectively meeting the future needs of people who have a learning disability and cannot be achieved without the active involvement not only of all relevant departments and organizations but also people working at all levels within and outside healthcare.

Whilst the collation of such data has been an acknowledged function of public health departments, for many years the information that has existed within any locality regarding the health needs of people who have a learning disability has been fragmented. In those areas where information does exist, it is often located within provider organizations across both health and social care and is often not collated to form a comprehensive picture.

ACTIVITY 5.2	Identify and collate information regarding the needs of the learning disability population with which you work. What population trends does this information identify? Are there any obvious gaps in this information? How might this affect the analysis of this information?

You may now have realized just how fragmented the data about people who have a learning disability actually are and how difficult it is to acquire a comprehensive picture or to identify any trends. You may, however, have acquired information through contacting your local public health department, community team, local libraries and local authorities. From these sources you may have accessed the following information: census data, community team databases, case registers, educational statements and epidemiological data. Analysis of this information should allow you to begin the process of identifying the needs of your local population of people who have a learning disability.

Having accessed data about the needs of your local population, it is important to consider your role and responsibilities with respect to the identified trends, as well as exploring the roles of other practitioners in achieving the goal of 'health for all'. This collective approach to improving the health of communities is at the heart of the new public health agenda. This agenda does, however, bring particular difficulties in relation to moving the perception of healthcare workers from that traditional understanding of public health as focused upon tasks, populations, lifestyle, individual responsibility and well-being to one that is about processes, partnerships, communities, life chances and reducing inequalities.

ACTIVITY 5.3

What contribution do you make to improving the health of the community in which you work? What other areas could you influence?

When considering this activity you may have identified areas such as building inclusive communities, creating opportunities for valued employment, supporting people to speak up for themselves and others and meeting the health needs of people who have a learning disability.

HEALTH INEQUALITIES AND THE UNDERLYING CAUSES OF ILL HEALTH

The issue of inequalities in health is fundamental to any work that aims to achieve improvements in the health of any given community. The Black Report (1982) and more recently the Acheson Report (1998) clearly identify the links between inequality and poor health. The increased health needs of people who have a learning disability have been well documented (Band 1998, DoH 1998a, Moss & Turner 1995).

However, not until the publication of *Our healthier nation* (DoH 1998b) did the country see any overt political acknowledgement of the relationships between health and the inequalities that some people experience. This document noted that health inequalities were widening, with the poorest in society often being more affected by the major causes of death than those who are well off. Consequently, the aim of government policy in improving the health of the whole nation was stated to be better health for those who are the least well off (DoH 1998b).

Health inequalities are typified by the fact that some groups within society experience a better quality of life in health terms and live longer than others. Evidence does suggest that there are many possible reasons for this, which may, for example, be related to sex, genetic make-up or ethnicity. However, the most significant reason for inequality in health is the socioeconomic circumstances of any given population. This is illustrated by the fact that increasing national prosperity does not appear to result in direct improvements in the health of the whole population. *Our healthier nation* states that health improvement will only be achieved when the gap between the highest and lowest income groups is lessened. One of the key areas in which significant progress in improving public health can and should be made is that of poverty. Within the context of this chapter it is not possible to discuss all the causes and impacts of poverty but the next section will consider particular issues for people who have a learning disability.

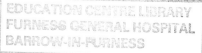

Poverty

People who have a learning disability are not always seen as people who experience poverty, primarily because society perceives that such people are cared for, have three meals a day, a roof over their heads and no worries about where the money is coming from. Within this there are, however, a number of anecdotal examples that demonstrate the misguided nature of this belief. Examples do exist of properties where people have less than £3 per day to feed themselves; this can result in the bulk buying of food and other commodities. This situation can not only result in service users not engaging with their community but can also affect the dietary intake of each individual within the household.

In addition, many people who have a learning disability can be excluded from the world of work as a consequence of living within residential care services. This is particularly relevant where significant fees are levied for their day-to-day care. This can result in people needing to enter the world of work on a salary scale of above average earnings (espie 2000). This is not always achievable and can result in difficult decisions needing to be taken, essentially about whether people continue to live within residential care or move out and achieve their aspirations for valued employment. Whilst this may seem an acceptable choice, the reality does not always support this as many people are unable to move out of the home they live in. This can be because they are caught up in care systems that are reluctant to support them to leave or because their request for accommodation may not be a priority for many care managers, particularly as they would not be regarded as homeless.

All these scenarios can also be influenced by the confidence that an individual has to challenge some of these constraints in order to achieve a better quality of life. The fact that many people who have a learning disability are consequently forced into a position of dependence upon state benefits does mean that this group of people are subject to similar difficulties that other parts of the population experience when in receipt of welfare payments.

ACTIVITY 5.4   As a practitioner working in the area of learning disabilities, what might you do about issues like the one noted above?

You may have considered issues around raising the public's awareness of the importance of work to people who have a learning disability and their strengths as employees. There is a great deal of evidence to suggest that poverty and poor health have a direct link to the employment status of an individual. Indeed, areas that have high rates of unemployment often have significant deprivation and suffer increased ill health. Whilst evidence suggests that people who have a learning disability make excellent employees, they are more affected by variations in the economic climate than many other groups of people. When the economy is not buoyant and jobs are scarce, then people who have a learning disability appear to find it more difficult to gain valued employment. Alternatively, you may have thought about work that you could do in schools to increase the understanding of school children about the issues facing people who have a learning disability.

Having noted the impact of poverty and unemployment on a person's health status, we will briefly consider other factors that influence health. Dahlgren & Whitehead (1991) (Fig. 5.1) identified a range of factors that they felt influence the health of individuals. Within this model they identify individuals and their fixed characteristics of age, sex and genetic make-up as central to all other factors and variables. This model represents each of these influences as concentric layers, each of which interfaces with the other factors and the fixed characteristics of the individual. They also suggest that whilst the inner 'circle' cannot be modified, many of these outer layers can be influenced by behaviour changes and life experiences. However, it must be acknowledged that the outer circles, in particular the socioeconomic and cultural factors, are less easily influenced by the individual.

The following case study utilizes Dahlgren & Whitehead's (1991) model to identify the factors which may affect the health of Sarah, a teenager with Down's syndrome.

FIGURE 5.1   *The main determinants of health (reproduced with permission from Dahlgren & Whitehead 1991).*

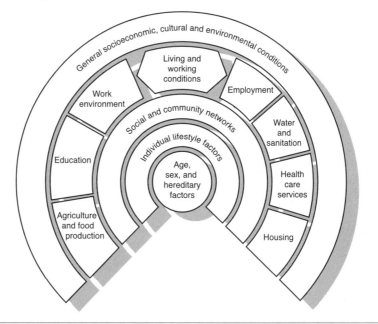

CASE STUDY 5.1   ### Age, sex and hereditary factors

Sarah is a 17-year-old who has Down's syndrome. In the context of Dahlgren & Whitehead's model, her genetic make-up will have significant implications for her future health status. As a young woman with Down's syndrome, she has an increased susceptibility to a number of conditions. These include chronic heart disease, leukaemia, thyroid dysfunction and Alzheimer's disease. Each of these may be subject to specific health screening in order to proactively manage Sarah's health. In addition, she will also have a greater likelihood of experiencing chronic eye infections, halitosis and obesity.

CASE STUDY 5.1 *(Cont'd)*

Individual lifestyle factors

As a teenager, many of these issues will be extremely important to her. She may find the fact that she is overweight difficult to deal with as she is becoming increasingly aware of her body image and her sexuality. When considering her lifestyle factors it may be apparent that Sarah does not do much physical exercise and does not always eat a healthy diet.

If Sarah was interested in improving her health, two possible courses of action could be taken: education about healthy eating and an increase in the amount of physical exercise she takes. The physical exercise option is important and will need careful assessment as a consequence of Sarah's genetic make-up which may impact upon this in a number of ways. First, she may have a congenital heart defect; approximately 50% of people who have Down's syndrome have such health problems. This is obviously important if she is going to engage in aerobic-type exercise and will require assessment regarding appropriate forms of activity. Second, she may have atlantoaxial instability. This condition also requires assessment when identifying appropriate forms of physical activity. Finally, she may have poor muscle tone that may mean she is unable to maintain the same level of physical activity as other people. The impact of this cumulative picture will also need to be considered in the context of her mental health and well-being.

As Sarah is also becoming interested in her sexuality, she is beginning to show an interest in young men. This means that it is important to consider her knowledge base about her own body, about relationships and about herself as an important person within those relationships. In considering Sarah's sexual health needs, it may be important to provide her with sex education and with the support structures to enable her to discuss these issues openly. This may mean interfacing with generic services as well as confronting a number of stereotypes and prejudices that can exist. Generic services will be particularly important in the context of health screening for Sarah.

Social and community influences

As a teenager, Sarah may also begin to experience peer pressure to conform to certain ways of behaving. Some of these pressures can be positive and allow people to formulate their own personality in a way that is different from their parents; others may be potentially negative, for example the pressure that may be exerted to start smoking or use drugs and alcohol. Lifestyle choices such as this can, if they are taken up, result in increased risks of cancer and coronary heart disease.

From the perspective of the social and community influences upon Sarah's health, it is also important to consider the impact of social networks. If Sarah has developed many friendships as she has grown up, and has plenty of people other than her parents and professionals to support her, she is likely to develop a positive sense of herself and subsequently will experience good mental health and well-being. However, if she has few friends or does not see people when she is not at work or the day service then her mental health and well-being may suffer. This will not only affect her now, for example through not developing a distinct persona separate to that of her parents or carers, but also later in life, as the divide between her life experiences and those of other members of society grows wider. A crucial point in this process could be when Sarah loses her final parent due to old age and potentially loses her home and friends at the same time.

Living and working conditions

Employment opportunities or the lack of them can also influence Sarah's health and well-being, particularly in the context of meeting friends, developing long-standing relationships and finding a future lifetime partner as well as the potential to create financial stability or welfare dependence.

General socioeconomic, cultural and environmental conditions

This section refers to the political and cultural environment in which Sarah lives. Every time the British or European government changes a policy or a law then there are impacts upon Sarah's life and potentially her health status. A clear example of this can be seen in the way that the needs of people who have a learning disability appear to have been politically constructed as social in origin. It is not our intention to suggest that Sarah's needs are not social in context but to acknowledge that she does have health needs that should be met in order to maximize the quality of her life. Many recent reports have clearly demonstrated the need to provide healthcare to people like Sarah. The difficulty, however, appears to be that the construction of Sarah's needs as predominantly social has allowed many health service providers to potentially avoid their responsibilities for meeting her health needs.

From a cultural perspective, society still appears to operate from the paternalistic viewpoint that people who have a learning disability need the protection and support of society. This means that they are unable to assert themselves and live everyday lives with the risks, rights and responsibilities that we all take for granted. Essentially, this can mean that the lifestyle choices made available to Sarah, as well as the working and living opportunities and experiences she is able to engage with, will be significantly affected.

ACTIVITY 5.5   What public health roles would you undertake with Sarah? How could these be utilized to improve the health of the wider population of people who have a learning disability that you work with?

The roles you may have identified could include developing the partnerships that would be useful in meeting Sarah's needs as well as those of other individuals who have a learning disability. The above case study may have prompted you to think about the services that you deliver to individuals and subsequently how you may meet the needs of service users in the context of each of the concentric layers identified by Dahlgren & Whitehead (1991). You may have identified functions in relation to health screening and health protection, health education, health promotion, acting as an expert resource and the need to stimulate local services to more appropriately meet service users' needs. Figure 5.2 elaborates upon this principle and may provide some guidance when considering your own actions.

FIGURE 5.2

Layer	Layer descriptor	Layer description	Public health roles
Layer One	Individual lifestyle factors	These are behaviours which may be either health damaging or health promoting, e.g. diet, smoking and physical exercise	Health promotion, health education, health screening, health protection, expert resource
Layer Two	Social and community influences	These include the presence/absence of support networks, peer pressure from friends and family. These factors also influence individual lifestyle factors in layer one, e.g. peer pressure about the use of drugs, alcohol and cigarettes	Community building, developing partnerships, health education, health promotion, expert resource, awareness raising
Layer Three	Living and working conditions	These include housing, education, employment and access to health services. Our occupation and where we live determine to a significant degree factors operating at layer two, e.g. support networks, which in turn influence individual lifestyle factors	Health needs assessment, community building, developing partnerships, developing services to meet local needs, operationalizing local health policy
Layer Four	General socioeconomic, cultural and environmental conditions	These operate at national, regional and other higher levels and include policies which affect employment, taxation, transport, housing, education and health. These influences exert a major impact on living and working conditions, social and community conditions, individual lifestyle factors and consequently the health of an individual	Influencing policy agenda locally and nationally based upon data collected through health needs assessment and other information gathered through carrying out other public health roles and responsibilities

Source: based upon the work of Dahlgren & Whitehead (1991)

ACTIVITY 5.6

Think about a person with whom you are currently working and identify factors that affect them in relation to each of these layers of influence. Note how each of the layers interfaces with previous levels. What strategies and interventions do you need to consider from a public health perspective in order to address the issues you have identified?

The factors you list are likely to be extremely personal to the individual you had in mind as you did the activity. You may, however, find it useful to re-read Case study 5.1 and relate the information within it to the issues noted in Chapters 2, 3, 4 and 8. One major area of activity you may have noted within your reflections is the importance of developing a range of partnerships with service users, professionals and other agencies.

The concept of upstream and downstream action within the public health agenda has considerable relevance in the context of appropriate and relevant partnerships and demonstrates the need for different approaches at different levels within society in order to meet the health needs of people who have a learning disability. Macro or upstream approaches include policies which aim to reduce inequalities in income, regeneration of communities, creation of jobs and the training initiatives to support people to access those jobs. Conversely, micro or downstream activities have a much narrower range of influence and are often aimed at the individual level; for example, nicotine replacement therapy on prescription and improving access to physical exercise.

From Sarah's perspective, upstream activity would involve the formulation of government strategies and policies that placed her as central to service delivery and noted the positive and negative interrelationships between the actions of different government departments upon her actual lifestyle. This partnership approach also needs to be mirrored at regional and local levels. Currently, this is typically achieved through the development of health improvement programmes (HImPs) but unfortunately many of these documents fail to include people who have a learning disability in an overt manner. There is therefore a clear need to ensure that HImPs do include this group of people and do so in a way that is inclusive rather than exclusive or unnecessarily segregationist. Additional upstream activity would also take the form of public education about the needs and wants of people like Sarah; this could typically take place during school years and could form part of the inclusion agenda. Downstream activity would include direct interventions with Sarah. These could be either on an individual basis or as part of a group and would relate directly to her needs and the lifestyle choices that she is making.

PROMOTING POSITIVE HEALTH

Having identified many of the influences on health and the resultant inequalities, it is important to consider ways in which these can be addressed. The 'how' of reducing inequalities in health inevitably requires a localized approach as each geographical area and each community will have different issues to address. Essentially these needs should be reflected in the priorities identified within the local HImP. Good health is the foundation of a good quality of life. It is something that most people hope for, both for themselves and those who are important to them. Within learning disability service provision, the attainment of a good quality lifestyle tends to be related to person-centred approaches to care delivery and all the principles and philosophies that underpin this.

From the perspective of people who have a learning disability, positive health is also important. Many people have, however, recently identified their lack of knowledge and understanding in relation to their own health needs. This is demonstrated aptly in the chapter on accessing health information in which the authors

8

talk about the difficulty they had in finding appropriate information. This is further compounded by the difficulties that people who have a learning disability experience in accessing this information and also some of the prejudices that abound, for example in relation to sex education. As for all members of society, the health of people who have a learning disability is influenced by the way in which governments, public bodies/agencies, communities and local groups engage with one another. Fundamental within this is the development of effective partnerships.

Partnership

Earlier in this book, Turner describes the range of health-related issues that people who have a learning disability may experience. Current philosophies indicate the expectation that these needs will be met by the services best placed to do so. Essentially, this means that if a person needs health screening of any description then this should be provided in the same way as it is provided to any other member of that population. Equally, if a person requires acute healthcare then the expectation once again is that this should be provided within the same setting as other people. This is not to suggest that if people require services in addition to those available within those environments or support to access those generic services, that they too should not be provided. It does, however, place a responsibility on all sectors of healthcare provision to adequately meet the needs of this group. This agenda is also important within other sectors which impact upon the health of a given community.

In relation to the public health agenda and people who have a learning disability, the local agencies and government departments involved in care delivery will include a diverse range of organizations. This may include housing, education, employment and environment agencies as well as the probation and criminal justice services. The issues of partnership working in order to promote the health of this and other parts of the population therefore become crucial to the achievement of the overall goal of healthy communities.

In addition, partnership is a fundamental theme in current government initiatives and is seen not only as the way to modernize statutory services but also as a catalyst to challenge the existing cultural mores within which our society operates. Within this, partnership is about developing and acknowledging our collective responsibility for the health and well-being of the community to which we belong. Initiatives such as Health Action Zones and Healthy Living Centres are clear attempts to improve health by placing the local community and the local health needs at the centre of the process of health improvement.

Furthermore, the partnership agenda neatly reinforces the priorities identified within *Our healthier nation*, which aim to reduce the gap between the poorer sections of our society and others. Within this, the work of the Social Exclusion Unit is of crucial importance and holds many opportunities for people who have a learning disability, particularly as social exclusion has been an inherent outcome of the lifestyles made available to many learning-disabled people in the past. Whilst social exclusion has not always been associated with poor health, consideration of the impact that limited social networks may have upon a person's mental health clearly indicates the importance of social contacts to our lifestyle and subsequently to our health. It is also possible to note the link between employment status, poverty and social inclusion, as work colleagues and leisure contacts can form the basis of a person's social network and subsequently their inclusion within their community (Thompson & Pickering 1998).

Although there have been many efforts to improve the lifestyle and consequently the quality of life of vulnerable members of society, these have focused upon the use of regeneration schemes as the key to achieving this. For a variety of reasons, many of these schemes have failed. These reasons include:

- the absence of effective national policies to deal with the structural causes of decline
- a tendency to parachute solutions in from outside rather than engaging local communities
- too much emphasis on physical renewal rather than better opportunities for local people
- the need to address the problem in a way that acknowledges the complexity of the issue and the need for creative solutions that are not compartmentalized based upon traditional structures and systems (Social Exclusion Unit 1998).

Essentially, other difficulties can be ascribed to a failure to listen to all groups within the community and an absence of active partnerships with and within these communities. Consequently, the national strategy for such neighbourhoods reflects these issues and identifies the following principles:

- investing in people, not just buildings
- involving communities
- developing integrated approaches with clear leadership
- ensuring mainstream policies really work
- making a long-term commitment with sustained political priority.

The principles upon which neighbourhood regeneration is focused are clearly important when working with people who have a learning disability. Of particular relevance is the agenda for building inclusive communities. Effort in this and other areas has resonance with the concepts underpinning social role valorization (Wolfensberger 1983), O'Brien's (1987) accomplishments, person-centred planning and circles of support. It is in this context that building community participation and the development of inclusive communities becomes fundamental to the health of any community.

BUILDING COMMUNITY PARTICIPATION

Community building is clearly acknowledged as a key role within a public health context. This is typified in many recent initiatives such as health improvement programmes, health and education action zones, joint investment plans (JIPs) and community care plans, etc., all of which identify a key responsibility for organizations to engage the local community in developing strategies to meet their identified needs. Within this context there is a fundamental need to empower the local community to become genuinely involved in the 'business' of that community. The NHS Executive, in conjunction with the NHS Confederation and the Institute of Health Services Management, suggests four models or approaches to making this a reality:

- community development
- direct participation of users
- informed views of citizens
- local scrutiny and accountability

(NHSE, IHSM, NHS Confederation 1998).

Community development

Both the United Nations (1948, cited in NHSE, IHSM, NHS Confederation 1998) and the World Health Organization (1986) have defined what is meant by community development and created the focus for action in engaging local communities in health issues. The United Nations defines community development as a movement to promote better living for the whole community and highlights the need for active participation of the community within that process. It also notes the importance of the initiative coming from within the community but does refer to the need to identify appropriate strategies to stimulate activity if this is not forthcoming. The WHO (1986) suggests that community development is about utilizing the existing human and material resources in any community to enhance self-help and social support to develop systems for strengthening public participation and the direction of health initiatives.

The fundamental principle that community development espouses is the belief that people should have control over their lives and a say in what happens to them. What is obvious is that some people are extremely capable of contributing in this way whilst others find it much more difficult. People who have a learning disability can in many ways be included within the latter group. This is not to say that all people who have a learning disability find it difficult to express themselves but that they are not automatically seen as a group who should be consulted regarding issues that are not directly related to having a learning disability. In addition, the information that is available for consultation is not always presented in a manner easily accessible to this group of people; for example the use of plain English (see Box 5.1).

From the perspective of health, community development aims to mobilize and engage communities in order to:

- provide a more effective and accurate health needs assessment of the local community
- increase the uptake of more accessible and appropriate services for that community
- create dynamic relationships between the public, providers and users
- develop healthy alliances which help to facilitate interagency work.

From the perspective of people who have a learning disability, the important groups to consider would be the local advocacy groups, either citizen advocacy or people first groups, as well as other local user groups that may exist. By connecting with these groups, service providers and public health specialists would both empower the people involved and facilitate meaningful consultation with some of the most devalued members of society. A useful advantage in utilizing these existing structures would be the support and expertise that could help those professionals not confident in engaging with people who have a

BOX 5.1	*Using plain English*

- Put all information in a logical order.
- Use typed rather than handwritten information.
- Use big print (14 point or above) and a clear typeface.
- Leave plenty of space around the text.
- Use symbols or pictures if appropriate.
- Use short sentences and simple statements.
- Do not use technical jargon.
- Include only one idea in each sentence.
- Write active positive sentences.
- Avoid abstract thought.
- Be direct and talk to your reader. Use 'I, we and you'.
- Be consistent and repeat words rather than use different ones.
- Don't use all capitals as this is difficult to read.
- Read your notes out loud; if it is hard to say it is probably hard to understand.

(Townsley & Gyde 1997)

learning disability. A cautionary note may be that these groups cannot always be seen as totally representative of the needs of all people who have a learning disability. However, as with other strategies for engaging members of the community, it is important to identify a start point and not to use the lack of representation as an excuse for non-action (Simons 1999). Successfully engaging with service users enables policy makers and politicians to identify the needs of people who have a learning disability in order to more appropriately support the community to meet the needs of this group.

Crucially, the principles that underpin the concept of community development demonstrate two fundamental requirements:

- that the community has a commitment to tackle inequality and discrimination
- that the community recognizes the need to give people more power over their lives so that they can control the social, economic, political and environmental factors which impact upon the community's health and well-being.

Whilst some public health specialists argue that community development is the active involvement of people in those issues that affect them, this approach can be seen as undermining the overall goal of inclusive communities and social inclusion. This is predicated upon the belief that for a community to be genuinely inclusive, its members need to act on issues that affect the whole community, not just those that impact upon them as individuals. Failure to operate from this perspective risks leaving people who have a learning disability isolated as few people will have an interest in the issues that affect this group. However, the growing interest in inclusion reflects the growing awareness of exclusion as a problem rather than a natural state of affairs. This awareness has developed from a sense that something is unnecessarily lost when people grow up excluded from the connections that define community life. Within this is a clear acknowledgement that this is a loss not just from the perspective of the 'excluded individual' but also from the perspective of that person's community. This acknowledgement can be clearly seen to have connections to the apparent increasing interest within society of the need to regain a sense of civic responsibility.

Direct participation of users

The aim of direct participation is to engage user and voluntary groups in decision making at all levels and to build partnerships between healthcare workers and service users. This is based upon the principle that user/carer perspectives have credibility and authority at least equal to those of the people who provide healthcare. In addition, it is founded upon the belief that the expertise and knowledge of those who use services can make an important contribution to needs assessment, service planning and delivery at a local level. The engagement of voluntary, self-help and advocacy groups can enable the collective accumulated expertise of service users to influence this agenda.

This strategy can be particularly difficult for professionals as it challenges the knowledge, expertise and power base of staff groups. Whilst significant progress has been made in service user-led groups contributing to the development, delivery and evaluation of learning disability-specific initiatives, there is still much progress to be made. This is especially apparent when considering the degree to which people who have a learning disability are being consulted on developments such as the building of a new hospital or the establishment of primary care groups. Often the process underpinning developments of this nature can exclude this group. In addition, there is an issue with regard to the development of service users' skills to genuinely engage in this process. Not only is this a difficult process in terms of time and commitment by practitioners, but resources also need to be available to fund and support this process.

Informed views of citizens

This strategy is one that is based on local populations. It aims to give citizens more information so they are more informed about health and health service issues, thus facilitating more effective strategic decision making between professionals and service users. Strategies for achieving this include citizens' juries, standing citizens' panels, deliberative opinion polls and citizen focus groups (Box 5.2).

Engaging people who have a learning disability in discussions such as these necessitates a significant amount of preparatory work. It is important to identify the structures that are already in place and to provide support to people who have a learning disability to develop their skills and confidence in order to enable them to make a valued contribution to any discussions they engage in.

In addition, it is crucial to provide appropriate support for their input before, during and after meetings. This might include practical input such as accessible venues, communication aids or interpreters as well as more process-based assistance such as helping the person to prepare what they wish to say and then enabling them to say it.

BOX 5.2		
Citizens' juries		Representative group of 12–15 people to consider an issue, where a recommendation is required, in depth. Usually meet for 3–5 days and receive information from witnesses and experts.
Standing citizens' panels		These meet on a regular basis to discuss issues on which an organization or authority wishes to receive the views of a cross-section of the public. Size of panels, membership and frequency of meetings vary.
Deliberative opinion polls		These involve more people than citizens' juries but the level of deliberation is less intense. There is usually a poll, then a discussion of the issue and then a re-poll.
Citizen focus groups		Generally, discussion groups designed to identify issues requiring more detailed exploration using other methods.

ACTIVITY 5.7

Think about the people with whom you work who have a learning disability. How could you help them to engage in any discussions taking place about local healthcare developments? How would you structure meetings that include people who have a learning disability?

Whilst engaging in this activity you may have considered the following action points:

- Don't use jargon or words that are hard to understand.
- Check that everyone understands what is being talked about at key points and before moving on to new items.
- Ensure that there are no interruptions when people are talking.
- Ensure that only one person speaks at any one time.
- Have frequent breaks to allow people to refocus and to check their understanding with supporters.
- Audio tape or video each meeting to allow people to re-engage with the material at a later date should they wish to do so.
- Make sure the notes of the meeting are short, concise, easy to understand and in plain English.
- Ensure that the agenda and any papers for discussion are set out in a way that service users can understand and sent in sufficient time for service users and their supporters to prepare for the meeting.

■ Create a positive and comfortable environment. Factors such as accessibility, lighting, space and what professionals wear can be important.

(Mencap 1997)

Participation in scrutinizing and regulating health services

The current policy agenda relies heavily upon the need to involve service users not only in their own care delivery but also in the planning, development, delivery and evaluation of local services. This focus upon evaluation is beginning to address the issue of the need for accountability. Recent proposals recommending changes to the monitoring of professionals within the welfare services also give the lay person an increasingly high-profile role in the quality agenda. This role is manifesting itself in a number of different ways within learning disability services, particularly as much of service delivery in this area is at the interface of both health and social care. Within health care the Commission for Health Improvement has lay membership, whilst within social care the Care Standards Commission and the Registration and Inspection teams also have such representation. Within some of the more innovative services, people who have a learning disability are acting as lay inspectors within residential care services. Whilst much progress can still be made, these small initiatives indicate a positive step in the right direction and could themselves be seen as promoting health.

DEVELOPING SKILLS IN PUBLIC HEALTH

The implications of the issues identified in the chapter thus far are that people working within both learning disability services and public health will need to have a significantly different range of skills from those that may have been necessary in the past. The skills that will be required by all practitioners can be considered under a series of broad headings that include:

■ interpersonal and communication skills as demonstrated in client interventions
■ knowledge of public involvement and its various methodologies
■ partnership practice
■ community development skills.

The following are some of the skills you may have identified as being relevant within each of the areas discussed:

ACTIVITY 5.8

Identify the skills you feel are relevant within each of these areas. Analyse your strengths and development needs in the four areas. Think about the skills that you have identified as development needs and, where appropriate, formulate your own personal development plan to further enhance these skills. For other areas, explore whether your development needs are areas of strength for other members of your team. Identify strategies that facilitate using the team's strengths to achieve collective goals. You may also need to think about skills available in other parts of your service or in other agencies.

- Research skills
- Critical appraisal skills
- Information management skills
- Leadership
- Media management
- Negotiation
- Augmented and facilitated communication skills
- Health needs assessment
- Risk assessment/management
- Planning skills
- Enablement and empowering skills
- Facilitation skills.

Many of the above skill sets are required in all practitioners working in this area, as are some of those noted within the section below headed Interpersonal and communication skills. The levels of expertise required may, however, vary in relation to each of these areas. With regard to the remaining skill sets, these may be used less frequently and consequently may only be available in very specialist areas.

Interpersonal and communication skills

Fundamental to any public health intervention is the relationship that exists between practitioners and the people they are working with. The quality of that relationship is heavily dependent upon the skills, knowledge and attitude of the professional. Essentially, therefore, each person needs to develop skills such as listening, questioning, presentational and teaching skills to a high level of proficiency.

Public involvement

Essential to any effective public involvement strategy are well-developed interpersonal skills which will be necessary for professionals to be able to run initiatives such as advocacy groups, citizens' juries and standing panels. In order to manage such groups practitioners require excellent presentation and group work skills. It may also be important to consider the skills required for involvement in such initiatives and for supporting people who have a learning disability to engage in these groups.

Partnership practice

In order to ensure that the true experience of the service user is reflected in the care provided, individual practitioners need to have skills in partnership practice. These skills are broader than traditional interpersonal skills as they include the need for the client to be placed at the centre of any consultation. The principle underpinning this approach is that the service user is as expert, if not more expert, than the professional. Although this principle is well embedded within learning disability services, the need exists to integrate this philosophy even further and to promote the centrality of people who have a learning disability within generic services.

Community development skills

Community development is essentially about working with groups and communities and practitioners need skills that enable them to work effectively in that context. These skills include:

- networking
- dealing with community conflict
- building a community's skills and capacity
- identifying other key individuals who are able to facilitate community development
- leading and managing projects.

CONCLUSION

Within this chapter parallels have been drawn between the current public health agenda and contemporary learning disability practice. Fundamental to this interface is the drive to reduce inequalities in health and therefore to promote positive health. The achievement of improved public health is of crucial importance in meeting the targets identified within *Our healthier nation*. This is particularly relevant to people who have a learning disability as they are clearly a group who have increased health needs (Band 1998a, DoH 1998a, Moss & Turner 1995, Singh 1997).

A further area of congruence is the focus within both public health and learning disability services upon building communities. From the public health perspective, this centres upon enabling communities to maximize their health through promoting healthy lifestyles. This agenda is equally important for people who have a learning disability, principally in the context of building inclusive communities. This is crucial with respect to the mental health and well-being of individuals, as well as an improved quality of life. It is only through achieving this that we will improve the health of some of the worst-off in society and meet the target of increasing the length of people's lives and the number of years people spend free from ill health (DoH 1998b).

FURTHER READING

Annual Report of the Director of Public Health for your Regional Office and Health Authority
These documents tend to identify statistical data in demography, mortality and morbidity, particularly for local health priorities. In addition, they will inform you about local progress towards meeting the national priorities and may cite examples of good practice. They can be acquired from local libraries and local health authority offices.

DoH 1998 Signposts for success. Department of Health, London
This document gives an overview of the health needs of people who have a learning disability and identifies standards of good practice for all parts of the NHS when working to meet the needs of this group.

DoH 1998 Our healthier nation. The Stationery Office, London
This document identifies the context within which much of the government's health policies are based. Also, it provides national statistics for each of the key target areas. This can provide useful benchmarks against which to set the comparative data for the learning disability population.

Health Improvement Programmes
These are available through local health authority offices. They set the programme of activity for meeting local health needs in the context of the national priority areas.

Moss S, Turner S 1995 The health of people with learning disability. Hester Adrian Research Centre, Manchester
This gives a comprehensive account of the health needs of people who have a learning disability.

REFERENCES

Acheson D (Chair) 1998 Independent inquiry into inequalities in health. DoH, London

Band R 1998 The NHS: health for all. Mencap, London

Billingham K 1997 Public health nursing in primary care. Br J Comm Health Nursing 2(6):270–274

Black D, Morris J N, Smith C, Townsend P 1982 Inequalities in health: the Black Report. Penguin Books, London

Dahlgren G, Whitehead M 1991 Policies and strategies to promote equity in health. WHO Regional Office for Europe, Copenhagen

DoH 1998a Signposts for success. Department of Health, London

DoH 1998b Our healthier nation. The Stationery Office, London

DoH 2000 Midwives and the new NHS: Paper 4 Public health. Royal College of Midwives, London

espie 2000 www. scotland.gov.uk/ldsr/espie.pdf

Ewles L, Simnett I 1995 Promoting health: a practical guide, 3rd edn. Scutari, London

French J 1990 Models of health education and promotion. Health Educ J 49(1):7–10

Lessof S, Dumelow C, McPherson K 1998 Feasibility study of the case for national standards for specialist practice in public health. A report for the NHS Executive. School of Hygiene and Tropical Medicine, London

Mencap 1997 Guidelines for working in meetings with people with a learning disability. Mencap, London

Moss S, Turner S 1995 The health of people with learning disability. Hester Adrian Research Centre, Manchester

NHSE, IHSM, NHS Confederation 1998 In the public interest: developing a strategy for public participation in the NHS. NHSE, London

O'Brien J 1987 A framework for accomplishment. Responsive System Associates, Decatur, GA

Simons K 1999 A place at the table. BILD Publications, Kidderminster

Singh P 1997 Prescription for change. Mencap, London

Social Exclusion Unit 1998 Bringing Britain together – a national strategy for neighbourhood renewal. NHS Confederation Briefing Paper 19. Social Exclusion Unit, London

Thompson J, Pickering S 1998 Social networks in old age. In: Pickering S, Thompson J (eds) Promoting positive practice in nursing older people: perspectives on quality of life. Baillière Tindall, London

Tones K, Tilford S 1994 Health education: effectiveness, efficiency and equity, 2nd edn. Chapman and Hall, London

Townsley R, Gyde K 1997 Plain facts: information about research for people with learning difficulties. Norah Fry Research Centre, Bristol

Twinn S 1996 Introduction – nursing for community health: changing professional issues. In: Twinn S, Roberts B, Andrews S (eds) Community health care nursing: principles for practice. Butterworth Heinemann, Oxford

WHO 1986 Ottawa charter for health promotion. WHO, Copenhagen

Wolfensberger W 1983 Social role valorization: a proposed new term for the principle of normalization. Mental Retard 21(6):234–239

6 The assessment of health needs

Elizabeth Newbronner

KEY ISSUES

- Health needs
- Supply and demand
- Health needs assessment
- Aproaches to health needs assessment
- Implementing health needs assessment in practice

INTRODUCTION

Health needs assessment is not a new idea. Individual needs assessment has always been part of the role of nurses and other healthcare professionals working with people who have a learning disability (Billings & Cowley 1995) and for many years health service managers have attempted to examine the health needs of the population to plan services and predict resource use. However, the changes in the organization of the health service which have taken place over the last decade, in particular the changing role of health authorities and the establishment of primary care groups (PCGs) and primary care trusts (PCTs) (DoH 1997), have led to increased emphasis on the use of health needs information to underpin commissioning decisions. The need to contain costs and target limited resources more effectively has also drawn attention to the value of population health needs assessment for providers of services, including those who provide services for people who have a learning disability. For individual healthcare professionals and their teams or practices, health needs assessment can provide a framework for changing clinical practice or service delivery, particularly where information about health need is considered alongside evidence of clinical and cost-effective practice. It enables those working with people who have a learning disability to understand more about the needs and priorities of their clients, including highlighting areas of unmet need.

This chapter introduces a number of key concepts in health needs assessment. It outlines the main approaches to health needs assessment and offers a practical guide to health needs assessment for those working with people who have a learning disability, in both specialist and general healthcare areas.

HEALTH NEEDS AND HEALTH NEEDS ASSESSMENT

Health needs assessment is essentially a way of systematically examining the health needs of the population or community in order to ensure that health services are planned and delivered to meet those needs effectively, but what do we mean by 'needs'? Health economists, public health doctors and sociologists have all contributed to the debate about what 'needs', 'health needs' and 'healthcare needs' are. In his work on the 'taxonomy of social need', Bradshaw (1972) talks about four types of need: normative need (i.e. need defined by an expert or professional), felt need, expressed need and comparative need. Epidemiologists have often focused on the idea of an iceberg of unmet needs, where only the most severely ill are seen by health services, whilst health economists have tried to integrate the concepts of need, demand and supply (Wright et al 1998).

Needs, health needs and healthcare needs

In recent years the ideas of the health economists have prevailed and *need* in healthcare is now often defined as the 'capacity to benefit from healthcare' (Culyer 1976). In the same way, population health need has been defined as 'the population's ability to benefit from healthcare' (NHSME 1991). The assumption underlying these definitions is that if health needs are to be identified, there should be an effective intervention available to meet those needs. These interventions might include diagnosis, treatment, disease prevention, rehabilitation and palliative care. Healthcare professionals often think about meeting healthcare needs in terms of the health services that are available to meet those needs but clients and communities are likely to identify wider determinants of health such as housing, social activity and employment. Within this concept, it has to be noted that when a service user has a healthcare need, there is a demand for healthcare services. The issue of demand is explored in the next section of this chapter.

Demand

Put simply, *demand* is what clients ask for from healthcare services. It is sometimes referred to as 'derived demand' because the demand for healthcare is based on the desire to be healthy, without the relationship between health and healthcare being well understood. It is also complicated by a number of other factors, such as the information available to clients, the social or educational background of the patient and the influence of doctors, particularly where they act as a gatekeeper to other services.

Supply

The term *supply* means the healthcare services provided. The supply of services is influenced by many factors, including resource constraints, historical patterns of provision and pressure from healthcare professionals and the public. However, there is growing emphasis on the need to demonstrate the effectiveness of new and existing interventions. National initiatives such as the National Institute for Clinical Excellence and the NHS Health Technology Assessment programme are highlighting the importance of both health authorities and their

PCGs and trusts assessing new services and treatments before they are commissioned or provided.

Approaches to health needs assessment

In an ideal world then, a health authority, PCG, community team or practice would examine the incidence and prevalence of health problems in the population, consider which interventions or treatments would be most effective for addressing them and then supply healthcare services which provide these interventions and treatments. This approach to health needs assessment is often referred to as an epidemiological approach (Stevens & Raftery 1997). Whilst it is rigorous it is also very time consuming and so two other broad approaches have come to be used in the NHS: the 'comparative' approach and the 'corporate' approach. Early guidance from the NHS Executive (NHSME 1991) describes each of them briefly as follows:

- *The epidemiological approach* which defines healthcare need as the ability to benefit from healthcare and is based on information about incidence, prevalence and the effectiveness of treatments, including cost effectiveness.
- *The comparative approach* which contrasts the services received by the population in one area with those elsewhere and is based on information about utilization rates, service performance and cost.
- *The corporate approach* involves the structured collection of information on healthcare services and needs from a range of stakeholders, including healthcare professionals, clients and the wider public.

HEALTH NEEDS ASSESSMENT IN PRACTICE

Many different frameworks for health needs assessment have been developed, according to the purpose of the assessment and the context in which it is being undertaken (Stevens & Gabbay 1991). Advocates of epidemiological approaches to health needs assessment argue that needs are best described in terms of diseases rather than population groups or services. However, much of the literature on health needs assessment in primary and community care emphasizes a more focused approach (Scottish Needs Assessment Programme 1998, Wilkinson & Murray 1998) and in practice, health needs assessments are often undertaken at one of three levels.

Generic or *population level assessments* examine the overall health needs of either a whole population (e.g. all the people who have a learning disability in the population of a GP practice) or a particular community (e.g. a town or a housing estate). They are often used to identify the key areas of health need and can help to focus further, more detailed needs assessments. These key areas can be defined in a number of ways; for example, the prevalence or incidence of a health problem, the number of consultations or contacts associated with a problem, the most common reasons for referral to secondary care, the frequency and cost of procedures or the health problems perceived to be of most importance by clients, their carers or the professionals working with people who have a learning disability.

Client group-specific assessments are used to examine the health needs of a specific group within the main population; for example, older people who have a learning disability, people with mental health problems and a learning disability. They are often undertaken where a team already has an indication that the needs of a particular group are not being met effectively (e.g. poor services for people with a sensory impairment) or perhaps because the group appears to be using a disproportionate level of the team's resources.

Disease or *intervention-specific assessments* can be used to examine the level of need in a particular disease area; for example, how many people who have a learning disability in the area also have epilepsy or experience seizures. They can also be used to assess the need for a particular intervention or procedure; for example, corrective surgery for congenital heart disease. However, in disease or intervention-specific assessments it is important to remember that consultation, referral and prescribing rates do not equal need. As in the population at large, some people who have a learning disability who could benefit from an intervention may not consult or be seen by a doctor and if they do see a doctor, the health problems they are experiencing may not be picked up quickly or clearly (Howells 1986). Referral and prescribing rates can also be affected by doctors' understanding of learning disability, their knowledge of a particular disease area or the availability of services. It is often important in this type of assessment to compare the information from your team or practice with information from other sources; for example, national and local prevalence and incidence figures or activity data from another locality

These levels are not mutually exclusive. You may decide to begin with a broad assessment at community or practice population level and then move on to examine the needs of a specific group in more detail. Alternatively, an assessment that focuses on a specific disease area such as Alzheimer's disease may raise wider questions; for example, about the way the needs of older people who have a learning disability are being met.

Set out below is a practical step-by-step approach to conducting a health needs assessment in your own team or practice. It highlights the issues you will need to consider and provides guidance on data collection and analysis.

CONDUCTING A HEALTH NEEDS ASSESSMENT

Step 1: Decide on the community, group or disease area on which you wish to focus

In deciding whether you want to focus your health needs assessment on a community, a group or a disease area, it can be helpful to ask yourself three key questions.

- What are the reasons for undertaking the needs assessment?
  It is important to be clear about why you are undertaking the health needs assessment, as this will influence all the other steps in the process, including who you involve, the information you gather and the way it is presented. For example, you may want to make a case to your health authority or PCG to invest in improved services for people who have a learning disability and

mental health problems. Alternatively, you may suspect that the health needs of people who have a learning disability who are living in long-term residential care in your area are not being met effectively and so you may want to examine how your team or practice can improve the situation.

- How can we build on local knowledge and interest?
  Health needs assessment can sometimes be complex and difficult, so try to use local knowledge and interest to give your work a head start. For example, if improving services for people with physical disabilities is a health improvement programme (HImP) priority for your health authority, an assessment which focuses on the needs of people who have a learning disability and a physical disability should be well supported and more likely to lead on to action.

- How much time (and resources) can we commit to the assessment?
  Health needs assessment can be time consuming but it is often a very cost-effective use of time, because it can not only produce demonstrable improvements in services, it can also help professionals to work together more effectively. From the outset, it is important to be realistic about the time and resources you and your team or practice can commit to the work. If you know that time is very limited then you may need to limit what your assessment covers. Alternatively, if the assessment is being undertaken as part of a wider project, e.g. a health authority-wide review of learning disability services, it may be possible to set aside more time. Either way, it is helpful to create some protected time and set aside a small budget for expenses such as obtaining a few key books and papers and extra travel or photocopying.

Step 2: Establish your health needs assessment team

Health needs assessment should never be a solitary activity. Working in a small team with colleagues from different professions or even different organizations will almost certainly result in your assessment being more comprehensive and more relevant and it will enable the workload to be shared. It can also help to make any changes in practice or services which take place as a result of the assessment more acceptable.

The size and composition of your health needs assessment team will vary according to the type of assessment you are planning to undertake and the context in which you are working (e.g. a community team working with people who have learning disability, GP practice, etc.). There are no hard and fast rules but teams of 3–6 people from different professional backgrounds, including clinicians and managers, often work well. If you are keen to look at the needs of a particular group or disease area, then it may be helpful to work with a practitioner knowledgeable in that area. For example, if you are looking at the needs of people with both a learning disability and mental health problems, you might involve staff from your local mental health services. Whatever the size and composition of your team, it is important to make sure that all the team members are keen to get involved in assessment and are committed to using the results of the assessment to improve services or practice.

Step 3: Decide what information you require and how to collect it

There is no such thing as a standard set of information for health needs assessment so when you are thinking about the information you will need, there are a few important points to remember.

It is vital to keep in mind why you are undertaking the assessment and how you hope to use the results. There is no point in collecting information simply because it is available or it might be generally interesting. Although it is the quality not the quantity of information that is important, you may want to consider obtaining data on the same issue from different sources so that you can validate or cross-check it. You may also want to think about the balance between quantitative information (e.g. how many people known to your community learning disability team (CLDT) have a sensory impairment) and qualitative information (e.g. how well do those people, their carers and their key workers feel their needs are being met). Finally, be sure that the information will actually tell you something about needs and is not misleading. For example, information about utilization rates for acute services may tell you more about the availability of a service or the accessibility of that service to people who have a learning disability than about the need for it.

It is likely that much of the data you are interested in already exists but getting hold of it in a usable form may not always be easy. There are three important sources of data for health needs assessment.

Service, team or practice-based data

There is often a great deal of information held within your own service, team or practice which you can use in your assessment. Some will be available from the service or practice information system but other data may need to be obtained from the nursing or medical notes and discussions with colleagues. There are three main categories of information you may want to look at.

- The use of community and primary care services, e.g. contacts with the CLDT or GPs and other primary healthcare team members, prescribing information, use of day services.
- The use of secondary care services, both specialist learning disability services and general healthcare services (e.g. referrals to outpatients, number of relevant procedures undertaken).
- Local epidemiological information, e.g. the incidence of acute illness or prevalence of chronic disease or physical disability amongst the people known to your team or practice.

Organizational data

There are several sources of this type of information and your local health authority, trust and local authority should hold most of what you need. The health authority's public health, information or commissioning departments will hold activity and epidemiological information for their population. They may also have details of other relevant studies or research. Local authorities usually hold the data collected in the National Census that applies to their area (e.g. demographic profile in 5-year age bands), including the Small Area Statistics.

National reports and papers can also be important, both to provide a comparison with locally held data and as a basis for making local estimates of prevalence and incidence, where a local study is not feasible or appropriate. For example, although the Health Care Needs Assessment series of epidemiologically based needs assessment reviews are now some years old, Review 19 'People with learning disabilities' (Felce et al 1997) still provides a useful baseline.

Health needs assessment data

Although there is often a great deal of existing information that you can tap into, you may find you do need to collect some information especially for the assessment, particularly if you want to look at the needs of a specific group of clients in some depth, map the services available in an area or canvass the views of people who have a learning disability and their carers. If you do decide to collect your own information, then it is important to take some time to decide on the most appropriate and practical approach to getting that information. Here again, you will need to consider the time and resources you have available. If you just want quantitative information (e.g. the number of residential places for people who have a learning disability in your PCG's area) or largely factual information (e.g. the type of support and accommodation they offer) a postal survey may be appropriate. However, if you wish to find out more about people's views and wishes, you might decide to use group discussions or interviews. It might be difficult or even impossible for some people who have a severe learning disability and/or significant sensory impairments to express their wishes directly but carers and staff may be able to offer an insight.

Finally, if a particular piece of information is likely to be difficult or time consuming to collect or extract, you may have to consider using a proxy or applying national estimates to your local population.

Once you have decided how to collect the information you want, you need to plan your fieldwork. It is important to decide at the outset who is going to be responsible for obtaining the different pieces of information. If you can, try to make use of the skills or connections of your team members. For example, if you have decided to use interviews and a member of the team has experience in writing interview schedules, they may be the best person to lead this part of the work. Alternatively, one of the clinicians in the team may have good links with the Public Health Department in the health authority and so may be well placed to obtain the data you require from them.

In this stage you should also think carefully about timescales. If you plan to undertake a survey you will need to allow time to pilot or at least test the questions with people outside the team. Where you are asking other organizations to supply you with existing data you may need to give them some time to compile it in the form you want. You will also have to allow for the possibility that some of the information will not be available and so you will need to consider alternatives. It can be helpful to use the process of collecting the information as a chance for the team to learn new skills and get to know colleagues in other organizations.

Finally, information about the health of a population can also provide an opportunity to learn from and involve people who have a learning disability and their carers. This process can be almost as important as the information itself and, if handled well, can lay good foundations for future work and relationships.

Step 4: Analyse the information

The approach you take to analysing and reviewing the information you have collected will depend very much on the type of health needs assessment you have undertaken. Again, there are no hard and fast rules but it is important to take a systematic approach. It is often helpful to group the information you have obtained into categories. For example, if you have been looking at the general health needs of people who have a learning disability, you may want to begin by using four groupings: demographic information, data on the use of primary and community care resources, referrals to secondary care or specialist services, and the perceptions and priorities of clients themselves. Using such categories can be particularly important if you have a lot of qualitative information to analyse.

When analysing and presenting quantitative information, it is helpful if you can express the information in three basic forms: the total number, the number as a percentage and the number as a rate (where appropriate). For example, if you are looking at the health needs of people with a sensory impairment, you may have established that there are 72 people known to your team who are visually impaired and that this group represents 10% of your team's caseload. You could also say that on average each person known to the team will have 13 contacts/visits per year but those people with visual impairments have an average of 15 contacts per year. Analysing and presenting information in this form helps to set the numbers in context but it also provides a basis for comparisons with other teams, practices or localities as well as regional and national figures. Such comparisons are often very illuminating and they can point you to issues that require further investigation.

Finally, don't feel that you have to undertake sophisticated statistical analysis. Your aim should be to use simple approaches well and produce information that is relevant and readily understood by colleagues and other organizations you work with.

Step 5: Share your findings and agree priorities

You will probably find that as you have collected and analysed the health needs information, your ideas about the key issues to be addressed have developed. You may even have started to identify possible solutions to any problems that emerged. How you take these ideas forward and agree priorities will depend on the original aims of the assessment. If, for example, the results of the assessment will be used to improve the care and support given to people with both a learning disability and mental health problems, you will want to share your findings with colleagues from mental health services and agree priorities for change. To help you compare or judge the proposed changes, it is helpful to agree a simple set of criteria against which they can be measured. Again, these will vary with local circumstances but they are likely to cover issues such as the health benefits that will be gained, the cost and the feasibility of achieving the change.

Step 6: Make an action plan and audit progress

In drawing up your action plan it is important to set measurable targets and agree realistic timescales in which to achieve them. Where possible, try to describe the outcomes you are hoping to achieve; for example, a reduced rate of self-harm amongst people with challenging behaviour. You should be able to quantify the outcome in some way, even if this is expressed in qualitative terms such as a perception of reduced stress for carers. You should also agree who is going to lead each action and identify the resources required to achieve it. Health needs assessment is all about making the best use of resources and improving services for people and their families. It is therefore vital that you set a date in the future to review the effect of the changes you have implemented.

CASE STUDY 6.1

Community learning disability team – the mental health needs of people who have a learning disability

The Walkington Community Learning Disability Team is based in a health centre near the middle of a large town. The town has a number of run-down housing estates as well as some more affluent areas and the team provides support to people who have a learning disability and their families across the town.

In recent years several members of the team, and some local GPs, have raised concerns about the coordination and quality of services for people who have a learning disability and mental health problems. Two recent incidents have highlighted the issues once again. In the first a middle-aged man, who had been living in a small residential home, attempted suicide. His family expressed a concern that his mental health problems had not been picked up sooner. In the other incident, a young woman who has a moderate learning disability and who was living on a local housing estate with her boyfriend, was picked up several times by the police for causing disturbances on the estate. Her GP and her key worker both felt she needed mental healthcare but the local acute psychiatric ward felt that they could not take her. Finally she was placed on a section of the Mental Health Act and admitted to a private secure hospital some 40 miles from her home. The local advocacy group took up the young woman's case and raised a complaint about the lack of mental healthcare available to her locally.

As part of its contribution to implementing the mental health objectives set out in the local Health Improvement Plan, the team has decided to look at ways of improving joint work between the learning disability service and mental health services. However, they are not sure how many clients might need mental healthcare in an average year, what sort of problems they might experience or how best to deal with them.

The team invited one of the community psychiatric nurses from the local community mental health team to be part of the project and a consultant psychiatrist from adult mental health services, who had occasionally assessed clients who have a learning disability and a mental health problem, also agreed to take part. The health needs assessment group began by asking all the key workers within the community learning

CASE STUDY 6.1   *(Cont'd)*

disability team (CLDT) to identify all the clients on their caseload who had experienced mental health problems in the last year. They also asked them to record the type of mental health problem the client had experienced (e.g. depressive episode), the treatment they had received, if any, and any referral made or additional services received (e.g. referral for assessment by a psychiatrist). They then compared the figures from this work with national estimates of the prevalence and incidence of mental health amongst people who have a learning disability and found that they were very low. This might suggest that mental health problems amongst people who have a learning disability are not being picked up as they should be. They decided that further work was needed to establish why this might be the case and so they contacted the trust's Research and Audit Department, to see if they might be able to assist the group with setting up a small study.

Of the clients who had experienced mental health problems, 17 had required specialist support or treatment (i.e. treatment not available from their GP or from the CLDT) and five clients had required inpatient care, although not all had received it. The health needs assessment (HNA) group decided that they needed to examine how well or otherwise the needs of this group had been met. They decided to look in depth at the experiences of five clients who needed specialist treatment and those of all five clients who had required in patient admission. They devised three interview schedules: one to be used with the client, one with the carer and one with the key worker. Where possible, they also arranged to talk to other key people (e.g. the key worker or psychiatrist from the ward). The interviews were conducted by four members of the HNA group over a 1-month period and then analysed by two members of the group. The findings from the interviews were presented to the CLDT and key staff from adult mental health services, at a lunchtime workshop.

CASE STUDY 6.2   **A GP practice – assessing the physical health needs of the people who have a learning disability registered with the practice**

Dr Johnson and partners are a large and quite go-ahead GP practice. They have seven partners and a practice population of just over 12 000. Most of their clients live in the large market town where their surgery is located but they also have clients from the surrounding villages. Ten years ago a learning disability hospital on the outskirts of the town closed and a number of former residents settled in the area and are now registered with the practice.

The practice is part of the Green Hills PCG and one of the senior partners is on the PCG board. The PCG has identified the need to improve services for people who have a learning disability as one of its priorities for the coming year. As part of this initiative, they are encouraging the practices within the PCG to examine how well the general health needs of all the people who have a learning disability registered with their practice are being met. Also the practice has recently recruited a new partner whose brother has a learning disability and she is keen to get involved in this initiative. She has suggested that the practice should establish a health needs assessment team to take the work forward.

The team began by identifying all the clients registered with the practice who have a learning disability. They also tried to identify their carers but found that in many cases there was no clear record on the person's notes or those of the carer. At the next practice meeting they agreed that over the coming year, in line with the National Carers Strategy, they should try to identify all carers.

They then looked at the consultation rate for people who have a learning disability and compared this to the overall rate for the practice population. They tried to see whether any particular groups consulted more than others (e.g. older people or people living in residential care). The practice had had a new computer system installed just over a year ago and so they were able to look at the main reasons for consultation and what had happened as a result of the consultation (e.g. medication prescribed, referral for treatment, etc.). The analysis of this information showed that there were two GPs who had significantly fewer people who have a learning disability on their list than the other five. These GPs also had a lower rate of referral and treatment for the people they did see. In discussing this finding, the GPs acknowledged that they felt their understanding of learning disability was not as good as it should be and they were perhaps a little out of touch with current thinking. The new GP with an interest in learning disability agreed to run a training session before the next practice meeting.

When the data was compared to national estimates of general health problems amongst people who have a learning disability, it suggested that whilst the GPs were diagnosing and managing most general health problems well, conditions such as hypertension and obesity were treated less actively. Anecdotal evidence from the GPs and practice nurses also suggested that the care and treatment of people with epilepsy could be improved and so the senior practice nurse agreed to contact the nurse specialist to ask if they would be willing to come and talk to the practice team about this issue.

Practitioners working with people who have a learning disability can use the approaches and processes associated with health needs assessment to determine the range of interventions and types of service required to meet the needs of the service users. If health and social care professionals use such approaches it is possible to address the health needs of a given population much more effectively. This chapter has explored health needs assessment and some of the concepts that are associated with it. The notion of health needs assessment and how it can be applied to start to identify health needs of people who have a learning disability have been also discussed. The practicalities of health needs assessment have been illustrated through the two case studies within the chapter.

FURTHER READING

Felce D, Taylor D, Wright K 1997 People with learning disabilities. Review 19. In: Health care needs assessment, 2nd series. Radcliffe Medical Press, Oxford
Although this review is now a few years old, it remains a very useful reference document. The estimates of prevalence and incidence of learning disability in the population and of the healthcare problems experienced by people who have

a learning disability provide valuable comparative figures for local needs assessment projects. The review also contains useful sections on the effectiveness of services and models of care, as well as more than 60 references.

Newbronner E, Acton C 1998 Health needs assessment step by step. York Health Economics Consortium, University of York
This is a very practical guide to health needs assessment for GPs, practice staff and primary healthcare teams. It suggests a step-by-step approach to conducting health needs assessments and contains an HNA toolkit, including an information checklist, advice on conducting questionnaire and interview-based surveys, and a guide to downloading HNA information from practice computer systems.

Popay J, Williams G (eds) 1994 Researching the people's health. Routledge, London
The book considers two related issues: the role of social research in health services and the relationship between lay and expert knowledge in public health and healthcare. Part II of the book covers the theory and methods of needs assessment and there are a number of other relevant chapters in Part III, which addresses issues of public involvement in needs assessment and research.

Scottish Needs Assessment Programme 1998 Needs assessment in primary care: a rough guide. SNAP Primary Care Network, Edinburgh
This is a relatively short and clearly written guide, designed to help primary healthcare teams, Scottish primary care trusts and healthcare cooperatives practise health needs assessment. It contains a number of simple step-by-step guides to different approaches to health needs assessment and lists contacts and data sources, which would be particularly helpful to those working in Scotland.

Stevens A, Raftery J 1997 Introduction. In: Health care needs assessment, 2nd series. Radcliffe Medical Press, Oxford
This first chapter in the second series of epidemiologically based needs assessment reviews provides a very valuable introduction to health needs assessment. In particular, the authors define and explain the main concepts used in health needs assessment and outline a number of approaches currently used in the UK.

Wright J, Williams R, Wilkinson J R 1998 Development and importance of health needs assessment. BMJ 316:1310–1313
This is the first in a series of six articles, published during April, May and June 1998, describing approaches to and topics for health needs assessment. The authors also highlight some of the pitfall and problems of health needs assessment and suggest ways in which the results from health needs assessment projects can be used more effectively.

REFERENCES

Billings R, Cowley S 1995 Approaches to community need assessment: a literature review. J Adv Nursing Pract 22: 721–730

Bradshaw J S 1972 A taxonomy of social need. In: McLachlan G (ed) Problems and progress in medical care: essays on current research, 7th series. Oxford University Press, Oxford

Culyer A J 1976 Need and the National Health Service. Martin Robertson, London

Department of Health 1997 The new NHS; modern, dependable. Stationery Office, London

Felce D, Taylor D, Wright K 1997 People with learning disabilities. Review 19. In: Health care needs assessment, 2nd series. Radcliffe Medical Press, Oxford

Howells G 1986 Are the medical needs of mentally handicapped people being met? J Royal Coll Gen Pract 36(291): 449–453

National Health Service Management Executive 1991 Assessing healthcare needs. DoH, London

Scottish Needs Assessment Programme 1998 Needs assessment in primary care: a rough guide. SNAP Primary Care Network, Edinburgh

Stevens A, Gabbay J 1991 Needs assessment needs assessment. Health Trends 23:20–23

Stevens A, Raftery J 1997 Introduction. In: Health care needs assessment, 2nd series. Radcliffe Medical Press, Oxford

Wilkinson J, Murray S A 1998 Assessment in primary care: practical issues and possible approaches. BMJ 316:1524–1528

Wright J, Williams R, Wilkinson J R 1998 Development and importance of health needs assessment. BMJ 316:1310–1313

7 Health promotion with people who have a learning disability

Philomena Shaughnessy and Susan Cruse

KEY ISSUES

- Barriers to health promotion for people who have learning disabilities
- Elements of and approaches to health promotion
- The importance of self-efficacy in attaining health-promoting behaviour
- Assessing health promotion need in communities and individuals
- Designing and implementing health promotion
- Healthy alliances and project management
- Evaluation of health promotion interventions

INTRODUCTION

The need to remove the considerable barriers to health promotion for people who have a learning disability has long been recognized (Mental Health Foundation 1996, NHSE 1998). However, what has been lacking are practical suggestions as to how these barriers may be removed or reduced. This chapter, through an application of health promotion theory to the field of learning disability, explores ways in which health and social care professionals can work towards the provision of effectively assessed, targeted, implemented and evaluated health promotion interventions, for individuals, groups or communities of people who have learning disabilities.

PROBLEMS WITH ACCESS TO AND AVAILABILITY OF HEALTH PROMOTION

There are various groups in society who take up invitations to health promotion initiatives in much smaller numbers than the rest of the population. For example, individuals from low social class and black and ethnic minority groups fail to access many health promotion interventions which are freely accessed by the rest of the population (Arblaster et al 1996). The reasons for this are varied but often centre around the characteristics of the service offered to them; that is, that the service is inaccessible or is inappropriate to their expressed and felt needs. Some of the factors contributing to this situation, which have both professional and user/carer origins, are represented in

Figure 7.1. This poor access to health promotion for people who have learning disabilities has also been recognized at governmental level (DoH 1995), where attempts have been made to address it through the production of good practice documents. One example is *Once a day* (NHSE 1999) which provides guidance for health professionals on the provision of primary care services for people who have learning disabilities.

Problems with access to and availability of health promotion services and interventions are of some concern, due to the reorganization of health and social care for people who have learning disabilities away from secondary care towards primary care, which has been accelerated by the NHS and Community Care Act (DoH 1990, Emerson & Hatton 1996). This has meant that the majority of people who have a learning disability now live in the community (OPCS 1993) with parents, unsupported or supported by spouses, siblings or other carers and that some health needs that were previously met in residential settings are now in danger of being missed (NHSE 1998). It follows that opportunities for preventing ill health and promoting good health may also be limited.

The health consequences of unmonitored community care have been illustrated by Wilson & Haire (1990). Of 69 adults who have a learning disability

---

FIGURE 7.1   *Barriers to health promotion for people who have a learning disability.*

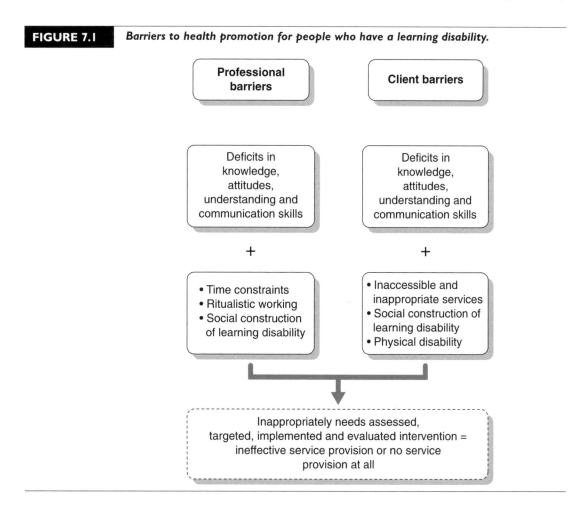

living in the community and attending a day centre, only eight did not have a significant, previously unidentified health problem brought to light by the study. The occurrence in the literature of similar accounts (see Cumella et al 1992, Mental Health Foundation 1996, McRae 1997, Stanley & Ng 1998, Vernon 1998) indicates that access to appropriate primary care and the health promotion interventions provided in this setting continues to be problematic for people who have learning disabilities. Because primary care is a frequently identified setting for health promotion activity (Stanley 1998, Stanley & Ng 1998), most discussion of health promotion in the learning disability literature tends to be medically focused. Although this is entirely appropriate for some interventions, for example immunization, an exclusively medical approach to health promotion can lead to reinforced dependency, with the power gradient between professionals and the individual emphasized. Also, this emphasis means that other forms of health promotion for people who have learning disabilities, for example community development, are either not identified as such, or not discussed.

The majority of people who have severe learning disabilities become known to service providers through their need for secondary and tertiary care as a result of associated multiple health problems (Moss et al 1993). Although local authorities are required to keep a register of learning-disabled clients (Thompson & Mathias 1999), registration is voluntary. Also the majority of GPs have not kept the practice registers of learning-disabled clients recommended by the National Health Service Executive (NHSE 1998). Therefore, it is extremely likely that only those people who have profound learning disabilities and who are known to service providers are registered with local authorities, leaving an unknown prevalence of mild to moderate learning disability in the community, with underidentification of need leading to inadequate service provision for this group (Kerr et al 1996). However, many of those who have mild to moderate learning disability may only require input from services from time to time or they may not be known to service providers (Mental Health Foundation 1996), reinforcing the importance of increasing the accessibility of mainstream health promotion services.

In the absence of reliable data on the prevalence of individuals who have a learning disability in the United Kingdom (Kerr et al 1996), estimates (based on below-average rating on IQ testing of samples of the general population) indicate that it is likely to be approximately 2% of the population. This equates to over 1 000 000 people nationally (Mental Health Foundation 1996, OPCS 1988) and 2000 per average primary care group population. The advent of Primary Care Groups heralded by the new NHS Act (DoH 1997) could have distinct advantages for people who have learning disabilities if health professionals are proactive in advocating for their needs. When viewed as a proportion of a Primary Care Group population, people who have learning disabilities become a sizeable 'minority' group, for which it is realistic to plan a health promotion strategy.

At the level of the learning-disabled individual, the characteristics of the learning disability, for example, communication and behavioural issues or associated physical disabilities and socialization into a passive role (Kinnel 1987), all inhibit access to health promotion services which generally have to be sought out, particularly those provided in health service settings such as primary care (Langan et al 1993, Wilson & Haire 1990). Sensory impairments and mental health problems have enormous implications for communication. In fact, communication difficulties confront almost every learning-disabled individual, with 48% having an impairment in one sensory domain and 18% doubly impaired (Kerr et al 1996, Stanley & Ng 1998). These disabilities often cause healthcare professionals and lay people to stereotype affected individuals negatively (Fitzsimmons & Barr 1997), which in turn can affect access to services. There is also a danger in totally relying on carers to seek out appropriate health promotion services for people who have learning disabilities, as many carers are as socialized into compliance as are their relatives, and may be unaware of the scope of preventive services (Kerr et al 1996).

Communication is also essential for informed consent and although fully informed consent is the ideal to which health professionals should aspire (Edwards & Bee 1992), cooperation may be all that is achievable (Haire et al 1992). This sits uneasily with the ethical position of many healthcare professionals, particularly nurses, who are obliged to promote client autonomy (UKCC 1996). Although the NHSE (1999) gives guidance on some areas, difficult ethical issues are unearthed when considering the provision of some preventive services, such as cervical screening (Shaughnessy 1999, NHSCSP 2000). Often these services are withheld on the basis of erroneous assumptions of a lack of need (Pearson et al 1998), the inability of the client to give verbal consent (Haire et al 1992) and the difficulty in determining whether the treatment is necessary or in the client's best interest.

The philosophy of normalization has been very influential in the design and delivery of all services to people who have a learning disability over the past 20 years, including the shift from institutional to community care (Emerson & Hatton 1996). The principle of normalization is concerned with ensuring that generic services are accessible to people who have a learning disability, helping to demonstrate to peers and others that this group is valued by the host society (Tyne 1981, Wolfensberger 1972). However, the misinterpretation and subsequent zealous pursuit of the ideology of normalization has meant that generic health promotion services are upheld as the ideal (Gates 1998), whilst specialist services for people who have learning disabilities have been eroded, or the need for them ignored (Cooke 1997). In addition, most healthcare professionals, with the exception of a few learning disabilities specialists, have little understanding of the concept of normalization and therefore of the philosophy upon which such services are planned (Cooke 1997). The idea that people who have a learning disability do not need services which are any different from the rest of the population can result in no service provision or in the provision of services which are inappropriate for the client group.

OVERCOMING BARRIERS TO HEALTH PROMOTION

Addressing and removing barriers to health promotion will ultimately promote inclusion and reduce inequalities in service provision. The main barrier to health promotion for people who have learning disabilities is difficulty with interpersonal communication. Unfortunately many primary healthcare professionals do not have the skills required to overcome such difficulties (Fitzsimmons & Barr 1997, Langan et al 1993, Thornton 1996). This results in people who have learning disabilities being less likely to receive lifestyle advice than those who do not have a learning disability (Langan et al 1993). People who have learning disabilities and their carers have recognized these communication difficulties as a barrier to healthcare and have highlighted the need for disability equality training and communication methods training for doctors and nurses, in order to address the situation (Mental Health Foundation 1996).

Learning disability nurses have a range of communication and observational skills, which could be usefully taught to other healthcare professionals (Cook 1998). However, community learning disability nurses are a largely untapped resource in assessing the health needs of, and planning health promotion for people who have a learning disability in primary care (Kay et al 1996, Thornton 1996).

One group of learning disability nurses has compiled guidance for health professionals working in primary care and other health and social care settings (Box 7.1). This guide to good practice is aimed at increasing the accessibility of primary healthcare to people who have learning disabilities.

Another barrier to effective consultation, which is rarely addressed, is the confounding effect of racism on people who have learning disabilities who are from black and ethnic minority groups (Bano et al 1993). The poor accessibility to and acceptability of services which are experienced by many black and ethnic minority groups are likely to be compounded further by the

BOX 7.1	*A guide to good practice aimed at increasing the accessibility of primary healthcare to people who have learning disabilities*

The following are examples of good practice that have been found useful in facilitating better clinic appointments.

- Allocating the first or the last appointment
- Allocating double appointments if needed
- Involving the family and carers (who are familiar with the person) may help in history taking and determining problem severity
- Acquiring background knowledge of the client through direct liaison with community learning disability nurse
- Providing access to quiet areas if they become distressed in crowded or noisy situations, or when kept waiting
- Being treated with friendliness, respect and dignity
- Providing physical access
- Checking understanding and not making assumptions about levels of comprehension
- Providing written instructions and regular follow-ups will help with treatment compliance
- Arranging appointments with friendly verbal reminders and signs written in large clear print, in simple language, colour coded and with symbols or pictures
- Prearranging for the use of an interpreter to sign or to translate from another language
- Making home visits

Source: North Hertfordshire NHS Trust Learning Disability Service

learning disability and it is important to remain mindful of the need to ensure that consultations and material are as culturally sensitive as that which should be available to other minority groups. This will mean prioritizing cultural issues and tailoring the approach of health promotion interventions to the needs of the targeted individual or group.

Perhaps for some of the reasons above, there is a tendency for people who have learning disabilities not to mention symptoms of disease to carers or members of the primary healthcare team. In addition, health promotion is rarely identified as a need by carers (Gates 1998). These needs are more likely to be identified if there is an opportunity for the client and/or carer to prepare for such an appointment. Such an opportunity could be facilitated through the use of a health promotion prompt sheet (Fig. 7.2) sent to carers or clients in advance of a planned meeting. The sheet can be adapted and could include space for agreed action to be written at the meeting. This approach may serve to enhance client satisfaction and positive outcomes from such interventions (Ley 1988).

FIGURE 7.2   *Example of a health promotion prompt sheet to be sent to the client/carer in advance of a meeting.*

How are you?

What makes you feel well?

What stops you feeling well?

What do you enjoy doing?

What else would you like to do?

Is there anything you especially want to talk about when you see the nurse?

PROMOTING HEALTH – SETTING THE SCENE

The World Health Organization's definition of health promotion as 'the process of enabling people to increase control over and to improve their health' (WHO 1984) has been formulated in the context of a social model of health which views the determinants of health more widely than just the absence of disease.

The recent government White Paper *Saving lives: our healthier nation* (DoH 1999) adopts this social model of health and recognizes health improvement as its key aim. In addition, it promotes a partnership approach as key to improving the health of the population. Such a partnership involves government, local communities and individuals all playing their part. However, as the WHO points out, in order for individuals to be able to play their part, people need to have sufficient control over their health. This inevitably entails obtaining particular knowledge and skills and fostering the belief in their ability to take control.

THE ELEMENTS OF HEALTH PROMOTION

Tannahill (1985) has proposed a model of health promotion (Fig. 7.3) which identifies overlapping elements of health promotion or 'spheres of activity'.

1. Health education

This is defined as:

> Communication activity aimed at enhancing well-being and preventing or diminishing ill health in individuals and groups through influencing the knowledge, beliefs, attitudes and behaviour of those with power and of the community at large.
>
> (Tannahill 1985)

FIGURE 7.3   *The elements of health promotion (reproduced from Tannahill 1985 with permission of the Health Education Authority).*

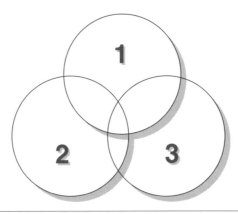

Also empowerment of individuals and groups is viewed as an important objective of health education. For example, health education might promote social inclusion through decreasing negative stereotyping regarding people who have learning disabilities, through valuing and respecting their needs. A participative educational process could involve people who have learning disabilities and professionals learning from each other.

2. Prevention

The prevention sphere focuses on the reduction of the 'risk of occurrence of a disease process, illness, injury, disability, handicap or some other unwanted event or state (such as pregnancy)' (Tannahill 1985). This incorporates primary, secondary and tertiary prevention and is generally medically focused. These activities are usually carried out in healthcare settings.

Primary prevention is the prevention of a disorder manifesting itself by removing or modifying a risk factor; for example, the prevention of obesity through health education and provision of an exercise regime and a healthy diet for people who have a learning disability. Secondary prevention involves identifying early signs of disease before they become symptomatic and preventing the disease occurring or advancing; for example, screening for breast and cervical cancer. Tertiary prevention involves preventing a disease which is already manifest becoming worse or preventing complications of the disease occurring; for example, preventing damage caused by repeated uncontrolled epileptic fits.

3. Health protection

Within the health protection sphere, are 'legal or fiscal controls, other regulation or policies, or voluntary codes of practice aimed at the prevention of ill health or the positive enhancement of well-being' (Tannahill 1985). These represent decisions by influential bodies, e.g. local or national government, which will positively protect health, one example being the legislation requiring the compulsory wearing of seat belts in cars. The aim of health protection measures is to promote health in whole populations, which are inclusive of people who have learning disabilities.

APPROACHES TO HEALTH PROMOTION

In addition to the elements of health promotion, there are differences in the ways in which health promotion can be conceptualized which affect its emphasis. Beattie's (1991) model can help health promoters to identify an appropriate strategy according to the social and political framework within which they are operating.

Beattie (1991) has developed a cross-classification device representing the paradigms of health promotion (Fig. 7.4). Two bipolar dimensions are considered to account for major ideological stances in health promotion:

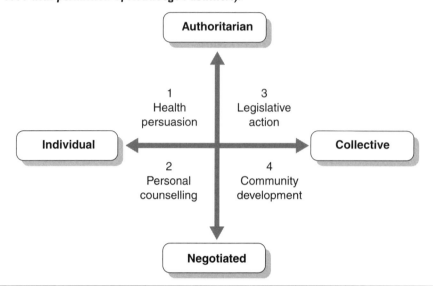

FIGURE 7.4   *The paradigms and strategies of health promotion (adapted from Fig. 7.1 in Beattie 1991 with permission of Routledge Publishers).*

- *the focus of intervention*, of which the bipolar opposites are an individual focus at one end and a collective focus at the other
- *the mode of intervention*, of which the bipolar opposites are an authoritarian, 'top-down', expert-led mode at one end and a 'negotiated' or participative mode of functioning (valuing individual autonomy) at the other.

The health promotion strategies generated through the interaction of these dimensions can be divided into those which are focused on the individual (1 and 2) and those which are collectively focused (3 and 4).

1. The individual authoritarian quadrant – health persuasion

Here responsibility for health lies with the individual. Individuals are conceived of as capable of making significant changes to their lifestyle or environment and success may be judged on the degree of compliance with advice from the health professional. This approach has been criticized for blaming the victim for non-compliance. In the case of people who have learning disabilities, the available evidence for the effectiveness of health promotion is limited as the social and health disadvantages that this group encounter may not be acknowledged. Mass media campaigns can be included in this quadrant, as their targets are individuals and their purpose is persuasion. An individual authoritarian approach may be justifiably used providing that the particular needs of people who have learning disabilities are considered and planned for.

2. The individual negotiated quadrant – personal counselling

In the individual negotiated quadrant the value base for health promotion work is person centred. This fits well with the service user consultation and partnership approach promoted within the philosophies of learning disability services and supported by the NHSE (1998), through the use of self-advocacy and advocacy services. Implementation is through counselling, education and group work. The relationship is more equal between the health promoter and the client, with the former working as facilitator, not expert. The health promotion intervention (both the topic and the mode) is negotiated and whatever the topic and mode identified, the goal is enhanced client autonomy and informed choice.

In order for people who have a learning disability to be able to engage in this more equal relationship, the generic health promoter may need support and guidance from a specialist practitioner, such as a community learning disability nurse, or an individual carer. This requires a fundamental respect for and valuing of those who have a learning disability, a willingness on the part of the health promoter to be guided, which is embodied in flexibility in ways of working.

3. The collective authoritarian quadrant – legislative action

The aim here can be expressed as the top-down redistribution of power by statutory authorities in favour of disadvantaged groups such as those who have a learning disability. This may be achieved through undertaking a formal consultation process regarding location and nature of accommodation prior to deinstitutionalization. A further example of this redistribution of power can be seen in direct payment schemes whereby the money and therefore the control in purchasing one's own services lies with the individual client.

4. The collective negotiated quadrant – community development

In the collective negotiated quadrant the aim is to redistribute power to disadvantaged groups through empowerment using action research, skills sharing, training and lobbying. This is particularly important for people who have learning disabilities who experience a much greater burden of disadvantage and disease than the rest of the population (NHSE 1998). The aim of health promotion is to assist people to identify and challenge the social structures which perpetuate their exclusion. An example of this would be a user group (usually supported by the expertise of health or social care professionals) who identify poor housing conditions as contributing to their ill health and poor social standing and negotiate improved standards of accommodation, leading to the benefit of being valued by the host society (Tyne 1981).

Examples of health promotion intervention classified according to this paradigm are shown in Figure 7.5.

It is a client-centred, empowerment approach, as exemplified by the individual negotiated and collective negotiated quadrants, that will ensure that a health promotion intervention is appropriate and acceptable to a client group. It is within these quadrants that the client's agenda predominates. In the context of people who have a learning disability, the focus is on the individuals and, where appropriate, their carers, facilitating in them a belief in their right and ability to

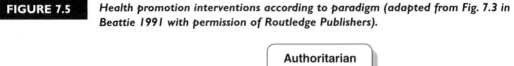

FIGURE 7.5   *Health promotion interventions according to paradigm (adapted from Fig. 7.3 in Beattie 1991 with permission of Routledge Publishers).*

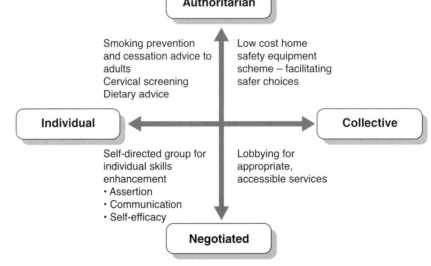

promote their own health through personal or networking strategies. The prime goal of a client-centred approach to health promotion is maximizing voluntary choice. This leads us to a belief in self-efficacy, which is a precondition for individual voluntary choice.

THE IMPORTANCE OF SELF-EFFICACY

Perceived self-efficacy, as defined by Bandura (1986), is the judgement of personal capability to organize and carry out a particular course of action. Efficacy expectations are based on several sources of information: performance, accomplishments, vicarious experience, verbal persuasion and states of physiological arousal (Bandura 1977). Efficacy expectations are strongest when informed by one's own personal experiences. Vicarious experience, seeing others perform activities successfully, can also lead to expectations in observers that they can do likewise, particularly if there are significant perceived similarities between observers and role models. Verbal persuasion involves persuasive suggestion as a means of leading people to believe that they can cope successfully in a particular situation.

An individual's level of physiological and emotional arousal will affect his or her perception of self-efficacy, with heightened levels of emotional arousal likely to debilitate performance. People who have learning disabilities may be especially at risk as all the sources of efficacy information outlined above may be negatively affected. In addition, performance accomplishments are likely to be more restricted than those of the general population. This may lead to self-efficacy being compromised, a situation that may be further reinforced by professionals and carers failing to support people who have a learning disability to achieve their personal goals.

Self-efficacy and health promotion

There is considerable evidence in the literature of the significance of the concept of self-efficacy for health promotion; in fact, it emerges as the strongest predictor of a health-promoting lifestyle (Gillis 1993). Self-efficacy is proposed as the key to a sense of control and to the ability for self-determination and is the condition upon which positive emotional and functional health depends.

The principal barrier to the promotion of self-efficacy is the social construction of learning disability. Self-efficacy belief will inevitably be restricted by a societal unwillingness to accept the learning-disabled person as an autonomous agent with a right to and capacity for self-determination. Verbal persuasion, to which people who have learning disabilities can be subject through social encounters, may also threaten self-efficacy beliefs where these emphasize limitations in capacities and capabilities. Therefore it is important to avoid negative stereotypes and judgemental attitudes that encourage segregation and reduced services and opportunities, i.e. exclusion.

The interaction between health professional and client presents an opportunity for strengthening self-efficacy belief and accurate appraisal of individual capabilities through situation- or issue-specific intervention. A health promotion approach, which has self-efficacy as its prime focus, will enable learning-disabled people to strengthen functional and emotional well-being and their facility for self-determination and so remove themselves from the socially constructed, stereotypical image of the learning-disabled person. This approach has been advocated by Dalley (1992), in which learning-disabled citizens are nurtured through mutual support, cooperation and equality of status.

ASSESSING THE NEED FOR HEALTH PROMOTION

The NHS and Community Care Act (DoH 1990) placed needs assessment firmly on the agenda of all those involved in delivering health and social care in the community, describing it as the cornerstone of high-quality community care. Since then a large literature base has developed on the subject, which attests the importance of systematic assessment of need in providing appropriate care to individuals and groups.

ACTIVITY 7.1

Why is it important to assess the need for health promotion?

- To identify and respond to specific needs of sections of the population who could benefit from health promotion interventions.
- To act as a basis for the appropriate design of health promotion interventions.
- To ensure that adequate resources, whether fiscal or human, are allocated to the intervention.

Although there are many different approaches to health promotion, which are discussed above, the primary concern of much health promotion practice is the proactive prevention of ill health and the empowerment of individuals and communities to adopt practices and lifestyles which *they* feel contribute to their health. Epidemiological and other health-related sources of data are of value in planning health promotion services to communities and groups but they have serious limitations. The exclusive use of such data may lead to the implementation of services that are professionally defined (Billings 1996) which may be inappropriate or even harmful; also such data disguise individual differences and needs. People who have a learning disability are not a homogenous group and there are large variations in the type and range of disability (Mental Health Foundation 1996). This can result in many areas of need remaining unidentified. This situation can in part be resolved by communicating with carers and significant others (Kerr et al 1996). All of this means that professionals, carers and users must collaborate in the assessment of health promotion need and that expressed need should heavily influence the provision of health promotion services. This is far more likely to result in a service which is acceptable and accessible to users and carers (Freeman et al 1997).

So far, we have considered health promotion as being individually or collectively focused but from the perspective of the health professional working with people who have learning disabilities, it is also necessary to consider health promotion on two planes – specialist and generic. The importance of ensuring that generic health promotion is available and accessible to people who have a learning disability is well acknowledged (DoH 1996) and the degree to which this is happening should form part of community health needs assessment. However, specialist health promotion services may also need to be provided at both a community (collective) and an individual level. At the community level, specialist health promotion interventions could be designed to counteract the isolation and poverty experienced by many learning-disabled individuals living in the community. The lack of meaningful activity during the day, opportunities for socializing and real hope for future change (McRae 1997) are areas in urgent need of attention. This could be tackled through a participative community-oriented approach (Freeman et al 1997) to health promotion.

Assessing community (collective) health need

Billings (1996) has demonstrated the use of a single embedded case study research design (Yin 1994) for the assessment of the health needs of a given community. The unit of analysis, or case, is identified as the community, with various sources of health-related data identified as subunits. The data contained in the subunits are used to arrive at an analysis of the case. Subunits can be added to the design or removed, although care must be taken to use only rigorous sources of data. Data sources may be quantitative or qualitative and may represent indicators of process (such as a service user survey on satisfaction) or outcome (Yin 1994) (for example, the number of women dying prematurely from breast cancer). Figure 7.6 shows such a design with the unit of analysis being the learning-disabled community. Although the subunits identified are comprehensive, they are not exclusive and you may know of other rigorous sources of local data which could form another subunit or be added to an existing one.

Obtaining data specific to those who have a learning disability may be difficult due to the dearth of such data and the limitations of the available data, discussed earlier. However, as people who have learning disabilities have the same underlying health needs as the rest of the community (Kay et al 1996),

FIGURE 7.6	*Single embedded case study design, identifying the learning-disabled community as the unit of analysis and other sources of relevant information as subunits (adapted from Billings 1996 with permission of EMAP Healthcare).*

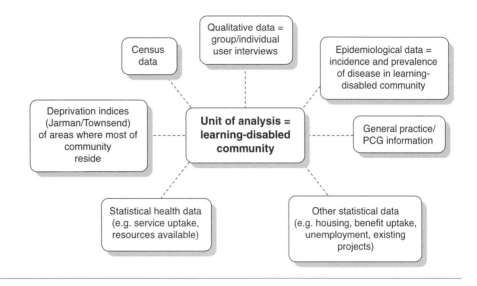

albeit compounded by the high prevalence of certain conditions, it may be appropriate to use sources of data extrapolated from the general population, using information specific to those who have a learning disability where it is available. For example, material deprivation indices which apply to a whole community, such as the Jarman Index (Jarman 1984), will be equally relevant to those who have a learning disability living in that community but if data on the number of people who have learning disabilities who are employed were also available, this would give a good indication of the socioeconomic standing of the learning-disabled community locally.

An assessment of this nature would be a useful exercise for a community learning disability team to undertake across a primary care group population, in order to assess socioeconomic influences on health, in addition to problems with access to and availability of health services. The resulting analysis provides the rationale for planning and implementing community-based health promotion initiatives, which will benefit this client group.

Assessing individual health promotion need

As we have seen, existing services need to be made more accessible to learning-disabled individuals. This is of particular importance to those who have mild learning disabilities and should be able to benefit from interventions available to the rest of the population. In addition, tailoring health promotion interventions to need is essential (Kay et al 1996). Most healthcare professionals will be working at the level of individual service users, which in turn will eventually impact at community level, as service users become more valued and gain health as a result of the interventions. Activity 7.2 illustrates the process of assessing the health promotion needs of an individual.

ACTIVITY 7.2

Assessing the health promotion needs of the individual client

Robert is a 21-year-old man who has a 'moderate' learning disability. He was living with his mother until recently when he became more and more unhappy with the situation and expressed a need for more independence. He and his mother have asked for help in ensuring that when he moves into his new home, he will be encouraged to be self-caring as far as possible.

■ You are aware that mental health and behavioural problems are prevalent in people who have learning disabilities, as evidenced by the NHSE (1998), DoH (1996) and Kerr et al (1996), and that the incidence of obesity is high (Beange & Bauman 1991). In relation to Robert it is important to identify whether these factors have any bearing on his perceived unhappiness.

■ Using the needs assessment tool (Fig. 7.7), structure a systematic health promotion needs assessment for Robert.

Tailoring health promotion to individual need

Multiple health promotion needs are likely to be disclosed by such an assessment. These may include sexual health needs, personal hygiene needs, educational needs, etc. which all need tackling separately. However, for the purposes of this exercise one of Robert's possible needs, regarding nutrition, is explored.

The result of your needs assessment shows that one of Robert's health needs is related to nutrition. You have found that Robert has a high Body Mass Index, has not been used to cooking for himself and has a preference for sweet and fatty foods.

As a result you propose that Robert joins a basic cookery class for people who have learning disabilities which runs at the local day centre. In addition, Robert will be able to join a group from the day centre on a weekly supported shopping trip. You discuss a staged approach to Robert catering for himself independently. You all agree that the approach will comprise three stages, all of which will require different skills and techniques in order to achieve them.

1. Robert's mother preparing food and explaining her activities, with Robert observing and asking questions.

2. Robert cooking and explaining his activity to his mother who observes and asks questions of him.

3. Robert cooking independently, whilst maintaining contact with his mother and participation in the shopping trips and weekly cookery classes at the day centre.

The tool used in Activity 7.2 could be applied in a variety of settings, to assess the health promotion needs of people who have learning disabilities. This tool is neither inclusive nor exclusive, being compiled from available information on problems faced by people who have learning disabilities. Therefore you may find that you need to adapt it by adding your own questions.

Nurses have a key role to play in much proactive individual assessment, by virtue of their knowledge base, and are ideally placed to involve service

FIGURE 7.7   *Individual health promotion needs assessment tool.*

Name _____ Date of birth _____ Date _____

1 What is the client's ethnic/cultural background?

_____

2 Does he/she have religious beliefs or customs which need to be taken into account in order to tailor interventions? *If so please specify.*

_____

3 What social support is available to the individual?

_____
_____

4 Does he/she feel able to:

• Attend to personal hygiene?   Yes ☐   No ☐
• Cook for him/herself?   Yes ☐   No ☐
• Talk to other people?   Yes ☐   No ☐
• Get on with other people?   Yes ☐   No ☐

5 How does he/she communicate?

Verbally ☐   Non-verbally ☐
Through a carer ☐   No communication ☐

6 If communication difficulties are present have the following been tested where possible?

Hearing   Yes ☐   No ☐
Vision   Yes ☐   No ☐

FIGURE 7.7	*Individual health promotion needs assessment tool.*

7 Is he/she in an intimate relationship?

Yes ☐   No ☐   *Go to Q8*

If yes, what contraceptive methods are in use? ----------------------------------

For women aged 20–60 years

Date of the last cervical smear -------- Result -------- Next smear due ----------

Are there any problems with other aspects of the relationship such as communication/sexual relationships? ---------------------------------------

8 How does he/she manage stressful situations on a day-to-day basis? For example, does he/she respond angrily, cry, become introverted, etc?

----

9 What activities is he/she engaged in during the day (work and leisure)?

----

10 Has general health screening been done within the year?

Yes ☐ Have the results been acted upon?

No ☐ Arrange health screen with primary health care team if client/carer wishes?

11 To what extent does health behaviour contribute to ill health/health?

Daily cigarette consumption ---

Daily alcohol consumption ---

Body Mass Index --

Waist circumference --

Nature of physical activity ---------------------- Frequency ----------------

FIGURE 7.7   *Individual health promotion needs assessment tool.*

12 What food does he/she eat regularly?

----

13 When was the last visit to the dentist?

----

14 *For women aged 50 onwards*

Has she attended for breast screening in the last three years?

Yes ☐   Next mammogram due _____

No ☐   Discuss and arrange if the client wishes

15 Are there any other expressed needs/wishes?

----

users, carers and advocates in determining priorities for intervention. Community learning disability nurses, with their understanding of the needs of people who have learning disabilities and their links to other agencies, are well placed to carry out or arrange such assessments (Kay et al 1996). Health and social care professionals working within community settings, particularly as care managers, are already conducting needs assessments and planning and coordinating packages of care (Harris 1996). When assessing need, there is an opportunity to include health promotion indicators in the assessment criteria, so that health promotion is not overlooked in commissioning packages of care.

DESIGNING AND IMPLEMENTING APPROPRIATE HEALTH PROMOTION

All health promotion involves the use of scarce resources, which may be wasted if there is no clear plan of what is to be achieved through the intervention. In addition, the recent emphasis on evidence-based practice and clinical effectiveness (DoH 1998) has meant that health promotion interventions, along with other healthcare interventions, will be judged and funded primarily on evidence of effectiveness, closely followed by cost effectiveness (McConkey 1998). It is the nature of this evidence that causes the most difficulty in the field of health promotion. Presently evidence is viewed hierarchically with the most highly prized being the quantitative evidence of outcome produced by randomized controlled trials, with qualitative evidence, often produced by asking questions about the process of interventions, valued far less (Naidoo & Wills 1994, Perkins et al 1999). These problems are amplified in the field of learning disability research because many services, including health promotion, have developed in response to local interest and are carried out with small populations, with limited or no evaluation undertaken (NHSE 1998).

For some time there have been calls for healthcare professionals working with people who have learning disabilities to set clear, achievable and measurable goals and to be able to demonstrate their positive impact on individuals who use the services (DoH 1996, NHSE 1998). There is no doubt that evidence-based health promotion requires the best quality quantitative and qualitative evidence available but the current absence of a robust evidence base should not induce paralysis through waiting for the results of randomized controlled trials (Perkins et al 1999). If well planned interventions based on the best evidence available are implemented and evaluated, this will go some way to preventing the antithetical situation of programmes being introduced on the basis of professional or lay whim (Kerr et al 1996).

Health promotion is a complex and wide-ranging activity, in which the possibilities for intervention seem almost limitless. The task of choosing and designing an intervention is made more achievable if a systematic approach is taken to planning. For health professionals, the planning process also has the important side effect of making health promotion a tangible work activity for which resources are required (Naidoo & Wills 2000), instead of it being viewed as something which is absorbed into other work activity. The planning process should also include a realistic appraisal of the timescale for the implementation and evaluation of the project, which may otherwise be overlooked and lead to the abandonment or failure of projects (Perkins et al 1999).

Ewles & Simnett (1999) have constructed a flowchart which represents the planning process (Fig. 7.8). The reason for representing planning for health promotion in this way is to highlight the need to keep the project under review as interventions may have to be modified at any stage, due to the fact that health promotion is conducted in unpredictable 'real-life' situations.

FIGURE 7.8   *A flowchart for planning health promotion interventions (reproduced from Ewles & Simnett 1999 with permission of W B Saunders Publishers).*

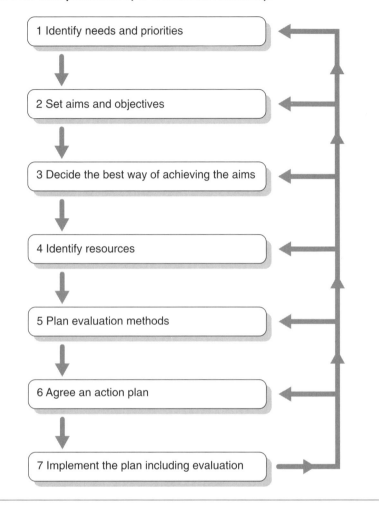

The flowchart is of particular use in planning health promotion interventions for groups, although the principles are equally applicable to interventions with individual clients. The first two stages involve assessment of need and identification of unmet need, an important part of the design, which is addressed in the previous section. Following this, general goals or aims of the project can be identified. The most crucial part of planning involves focusing on what is to be achieved and how this will be judged. If this is carried out with care, the intervention has a much greater chance of success. This revolves around setting objectives for the project which must be specific, measurable and realistic (Ewles & Simnett 1999, Naidoo & Wills 2000). These objectives provide the framework which will guide the precise planning of the intervention and also provide markers against which the project can be evaluated. Effectiveness in health promotion has been defined as the extent to which these objectives have been met and have led to the specified outcomes (Naidoo & Wills 2000, Tones & Tilford 1994).

Therefore, although planning the precise method of evaluation is carried out after the detail of the content of the intervention has been worked out, careful thought needs to be given to the indicators of effectiveness and method of evaluation at this stage.

ACTIVITY 7.3

A group of women clients who have learning disabilities and who attend a day centre have decided that they would like some information on sexual health. After collecting further information, it is clear that there are multiple unmet needs associated with this topic. These include advice and support on relationships, including assertiveness skills; awareness of anatomy and physiology; and information on choice and method of contraception. In conjunction with a local Primary Care Group, you decide to arrange a programme of group sessions in order to address some of these needs.

■ What aims and objectives could you set for the programme?

■ How would you measure success?

The aims will need to address the women's perceived need for information. The objectives or outcomes of the programme will encompass the precise ways in which these needs can be met. Therefore, the aims and objectives for such a programme may resemble the following.

Aim

To increase knowledge and understanding of the concept of sexual health.

Objectives

By the end of the programme the women will be able to:

1. identify male and female sexual organs

2. describe the basic principles of reproduction

3. understand basic contraceptive methods

4. demonstrate negotiation skills within relationships, particularly in terms of boundary setting

5. demonstrate assertiveness skills through role play

6. understand how to access family planning guidance.

The programme will therefore need to address knowledge and skills and, in order to do this, will need to be broken down into several topic areas. One of these areas revolves around assertiveness skills and interpersonal communication, with objectives 4 and 5 referring to this. This could be taught through role play, small group work, etc. with a view to expanding the vocabulary and practical strategies available to address feelings and wishes, which should lead to increased ability to negotiate boundaries regarding intimate relationships.

The before/after evaluation discussed below could be usefully employed in this situation, to measure success. One way of conducting this may be to give clients a 'case study' which focuses on assertiveness skills and interpersonal communication and record client responses before the input and again afterwards.

HEALTH PROMOTION AND HEALTHY ALLIANCES

The importance of professional coordination of care and the creation of 'healthy alliances' is stressed in *A strategy for people with learning disabilities* (DoH 1995) and this cannot be overemphasized. Healthy alliances have been defined as 'active partnerships between the many organizations and individuals who can come together to improve health' (DoH 1992). Healthy alliances can lead to more effective use of resources, broadened responsibility for health, the breaking down of barriers between organizations through promoting better mutual understanding, improving exchange of information and generating networks.

People who have learning disabilities are significant consumers of other services apart from those of the primary healthcare team; for example, social care support services. Coordinated health promotion packages integrated into health or social care provision will allow health promotion responsive to need throughout the lifespan. Generic primary healthcare services cannot be expected to develop sensitive services in isolation.

Where people come to work together from a variety of professional and lay orientations and representing a variety of organizational priorities, there is a need for close coordination of the process. The aim of such coordination is to minimize the risk of a breakdown in cooperative working through lack of a common purpose or misunderstanding of each other's roles, and to maximize the effectiveness of the health promotion intervention.

The project management of healthy alliances

A project management approach to healthy alliances will facilitate the formulization of agreed aims and objectives which will aid the successful implementation and maintenance of collaborative activities. This is particularly important in maintaining a cohesive approach to the project. In situations where, for example, an agreed philosophy and goals are missing, tension is likely to build up within an alliance with a potential reduction in willingness to cooperate, subsequently resulting in reduced effectiveness.

Within a project management approach, a project manager is responsible for ensuring that cooperative working is established and maintained and that the work is targeted appropriately, monitored and reviewed. Monitoring of the work includes providing regular feedback to member organizations on process and output indicators (Speller et al 1994). In a healthy alliance which has the aim of promoting the health of people who have learning disabilities, membership might include GPs, general practice nurses, specialist learning disability nurses, social workers (generic or specialist), clients, carers and voluntary organizations. The project manager might be drawn from any one of these groups. The most important elements of the leadership skills of a successful project manager have been identified as those of integrater, enabler, leader, motivater, effective communicator, organizer and decision maker (Baguley 1995). If a person who has learning disabilities wishes to steer a project, there may be a case for co-management or robust support mechanisms to be put in place such as support from an external consultant project manager or the service user may manage specific parts of the process, if that is the wish of the team.

The project manager guides the team through the five distinct stages of a project identified by Ward (1994a,b), which can be conceptualized as a reflective cycle, demonstrating its ongoing nature (Fig. 7.9). An explanation of each of the stages in this cycle is given in Table 7.1.

FIGURE 7.9   *Project management as a reflective cycle.*

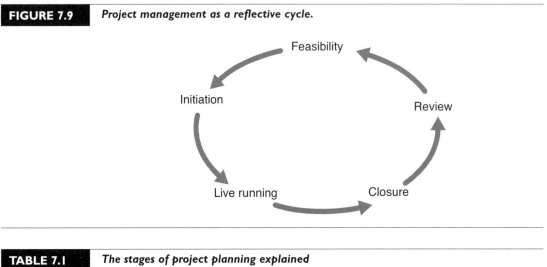

TABLE 7.1   *The stages of project planning explained*

Project stage	*Descriptor*
1. Feasibility	This phase precedes the formal opening of a project when the issues explored include whether the project is likely to meet an identified need and its likely costs, benefits and risks. The main purpose of this phase is to establish a solid foundation in the form of a rationale for the project and secure resourcing from which the project can go forward.
2. Initiation	At this point all necessary information and resources are to hand and a clear plan for the way forward is required. The who, what, why, when and how of the project is defined and documented. The 'who' involves roles and responsibilities being clearly identified; the 'what' implies a clear set of objectives and boundaries for the project; the 'why' is expressed as the rationale for the project; and the 'when' and 'how' constitute the project plan, detailing by which means objectives will be achieved, by which date and which resources are required. The initiation stage ensures that the project is brought under control from the outset.
3. Live running	The task of this phase is to produce planned outcomes using planned resources, within the planned timescale and to the preset quality standards and specifications. All processes are monitored and appropriate corrective action taken while organizational and environmental changes which bear on the project are addressed and managed.
4. Closure	The project and its team cease to exist or alternatively pause for review. It may be that the project is handed over to the clients, if empowerment was the goal, and if sustained self-help was the intended outcome.
5. Review	The degree of completion/attainment of project outcomes and therefore the effectiveness of the project management is examined. The review stage also permits ongoing project benefits and problems to be recognized and addressed.

A project management approach ensures regular timetabled reflection and stocktaking of the activities of a healthy alliance.

The following case study provides a practical example of how the project management approach outlined above can be used to develop and implement a smoking cessation project.

CASE STUDY 7.1

A group of clients and their carers have expressed a need for support for smoking cessation to a practice manager within the local primary care group/trust. This is communicated to the community learning disabilities team from the local NHS trust. The team reviews existing smoking cessation support and identifies an inadequacy in health education material. The learning disabilities nurse for the practice convenes a group comprising a practice nurse, a service user, a carer, a GP, a social worker, and a health promotion specialist. The learning disabilities nurse is identified by the group as the project manager.

The project management cycle is used to organize the project, with the various stages illustrated below.

1. Feasibility

The project planning group establishes a need for appropriate written material to reinforce verbal messages (Ley 1988) in both one-to-one or group settings. A team member obtains costings for design and printing of material from a local graphic design and print house. This is provisionally approved by the project manager who negotiates that the cost will be borne jointly by the primary care group/trust, the NHS trust and the specialist health promotion service.

2. Initiation

Who? Roles and responsibilities are defined. The learning disabilities nurse will provide specialist advice to the project team on the needs of people who have learning disabilities and the health promotion specialist will advise on effective health promotion regarding smoking cessation. The learning disabilities nurse will manage the budget as the project manager. The practice nurse, together with the service user, will lead the development of the resource.

What? A smoking cessation resource for people who have learning disabilities is developed, using a staged approach based on the Cycle of Change (Prochaska & DiClemente 1986) (Fig. 7.10). Guidelines for use of the pack are developed by the team along with a training schedule for primary care practitioners.

How? A participative approach is adopted, consulting with service users through the local user self-help group as the resource is developed.

3. Live running

The resource, an interactive teaching/discussion pack, is piloted with a group of service users at the first draft stage and is adjusted according to the findings from this pilot study. Production of the resource is then arranged in accordance with the budget and needs of local health professionals and service users.

4. Closure

The resource is produced and launched to primary healthcare teams, learning disability teams, NHS trusts and user groups, with one teaching/discussion pack allocated to each practice within the primary care group/trust. Training in the use of the

CASE STUDY 7.1   *(Cont'd)*

resource is delivered by the learning disabilities nurse, the practice nurse, the carer and the service user, as required by primary care practitioners. The project team's joint working is reviewed, recommendations for future healthy alliances are made and the project team is disbanded, with the project manager retaining responsibility for agreed evaluation beyond this point.

5. Review

The learning disabilities nurse as project manager conducts a process evaluation, which involves professionals and users in assessing the acceptability and usefulness of the resource, and recommendations are made for future versions (more detail on the evaluation of health promotion is covered in the next section). As a result, a new project team may be convened at a future date, demand, resources and organizational will permitting.

EVALUATION OF HEALTH PROMOTION

All evaluation involves making judgements about what is worth evaluating and what outcomes are of value from a project (Luker 1992, Øvretveit 1998, Perkins et al 1999, Tones & Tilford 1994). Evaluation is a research focused activity which, in common with all research, needs to be designed carefully in order to maximize its validity and, where possible, its reliability. This is particularly so in the context of evidence-based health promotion. In addition, it is also important to acknowledge the limitations of evaluative research designs, so that findings are not misrepresented as being more robust than they are in reality (Perkins et al 1999), especially as this could lead to interventions of dubious effectiveness being put into practice. At best, this can harm the credibility of health promotion and at worst, cause harm to clients.

The choice of the evaluation method and the questions asked of an intervention will be influenced by the nature of the intervention and the perspective of the interest group for whom the project is being evaluated (Øvretveit 1998). Most healthcare professionals working with people who have learning disabilities will be concerned with the interests of clients and carers, healthcare practitioners and managers. Managers are far more likely to be concerned with cost effectiveness than are clients, who in turn will be far more concerned with whether the intervention works for them. Health professionals may want to know under which conditions the intervention works for the most people (Øvretveit 1998) and possibly how much difference this will make to them in their working lives.

It is also likely that different groups may want different questions answered. However, to plan to answer multiple questions with a small-scale evaluation is unrealistic. Øvretveit (1998) sagely advises confining evaluative research to answering two or three key questions, clarifying exactly what is to be evaluated and over what time frame. So the key to successful evaluation is developing a focused approach rather than attempting the impossible task of trying to answer many divergent questions with one research design.

Evaluation designs range from descriptive designs through to randomized controlled trials and Øvretveit (1998) gives a succinct account of different evaluation designs and their relative advantages and disadvantages elsewhere. It is

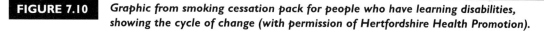

FIGURE 7.10   *Graphic from smoking cessation pack for people who have learning disabilities, showing the cycle of change (with permission of Hertfordshire Health Promotion).*

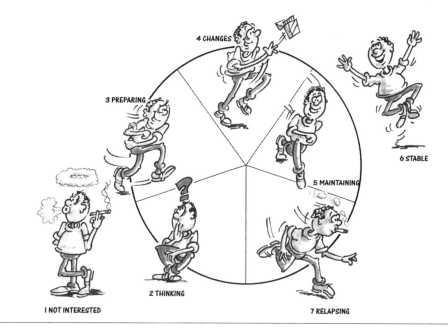

unlikely that most healthcare professionals trying to design small-scale health promotion interventions will have access to sufficient funds and expertise to conduct a randomized controlled trial; rather, it may be more realistic to conduct either a descriptive evaluation, an audit or a 'before-and-after' type evaluation.

The descriptive design

In evaluative research, descriptive evaluation, as its name suggests, sets out to describe the intervention, including the use of resources and the context of the intervention. It is often used to describe new interventions, perhaps where no evidence base exists. A clear account of what the intervention is and what it does may help others in project planning and enable users to make judgements about the value of interventions. The limitations of this design are that although it can give a description of outcomes, it cannot evaluate effectiveness because it does not take into account the situation before the intervention was implemented or any other factors which may have impinged on the result. Because of these limitations, some may dismiss the results as unscientific or worthless.

The audit design

The audit approach judges whether the intervention has met its objectives. If these objectives are evidence based, this can be a cost-effective method for improving practice. It does not aim to evaluate effectiveness, unless this is stated as a measurable objective of the intervention.

Auditing gathers data on practice, which will help to identify best practice. The emphasis on best practice constitutes a key element of clinical governance, which is central to monitoring the quality of local health services (DoH 1998, McCray & Carter 1999).

The 'before-and-after' design

The 'before-and-after' design measures the object of change before the intervention and again afterwards and although this does attempt to measure effectiveness, it does not allow for the multitude of other factors that may have had some effect on the results (Øvretveit 1998), partly because there is no means of comparing it to a group of individuals who are not exposed to the intervention. These would need to be controlled for in much more resource-intensive designs such as quasi-experimental designs or, if possible, the randomized controlled trial.

Given the stated limitations, which need to be made clear when results are published, these three designs are relatively cost effective and quick to perform and are those most commonly available to healthcare professionals.

Although there have been repeated calls to introduce annual health screening in primary care for people who have learning disabilities, there is little robust information on its effectiveness (Kerr et al 1996). The sorts of questions which would need to be asked of such an intervention, according to the evaluation design chosen, are shown in Box 7.2.

Often it is as important to evaluate the effect of the process of the intervention as it is the outcome. Donabedian (1969) has identified structure, process and outcome as equally important when evaluating services. Of these, process and outcome evaluation have attracted particular attention in evaluative research; indeed, process evaluation is germane to project management (Øvretveit 1998). Evaluation of the process of health promotion involves the collection of primarily qualitative data (Naidoo & Wills 2000); for example consumer satisfaction interviews and user consultation exercises. Indeed, evaluation of process fits well with the principle of normalization, where the process of raising the standard of services to people who have learning disabilities precedes raising their status in the community which is seen as being just as important as the outcome of the service provided (Tyne 1981, Wolfensberger 1972).

Outcome measures indicate the long-term effects of an intervention; for example, the decrease in deaths from lung cancer or suicide or a sustained decrease in obesity among learning-disabled adults. Evaluation of impact involves short-term indicators of the effectiveness of the service; for instance, the number of sensory disorders diagnosed on annual health screening. Evaluative questions which could be asked to gain information regarding the structure, process, impact or outcome of a service are given in Box 7.2.

Kay et al (1996) suggest that an important feature in evaluating best practice in providing services to people who have a learning disability is the degree to which the lifestyles of service users are prevented from regressing or show a sustainable positive movement from segregation through community presence and community participation to community involvement, which may be demonstrated through process, impact and outcome indicators depending on the questions being asked.

CONCLUSION

A strategy for meeting the health promotion needs of people who have a learning disability will involve change at individual (professional, service user and carer) level as well as at societal level.

An attitudinal shift at both individual and societal level will create the conditions for the prime aim of health promotion: self-determination facilitated by self-efficacy belief and not merely passive compliance. The starting premise for a health promotion strategy for people who have a learning disability is that such people possess full citizenship and the potential for development. This view is by no means universally held at present and needs to be addressed through professional and personal development processes. A response to the reality of low uptake of health promotion services is to address its root causes. Services which are based on adequate needs assessment will be accessible and appropriate. Health promotion needs assessment, which will lead to a supportive service, is conducted in collaboration with service users and carers and tailored to the expressed needs of the individual and of the learning-disabled community.

The health promotion interest of those who have a learning disability will be most effectively furthered in the context of collaboration. Interagency and interdisciplinary cooperation will create the conditions for a sensitive response to need and the mechanisms of healthy alliances, and a project management approach will facilitate this. The emphasis is not on whether a service should be specialist or generic but how specialist and generic professionals working together can best promote the health of people who have a learning disability. In order for effective, evidence-based health promotion to be designed and planned, the protagonists need a familiarity with, and an ability to apply health promotion theory to practice.

BOX 7.2

Evaluation of structure
- What is the availability of facilities and equipment?
- What are the staffing levels?
- What are the styles of management and the characteristics of the caregivers?

Evaluation of process
- How are interventions interpreted and responded to by clients?
- How was the intervention carried out?
- To what degree was the community involved?

Evaluation of impact
- What was the uptake of the service?
- How many health education leaflets were dispersed?
- Has intention to change behaviour occurred as a result of the intervention/s?
- Was there any change in attitudes as a result of the intervention/s?

Evaluation of outcome
- What is the long-term effect on the client?
- What is the long-term effect on the community?
- Are the community being involved in decisions regarding health promotion priorities on an ongoing basis?

Acknowledgements

We would like to thank the members of the Learning Disability Service, North Hertfordshire NHS Trust, for their advice and the use of material from their training guidance for primary care staff.

FURTHER READING

Billings J R 1996 Investigating the process of community profile compilation. NT Res 1(4):270–283
This article gives a good account of the process of community health profiling using the single embedded case study design. Whilst identifying the sources of data that could be used in assessing the health needs of a community, Billings also acknowledges their limitations. A useful article for any healthcare practitioner wishing to carry out a holistic health needs analysis at community level.

Ewles L, Simnett I 1999 Promoting health: a practical guide, 4th edn. Baillière Tindall, London
This popular and highly practical health promotion text gives guidance on hands-on health promotion. It is particularly strong on approaches to health education at individual and group level.

Haire A, Bambrick M, Jones J 1992 Cervical screening for women with a mental handicap. Br J Fam Plann 17:120–121
Haire et al give a rare insight into the real problems of consent and cooperation which abound in areas such as cervical screening applied to women who have learning disabilities.

Mental Health Foundation 1996 Building expectations. Opportunities and services for people with a learning disability. Report of the Mental Health Foundation Committee of Enquiry. Mental Health Foundation, London
This text gives a useful glimpse into the problems faced by people who have learning disabilities when they access various health services. The section on primary care indicates that poor communication is a barrier to accessing services.

Naidoo J, Wills J 2000 Health promotion. Foundations for practice, 2nd edn. Baillière Tindall, London
A comprehensive and usable health promotion text, which addresses health promotion at the level of the individual and the community. The use of vignettes and other exercises throughout the text encourages the application of theory to practice, which is so often missing in health promotion initiatives.

National Health Service Cervical Screening Programme (NHSCSP) 2000 Good practice in breast and cervical screening for women with learning disabilities. NHSCSP Publication no 46 and no 13, Sheffield
This recent government publication aims to increase the acceptability and accessibility of breast and cervical screening for women who have learning disabilties. It addresses all stages of the screening process from helping women to respond to screening invitations to carrying out mammography and cervical

smears. It gives much needed guidance on assessing capacity to consent to screening and the health professional's role in breast awareness in women who have learning disabilities.

Øvretveit J 1998 Evaluating health interventions. Open University Press, Buckingham
An excellent text on evaluation, which deals with six evaluation methods of varying complexity which can be applied to any health service intervention. The evaluation techniques range from simple description and audit to comparative experiments.

Tones K, Tilford S 1994 Health education: effectiveness, efficiency and equity. Chapman and Hall, London
A stimulating and thoughtful text which grasps the nettle of evaluating health education and health promotion interventions. It emphasizes the importance of evaluation being informed by well-founded theory.

REFERENCES

Arblaster L, Lambert M, Entwistle V, Forster M, Fullerton D, Sheldon T, Watt I 1996 A systematic review of the effectiveness of health service interventions aimed at reducing inequalities in health. J Health Services Res Policy 1(2):93–103

Baguley P 1995 Managing successful projects. Pitman Publishing, London

Bandura A 1977 Social learning theory. Prentice-Hall, Englewood Cliffs, New Jersey

Bandura A 1986 Social foundations of thought and actions: a social cognitive theory. Prentice-Hall, Englewood Cliffs, New Jersey

Bano A, Crosskill D, Patel R, Rashman L, Shah R 1993 Improving practice with people with learning disabilities. Antiracist social work education. Northern Curriculum Development Project. Central Council for Education and Training in Social Work, Leeds

Beange H, Bauman A 1991 Health care for the developmentally disabled: is it necessary? In: Fraser W (ed) Key issues in mental retardation research. Routledge, London

Beattie A 1991 Knowledge and control in health promotion: a test case for social policy and social theory. In: Gabe J, Calnan M, Bury M (eds) The sociology of the health service. Routledge, London

Billings J R 1996 Investigating the process of community profile compilation. NT Res 1(4):270–283

Cook H 1998 Primary healthcare for people with learning disabilities. Nursing Times 94(30):54–55

Cooke P 1997 Learning disability. In: Skidmore D (ed) Community care: initial

training and beyond. Arnold, London, ch 14

Cumella S, Corbett J, Clarke D, Smith B 1992 Primary healthcare for people with a learning disability. Mental Handicap 20:123–125

Dalley G 1992 Social welfare ideologies and normalisation. In: Brown H, Smith H (eds) Normalisation: a reader for the nineties. Routledge, London

Department of Health 1990 NHS and Community Care Act. HMSO, London

Department of Health 1992 The health of the nation. HMSO, London

Department of Health 1995 The health of the nation: a strategy for people with learning disabilities. HMSO, London

Department of Health 1996 Meeting needs through targeting skills. A guide to learning disability nursing for health and social care commissioners, GP fundholders, NHS trusts and the independent sector. DoH, London

Department of Health 1997 The new NHS; modern, dependable. Cm 3807. The Stationery Office, London

Department of Health 1998 A first class service. Quality in the new NHS. The Stationery Office, London

Department of Health 1999 Saving lives: our healthier nation. The Stationery Office, London

Donabedian A 1969 Some issues in evaluating the quality of nursing care. Am J Public Health 59(10):1833–1836

Edwards P, Bee D 1992 Screening, ethics and the law. BMJ 305:26–27

Emerson E, Hatton C 1996 Impact of deinstitutionalization on service users in Britain. In: Mansell J, Ericsson K (eds) Deinstitutionalization and community living. Chapman and Hall, London, ch 11

Ewles L, Simnett I 1999 Promoting health: a practical guide, 4th edn. Baillière Tindall, London

Fitzsimmons J, Barr O 1997 A review of the reported attitudes of health and social care professionals towards people with learning disabilities: implications for education and further research. J Learning Disabil Nursing, Health Social Care 1(2):57–64

Freeman R, Gillam S, Shearin C, Pratt J 1997 Community development and involvement in primary care. A guide to involving the community in COPC. King's Fund, London

Gates B 1998 A new health agenda for learning disabled people: reflections on platitudes and rhetoric. J Learning Disabil Nursing, Health Social Care 2(1):1–2

Gillis A J 1993 Determinants of a health promoting lifestyle: an integrative review. J Adv Nursing 18(3):345–353

Haire A, Bambrick M, Jones J 1992 Cervical screening for women with a mental handicap. Br J Fam Plann 17:120–121

Harris J 1996 (ed) Purchasing services for people with learning disabilities, challenging behaviour and mental health needs. Paper No 6. British Institute of Learning Disabilities, Kidderminster

Jarman B 1984 Underprivileged areas: validation and distribution of scores. BMJ 289(6458):1587–1592

Kay B, Rose S, Turnbull J 1996 Continuing the commitment. The report of the Learning Disability Nursing Project. DoH, London

Kerr M, Fraser W, Felce D 1996 Primary healthcare for people with a learning disability. Br J Learning Disabil 24(1):2–8

Kinnel D 1987 Community medical care of people with mental handicaps. Mental Handicap 15:146–150

Langan J, Russell O, Whitfield M 1993 Community care and the general practitioner: primary health care for people with learning disabilities (summary of the final report to the Department of Health). Norah Fry Research Centre, University of Bristol

Ley P 1988 Communicating with patients: improving communication, satisfaction and compliance. Chapman and Hall, London

Luker K 1992 Evaluating practice. In: Luker K, Orr J (eds) Health visiting: towards community health nursing. Blackwell, Oxford, ch 5

McConkey R 1998 Matching services to client needs: a research agenda for the new century. J Learning Disabil Nursing, Health Social Care 2(2): 57–59

McCray J, Carter S 1999 Access unrestricted. Nursing Times 95(23):47–49

McRae D 1997 Health care for women with learning disabilities. Nursing Times 93(15):58–59

Mental Health Foundation 1996 Building expectations. Opportunities and services for people with a learning disability. Report of the Mental Health Foundation Committee of Enquiry. Mental Health Foundation, London

Moss S, Goldberg D, Patel P, Wilken D 1993 Physical morbidity in older people with moderate, severe and profound mental handicap and its relation to psychiatric morbidity. Social Psychiatr Psychiatr Epidemiol 28(1):32–39

Naidoo J, Wills J 2000 Health promotion. Foundations for practice, 2nd edn. Baillière Tindall, London

NHSCSP 2000 Good practice in breast and cervical screening for women with learning disabilities. NHSCSP Publication no 46 and no 13, Sheffield

National Health Service Executive 1998 Signposts for success in commissioning and providing health services for people with learning disabilities. DoH, London

National Health Service Executive 1999 Once a day. DoH, London

Office of Population Census and Surveys 1988 The General Household Survey: informal carers. HMSO, London

Office of Population Census and Surveys 1993 1991 census for Great Britain. HMSO, London

Øvretveit J 1998 Evaluating health interventions. Open University Press, Buckingham

Pearson V, Davis C, Ruoff C, Dyer J 1998 Only one quarter of women with learning disability in Exeter have cervical screening. BMJ 316:1979

Perkins E R, Simnett I, Wright L 1999 Creative tensions in evidence based practice. In: Perkins E R, Simnett I, Wright L (eds) Evidence based health promotion. John Wiley, Chichester, ch 1

Prochaska J O, DiClemente C C 1986 Towards a comprehensive model of change. In: Miller W R, Heather W R (eds) Treating addictive behaviours: processes of change. Plenum, New York

Shaughnessy P 1999 Better cervical screening for women with learning disabilities. Nursing Times 95:44–45

Speller V, Funnel R, Friedli L 1994 Towards evaluating healthy alliances. Institute of Public Health Medicine, Winchester

Stanley R 1998 Primary healthcare provision for people with learning disabilities: a survey of general practitioners. J Learning Disabil Nursing, Health Social Care (1):23–30

Stanley R, Ng J 1998 Primary healthcare provision for people with learning disabilities: a survey of parents. J Learning Disabil Nursing, Health Social Care 2(2):71–78

Tannahill A 1985 What is health promotion? Health Educ J 44:167–168

Thompson T, Mathias P 1999 Evaluating learning disability – embracing change. In: Atkin K, Lunt N, Thompson C (eds) Evaluating community care. Baillière Tindall, London, ch 8

Thornton C 1996 A focus group inquiry into the perceptions of primary health care teams and the provision of health care for adults with a learning disability living in the community. J Adv Nursing 23(6):1168–1176

Tones K, Tilford S 1994 Health education: effectiveness, efficiency and equity. Chapman and Hall, London

Tyne A 1981 The principle of normalisation. A foundation for effective services. (Adapted for VIA from the work of J O'Brien.) Values Into Action, London

United Kingdom Central Council for Nursing, Midwifery and Health Visiting 1996 Guidelines for professional practice. UKCC, London

Vernon L 1998 Access to sexual and reproductive healthcare for people with learning difficulties. J Commun Nursing 12(2):10–16

Ward J 1994a Under the spotlight. Health Sci J (Health Management Guide) 28:1–3

Ward J 1994b All systems go. Health Sci J (Health Management Guide) 28:4–10

Wilson D N, Haire A 1990 Health care screening for people with mental handicap living in the community. BMJ 310(6765): 1379–1381

Wolfensberger W 1972 Normalisation. The principle of normalisation in human services. National Institute on Mental Retardation, Toronto

World Health Organization 1984 Health promotion: a discussion document on the concept and the principles. WHO, Copenhagen

Yin R K 1994 Case study research design and methods. Sage, Thousand Oaks

8 Accessing health information

Nicola Taylor with Susan Smithurst

We were delighted to be asked to contribute a chapter in this book, especially as we had been involved in a research project about health needs. The material in this chapter has been compiled by Nicola with assistance from Sue but there has also been an involvement by the Acorn Group.

KEY ISSUES

- Starting out
- Why it is important to involve people who have a learning disability
- Forming and running groups
- What is information
- Presenting information and ways of communicating
- Practicalities
- Ways to improve access to health information for people who have a learning disability

INTRODUCTION

The chapter sets out how we met and became the Acorn Group as part of a research study. The aim of the chapter is to inform the reader about us as a group and what it is like to access health information. Also to talk about the availability of health information, what we did and said to help others who have a learning disability learn about accessing adequate information about their health in order that they can make informed decisions.

Access to information about health is difficult for people who have learning disabilities. Production of material is often in a format that is not user friendly and interactions between professionals and users are sometimes difficult. For a person who has a learning disability, information can come from many perspectives; for example, general practitioner and other professionals (medical model), carer (medical/lay perspective) and other people who have a learning disability (lay perspective).

Currently more information is being produced and made available in places like the British Institute of Learning Disabilities (BILD). We wanted to know how easily people who have learning disabilities could access this information.

HOW DID WE START OUT?

Initially Sue was doing some research into why people who have learning disabilities weren't getting their health needs met either in long-stay mental handicap hospitals or within the community. A number of people have written about this, including Howells (1986) and Rogers (1994), who talked about communication presenting difficulties for people who have learning disabilities. Research has shown that explaining diagnosis or medication to a person who has a learning disability may lead to misinformation or misinterpretation. We feel it is important that this is not just blamed on the person who has a learning disability but that the professional should take some responsibility. Wilson & Haire (1990) also said that 'People with a mental handicap fit badly into a system of healthcare delivery in which no care is received unless it is asked for'.

The institutional medical model of care for people who have learning disabilities may have implications for receipt of appropriate care but other factors have to be taken into account such as social aspects, i.e. housing (Rodgers 1994). 'A learning disability label doesn't mean that we are ill or have any more health problems than anyone else; what it means is that perhaps we have conditions that may cause concern medically or that we can't communicate our needs as clearly as other people.'

WHY DO THIS RESEARCH?

From these studies we decided to find out what factors prevented people who have learning disabilities from receiving the same healthcare as other people. At the start of the study, Sue wanted to find out about information that went to the GP when a patient was resettled from long-stay hospital into the community because it was thought that they did not have enough information about us as patients. The point has been raised that some patient records may consist of a one-line letter whilst others contain a full psychiatric history but with little information about that patient's health needs. To find out what they wanted, Sue visited some GPs and asked what information they would like in a new discharge letter. She also wanted to know if they would like this information sent to them by computer. It had been thought that this may not be practical as many practices use different systems.

The results from this part of the study showed that GPs wanted a discharge letter that gave information about the patient, especially for the ones who had little confidence or felt that they couldn't talk about their past healthcare. They wanted that information given in a clear way. They did not want a long letter but one that would enable them to understand the health needs of the patient.

The next stage of the study was where we as a group came in. As the first part of the study was about information going to the GP when a patient was resettled to help them give better healthcare, it was decided to look at what healthcare was like in the community for people who have learning disabilities.

As part of the study, it was intended that Sue would look at what information was available to people who have learning disabilities about health. We also needed to look at other factors that prevented people receiving adequate care. We found a booklet called *Going to the doctor* had been produced by the St George's Medical Centre and Sue came round to show groups of people who have learning disabilities this booklet when she explained her study. Some people were keen to see changes made to this booklet from the perspective of a person who has a learning disability.

Although the booklet was very good and possibly a unique source of information, there were some comments made about the font size and the difficulties someone may experience if they had an additional physical disability. Therefore we requested that we produce our own illustrated booklet.

FORMATION OF THE ACORN GROUP

This group was set up to explore, with assistance from Sue and a facilitator, what kinds of health information they might need to enable them to receive better healthcare. Also the group was involved in all aspects of the research in this phase of the study. It is what is called an emancipatory model which means that the researcher puts her skills at the disposal of the participants to enable them to challenge discrimination and disadvantage at whatever level it occurs.

Before the group was set up Sue and Audrey (the facilitator) read up on different aspects of running a group. All issues surrounding feedback to the group, the relationship between the researcher and the group, time constraints, limitations, communications, confidentiality, language skills, methodology and the construction of a picture-prompted questionnaire were explored.

Next we looked at places where we could hold the group and the availability of dates and times. It was decided that we would hold the sessions at the local training centre, once a month and between 12.30 and 1.30pm on a Friday. This was because everyone was attending a training centre and finished for the weekend at lunchtime on a Friday. Although in the initial stages people came from other locations, eventually through shifts in placements (nothing to do with the research) all group members attended this centre on a daily basis.

Group members are both male and female (the group is still running as a health information group) and between 18 and 53 years old. There is a wide range of communication skills within the group and therefore we were grateful for the help of Audrey who has a lot of experience of not only working with people who have learning disabilities but also of facilitating groups like the Student Council for People with Learning Disabilities.

HOW DID WE RUN THE GROUP?

Sue met the group informally at the first session and explained about the research. She told us about different ways of doing research and the emancipatory model. She talked about our willingness to be involved and we helped to design a pictorial consent form. She told us about the rights that we had to withdraw at any time if we so wished and gave us a week to make up our minds. We all consented as we had self-selected as a focus group when being told about the project and seeing that booklet.

We looked again at research models in following sessions as well as ethical considerations. Then we started to talk about access to health information.

Most of us had little knowledge about health information or where we might go to find it so we set out to do a little bit of research ourselves. Those of us who were able to visit libraries and public places did so, looking for any leaflets, video, tapes with books or any media that might be available to help us.

When we came back to report at the next session there didn't seem much available. One group member found some leaflets about AIDS/HIV but it wasn't written in our language; that is, language that is user friendly. Other people had visited their doctors' surgeries and looked in the racks of information leaflets. Although the health information section was limited there were some interesting leaflets about welfare benefits.

In the next sessions we looked at what you might go the doctor or hospital for; interestingly, people didn't visit their doctors that often. This was because in the main the carer dealt with the 'less important illnesses'. When asked what a 'less important illness' was, we discovered things like 'bad chesty coughs', 'verrucas', 'athlete's foot' and others. When a person did go to the doctor, very often, due to the 'doctor not having the time to talk to me', the carer was involved in the main discussion.

We tried to enhance the group's concept of health and look at their perspectives so we did an exercise looking through printed material, magazines, health and fitness catalogues and brainstormed ideas. We also looked at ways of asking questions to access information that we either knew nothing about or had limited knowledge about. What came out of these sessions was that people had little or no notion of advocacy or self-advocacy although two group members were very knowledgeable, being self-advocates themselves. They were able to inform the group about a local self-advocacy group which other people are now considering joining.

To access information about health provision involves the individual requesting advice. For people who have learning disabilities this can present a problem as often they don't have the confidence or the ability to do so and therefore we felt one way of improving access to information would be to promote emancipation and advocacy. But we were not sure what the statutory health bodies are doing to further this emancipation and our health.

Within recent years it has become popular within the health service to involve patients. For example, the Patient's Charter has been very clear about the rights of patients regarding information that is given to them. Some people feel we need to be even more revolutionary in that this can be a circular concept where information is given and feedback received in order to improve access to health and health information.

Patient participation means that patients should know about the health system and the best way to use it. They should have their views and opinions listened to, to enable them to be instrumental in the planning and delivering of services. Theoretically this appears to be ideal but in the real world it means a large adjustment for both users and providers, especially as people who have a learning disability are not a homogenous group. Additionally people can have physical disabilities and also dual diagnosis (mental illness and learning disability). All these things affect the way people need to work with us.

From looking at the Patient's Charter, we can see that everyone has the right to receive healthcare on the basis of clinical need regardless of whether or not they can pay. In addition, they should be given a clear explanation about what treatment they are being offered and any risks they might encounter should be highlighted. Another consideration should be an alternative to treatment. Another important piece of legislation that has looked at the healthcare of people who have learning disabilities has been *The health of the nation: a strategy for people with learning disabilities* which sets targets and acknowledges the importance that must be placed on healthy lifestyles.

Taking all these points into account we, as a group, set out to design our own questionnaire designed by people who have a learning disability to be used in research or general practice with people who have a learning disability. First, we discussed the format and physical size of the book and font. It was agreed by the group that the booklet had to be large enough to be held comfortably by a person having an additional physical disability. The size it was decided would be A4 size and the font would be 16–18 point to enable those with visual difficulties to use it. It was considered appropriate that the booklet could be used in collaboration with the person who has a learning disability and the GP although, understandably, the consultation in this instance would take longer. It was believed, though, that some of the questions might not be relevant for some consultations and that would save some time. It certainly would help the concentration of the patient and enable the GP to develop a better picture of the individual.

The questions were quite open and asked 'What is it like when you visit your doctor?', 'Do you take any medicines or tablets?', 'Do you have a dietician?', 'Do you know about a healthy lifestyle?'. It might be argued that the GP or related health professional would know the answers to these questions but by carrying out this assessment with the patient, they would be able to identify where the patient had limited or no knowledge about their health needs or care.

WHAT IS INFORMATION?

We have talked about access to information throughout this chapter; first the information that a GP needs when a patient is resettled into the community and then the availability of information for people who have learning disabilities. But what is information? We have to be clear what we are talking about when we talk about health information. As McIver (1993) comments, information can be divided into three main types that don't usually overlap:

1. Knowledge can simply be facts passed from one person to another or by leaflets that are likely to have no effect on their behaviour.
2. Education, where some help is given in making sense of the information and fitting it into the individual's prior learning and lifestyle.
3. Empowerment in which, unlike the previous two, the enquirer's needs are always central and the individual determines the agenda of what information is shared and how.

From this we can see that health information could be a variety of things and if the person who has a learning disability is to be involved in the process then this will be different to providing them with whatever is available. With reference to the access to information for a new discharge summary, GPs were consulted and their views fed back into the production of a new discharge summary for those people being resettled. Therefore people who have a learning disability must be consulted about what information they need about healthcare and the most appropriate place/person to access that information from.

What's the best format for information? What do we think as a group?

By the time that most people become adults they can read and write and communicate with people at most levels. As people who have learning disabilities we may not have those skills. Some of us may have been in institutions or experience difficulties with communication. It is important to recognize that we are not all the same (not a homogenous group) and that to give us information might not be easy.

As many people who have learning disabilities have lived in institutions or been cared for by people who could speak up for them, their ideas have often been ignored or not taken seriously. What other people and the medical profession often fail to recognize is that some people who have learning disabilities have always lived in the community and have visited their doctors as much as everyone else; in some instances, and for some conditions, more. From this we can see they are a valuable source of information about what services are on offer and how good these services are.

The limitation of accepting that we are a valuable source of information is related to the fact that we are still seen as childlike by some people and as such, can't make informed choices. There are those who think that learning disability equates with vulnerability, which means that no information given by a health provider would be understood. Due to differing levels of disability, some people may need more help than others in understanding but this does not mean we cannot say what we think. Also there are those of us who are fully capable of sharing ideas about our health without the assistance of a carer or anyone else.

How, then, can we ensure that people who have a learning disability receive adequate information to enable them to make an informed decision, for example about a cervical smear test. There are GPs who feel uncomfortable with carrying out smear tests for a number of reasons (Stein 2000) and yet women who have a learning disability have as much right to this examination as non-disabled women. The following two case studies highlight the need for adequate information to alleviate the situation between health professionals and service users. The names of both participants have been changed for confidentiality.

CASE STUDY 8.1   **Jayne's story**

Jayne is a 30-year-old woman who lives semi-independently and has a learning disability. Jayne works part time in a local supermarket and attends a day centre 2 days a week. Jayne doesn't have a partner at the moment but says she would like to meet someone one day. She has not ruled out the possibility of having children although says she has been advised against this by members of her family. 'It's my learning disability see, I'm a bit mental and the baby might be.' Jayne has talked to her community learning disability nurse about the possibility of having a cervical smear test and says she would like to have one. As yet she has not been offered one because her mum and the GP believe that as she is not sexually active it is not a necessity. Jayne commented that the community nurse is excellent and they have had many discussions around this issue but she would like the doctor to talk with her in the same way and give her the opportunity to make that informed decision.

CASE STUDY 8.2   **Mary's story**

Mary is 28 years of age. She lives in a small group home with three other residents and attends a training/day centre. Mary has no partner and says she doesn't think that she will get married. When Mary attended the doctor about a cervical smear test her mother went with her. Mary believes that to be tested is essential especially as a cousin had died from cancer some 4 years previously. She says that on the day she attended she had no idea that the appointment was to have a smear test and was surprised when requested to remove her clothes. Once the doctor became aware that she had no knowledge of what the process involved, he very kindly explained it to her. She was able to make an informed choice to go ahead but as she was so tense the test had to be terminated. The whole situation distressed her so much she has not felt able to go back to complete her smear test and says she doesn't think that she will either in the immediate future or in the long term. What she says would have made things better would have been more readily available information, some user-friendly leaflets from 'a to z' about what would happen. Maybe a video she could have borrowed from the doctor's surgery or a community nurse present to 'lend a hand' when she became distressed.

USING DIFFERENT WAYS TO GIVE INFORMATION

Listening to those two stories led us to look at ways to transfer to people information that we considered of vital importance. For example, 60% of the people in the Acorn Group are women and as such could relate similar experiences. A lady in her 50s told us about her experience of having a mammogram after receiving no prior information; as we might predict, this lady would not go through the experience again. Another lady told us about misleading information about smear testing and dentistry. She was told 'This won't hurt' only to find herself in what she terms 'agony'. The group believe that if something is going to cause pain or be uncomfortable, they must be told, as they believe a non-disabled person would be told.

We have already mentioned our contribution to information giving but we had one session especially to explore different ways of giving information to people who have learning disabilities. In this session we talked about the kinds of things that are available and how useful they are. It is important to remember that apart from printed and visual/audio material there are different ways of passing on information. Also of significance in relaying information is the person's level of understanding. It is also important to keep an open mind and not fall into the trap of low expectation because the person is labelled as having a learning disability.

Those who work with people who have a learning disability can have low expectations and assume that these individuals would 'prefer pictures to writing, or even symbols'. Also, because the point is raised about higher expectations, 'Don't assume that we fully understand technical language, write in a way we understand but please don't patronize us'. Interestingly, McIver's (1993) study placed leaflets as the medium liked least by members of the general public, with TV and radio being considered the best way to transfer information. This does not always work for those of us who have a learning disability.

McIver also commented on the strength and weaknesses of audio-taped material, saying that literacy wasn't necessary to use this approach; people can rewind and fast-forward and thus proceed at their own pace or revisit places where they felt unsure. Additionally, more detailed information could be transferred.

One area where the Acorn Group readily agreed with McIver was with reference to relaxation tapes. Most of the group had used this kind of tape and were 'delighted with the results', 'It helped me to chill out after a hard day'. However, there were some limitations with audio material; for example, people with hearing difficulties could not access it, in some cases recordings are of poor quality, and people sometimes have to listen to the whole tape to find where they want to be. 'Can't they use something like CDs where there is a counter and you can move to number 10, for example?'

Nicola talked about the advantage of using videos to give people information about health. This is a favourite medium of hers. Video material has been reported to be valuable when used with younger people who have learning disabilities but there are some reservations. The video should be pitched at the right level and in an appropriate way otherwise the learning opportunity is lost and confusion can result. As Greenhalgh (1994) suggests, being involved in making a video can be stimulating and motivating for many people. This is something that the Acorn Group endorses and would like to be involved with in the near future, either videoing the health sessions with a speaker present or making a video to accompany the illustrated booklet *You and your health* which they hope to publish.

Photographs and pictures are a useful way to communicate information. The Acorn Group decided this was the way forward with the illustrated booklet 'and many session were spent looking at pictures, magazines and catalogues to determine what our booklet would look like'. We thought about symbols but decided that a pictorial guide was what we wanted. We engaged the services of a graphic designer (Margaret) who put it all together for us and listened to our ideas about how we wanted to improve the pictures. Sue took the draft booklet to Margaret Flynn from the National Development Team in Manchester. Margaret told Sue some ways we might like to change things but told Sue to consult with us first. Sue came back and told us what Margaret had said and we changed some things and kept others as they were.

It has been suggested that there is a wealth of information about health information and learning disability research on the Internet. Some of the Acorn Group commented that they could access the computer at home but that they had limited knowledge of technology and that they might be constrained by finance.

What we came up with from the sessions about media was that the most useful way forward is pictorial guides and leaflets geared to people who have learning disabilities pitched at an appropriate level, by which we mean not patronizing and not too technical.

WHERE ARE WE NOW?

The Acorn Group have been meeting on a monthly basis. The illustrated booklet has been produced and used in the research project for which it was intended. As a byproduct, it has come to light that many of the interviewees have limited knowledge about healthy lifestyles or where they can get that sort of information.

It would appear that GPs and health professionals are attempting to meet the needs of people who have learning disabilities, but the fact that studies are still being carried out into the inequitable distribution of healthcare suggests that something is not happening. Could it be that people are not accessing important information that could influence their decision to consent to medical interventions? On a recent visit to places where one might expect to find health information, we were sadly disappointed to find racks filled with out-of-date information designed for the non-disabled population.

Nicola was also sad about this as she found that there was nothing printed that would be useful to any of the group. 'Though I have to be honest and say that my carer and GP are excellent and that my GP gives me plenty of information, the sad part is I know this does not happen for everyone.'

PRACTICALITIES IN ACCESSING INFORMATION

Practical issues for people who have learning disabilities include the location of material – where is it? Material like some of the things that BILD publish (Sue told us about BILD and brought information for us to look at) aren't available to us. Where do we get it from if we aren't members? How do we afford it? Should the centre have it? Do people come from BILD to talk to us about their work? We don't know how to pay for information or even if we could afford it.

Other things to consider are what health information is. As a group we have discussed this and we feel that anything can be related to health. For example, what information is there about stress for people who have learning disabilities? Sometimes we feel that people don't think that we get stressed, we just have 'challenging behaviour' that needs medical treatment. Bereavement is another area that is low on information. Some well-meaning people involved in our lives think that we shouldn't be told when someone dies but we have a right to know and grieve like anyone else. We also would like to know about other therapies like hypnotherapy to stop smoking but these therapists don't provide information about their therapy for people like us. We don't know whether they would see someone who has a learning disability.

As a group we have researched the availability of information for people who have learning disabilities and have found it to be limited. Information of an audiovisual and textual nature can be purchased from the British Institute of Learning Disabilities but the prices can range from £5 to £35, more in some instances. However, some adult education and day centres are purchasing these materials and working with their attendees, which we think is good. However, this is not the picture for everyone and there are services that people would like to know more about that they are not getting to find out about; for example, some of the complementary therapies.

Within our sessions we have decided that as a way forward we will invite professionals from different fields to visit us and give us information about their particular specialism. After their presentation they will be asked questions by the group and their responses/information will then be shared with other health/self-advocacy groups.

For emancipation, self-advocacy seems the route forward. Some of the group members are considering joining the local People First organization. This group is expanding to a nearby seaside town which will give more people who have learning disabilities access to information, health workshops and the ability to find 'their voice'.

As a group we hope that people will find our contribution useful for accessing information. Perhaps these booklets could be used in consultation with professionals to enable them to build a relationship with the person who has a learning disability. And finally we as a group hope to give talks and presentations, perhaps write articles about health issues for people who have a learning disability from a learning disability perspective.

RECOMMENDATIONS

- We feel that to enable us to access health information, there must be an increase in leaflets and material that is user friendly. That is to say that the language is pitched at the right level; remember, we speak the same English language as the professionals, not their technical language. Also a suggestion is that the leaflets could be in brighter colours to attract the eye not only of people who have learning disabilities but also for the non-disabled population. This might encourage people from all walks of life to access important health information.

- Perhaps the leaflets could be placed on the receptionist's desk in waiting rooms rather than on hard-to-reach racks or racks that are overladen. When a non-disabled person knocks a rack over they feel silly; imagine what it feels like for someone like us!

- When information is produced for people who have learning disabilities by the BILD or other organizations, perhaps they could give local presentations so that people who have learning disabilities have the chance to view the work they have done and other organizations have a preview of what they might buy.

- Communication is an important part of accessing information. Therefore please remember that we don't know much about the medical model so talk to us in our language.

- Professionals planning care packages should consult with the person who has a learning disability. As people who have learning disabilities we feel that we are in a sense 'experts'.

- Don't have high/low expectations about learning disability; just talk with us or with an advocate and it will be easy to identify our needs.

- Don't forget that although people who have severe learning disabilities can't talk, this doesn't necessarily mean they can't understand. Use Makaton or enlist the help of an advocate to ensure that the individual accesses information.

- At regular intervals research should be carried out to find out if adequate information is being accessed and if not, why not. It will be useful to involve people who have learning disabilities in this research.

■ These are some of the things that we as a group believe will make accessing information easier not only for people who have learning disabilities but also for you, the professionals.

REFERENCES

Greenhalgh L 1994 Well aware: improving access to health information for people who have learning difficulties NHS Executive, Anglia and Oxford Regional Health Authority

Howells G 1986 Are the medical needs of mentally handicapped adults being met? J Roy Coll Gen Pract 367:449–453

McIver S 1993 Obtaining the views of users of health services. King's Fund, Nuffield Institute for Health Studies, London

Rodgers J 1994 Primary health care provision for people with learning difficulties. Health Social Care Commun

Stein K 2000 Caring for people with learning disability: a survey of general practitioners' attitudes in Southampton and South-west Hampshire. Br J Learning Disabil 28(1): 9–15

Wilson D, Haire A 1990 Health care screening for people with mental handicap living in the community. BMJ 301:1379–1380

3 MEETING HEALTH NEEDS

This section focuses upon meeting the health needs of people who have a learning disability. Identifying the areas for inclusion in this section was extremely difficult. It was, however, important for us not to simply reinforce the medical approach to labelling health needs. Not because it is not appropriate to meet those needs but because we have far more expertise in that area than some of those we chose to explore. In addition, we had the feeling that issues such as well-being, self-perception, employment or valued occupation, sexual and mental health as well as support to manage the difficult times in life were at least equally important.

SECTION CONTENTS

9 **Being well and my well-being**
Anya Souza with Paul Ramcharan

10 **Self-concept and people who have learning disabilities**
Mark Statham and Diane Timblick

11 **Valued occupation for people who have a learning disability**
Caroline Heason, Lynne Stracey and Dommie Rey

12 **Sexual health**
Damian Dunn

13 **Mental health**
Steve Moss and Pauline Lee

14 **Life transitions and personal change**
Jeanette Thompson and Sharon Pickering

Being well and my well-being

Anya Souza with Paul Ramcharan

A colleague who is putting together a book on learning disabilities asked whether I would like to work with a person with a learning difficulty to write an article about health issues. I said that I knew someone who might be willing to contribute an article and that I would contact Anya. After a phone call with one of the editors Anya agreed to contribute a chapter as long as she worked with me and as long as she was paid! I then visited Anya and we started to talk about issues tied up with her health and illness experiences as well as her ideas for other people with learning difficulties. I taped the discussion and went away and set out some themes which we discussed when we next met and on subsequent occasions. I then wrote up what Anya had said in the form of an article. We went through this together and Anya was able to add to things, take things out or to say she did not understand some ideas or words. I went away again and made changes and we conversed by phone until the final chapter emerged.

Paul Ramcharan

INTRODUCTION

Not many people ask me about my health. They do ask, 'Are you well?' or 'How are you?', but these are pleasantries. Nobody is really concerned about whether I am ill or not except when I *am* ill. Then it concerns the people close to me and it brings out doctors and others who can help me to get better. I am not ill at the moment and so it was a pleasant surprise to be asked to write something about my health and to think about it more closely.

When we started this article I didn't have much idea about health and illness but there are several ideas below which came out of the discussions we have had in putting together the article. These themes have been used as headings for the rest of the article.

HEALTH AND STAYING HEALTHY

A meaningful life is important to health

When I was asked in this article to think about health I thought about things like healthy eating, a healthy body and being fit. I usually don't think about them in this way. It happens differently. For example, some people very close to me will say something to me like 'Oh, you're putting on weight, Anya'. I know about food and dieting and I don't eat loads of chocolates or fatty foods. And it always makes me ever so angry because it is not them who have to do something about getting the weight off.

But then I think I'd better do some exercise or go on some sort of diet. But I'm just like a lot of other people and it never really works out like that. I also get upset when I've tried very hard to lose weight but then find I've lost none. It's hard to lose weight when you've got Down's syndrome and I know it can lead to health problems like heart disease. I mean I've been to yoga and swimming, I've eaten more vegetables and reduced the amount on my plate, but it hasn't made a difference.

I am happy being who I am really and sometimes I just don't think it's worth the effort to try and change myself and the way *I look*. But if I'm happy with the way *I look*, I'm often not happy about what my body allows me to do when I don't feel my best. I get tired more quickly. I find climbing steps harder and I can't do sports. I would like to do these things and know I would be able if my body would let me. So it's not really about how I look. It's more about whether my health allows my body to do the things I want to do.

And when I can't do the things I want to do it's not about being ill, it's about not being fit enough. Fitness is about making the most of what my body can do. Being ill is different altogether. Being ill means you have to get better first. Only then can you make your body fit enough to do what you want it to do.

The thing for people who have learning disabilities is that they often don't have much they want to do or are encouraged to do. People don't expect too much from us. For example, at a special school I attended they treated us without respect. There was no discipline and they did not help us to learn. Like in this school, many people who have learning disabilities don't have much to do during their days and are not actively involved in sports or leisure or paid work. So, many people have no aims. They just drift along and nobody really cares. And if I were to just drift along like this I would not need to be fit. I wouldn't want or need to get the most out of my own body. There would be no incentive or reason to make the most out of my body.

When I was very young my mother made a decision that I should be involved in things just like everybody else. As I have said elsewhere (Souza & Ramcharan 1997), if my mother had listened to the doctor when I was born, she would have treated me like a handicapped person for the rest of my life. She might have hidden me from the world and put me into schools for the 'mentally handicapped'. But from the very beginning my mum fought to get me into mainstream schools and helped me to find my own interests.

I followed in my mother's footsteps in some ways. She was an actress and I loved the stage from my very first experiences. My mother was pleasantly surprised when I was out of school at 19 years of age and wrote a letter to a local drama school because I wanted to act. Mind you, I've had to give up more recently because it's a long way to travel over London and I've got other things to do and to spend my money on.

Since leaving school and college with some qualifications I have fought to find paid work. When I lost a job at one organization run by and for people who have learning disabilities I was very upset, but I did not give up hope. My mum had passed away not long before but I have always had a second mum, a close friend of the family, June. June has been teaching me to make stained glass for as long as I can remember, as well as other forms of art. I can now sell the stained glass and I often have exhibitions where friends and others can come and see my work. If I ever go to conferences I also take items with me to sell.

So, unlike a lot of people who have learning disabilities, I have a very full life in terms of my creativity and in trying to earn enough to do the other things I want to do. If I didn't do these things I could imagine getting really bored and finding it difficult to get up in the mornings. I wouldn't need to be healthy. So I think making people healthy is something about making their lives meaningful first and foremost.

Friends are important to my health

Now there are other things that give my life meaning and I need the resources to do the things I want and like to do. Throughout my life I have met a great many people, lots of whom have become my good friends. I have kept a lot of friends despite moving from one school to another or from job to job. I have a qualification in Food Industry and Catering and there is nothing I like better than to entertain my friends. I also love a good dance or a party at home which I usually organize three times a year in February, September and then for my birthday in November. Parties and get-togethers cost money so I have to make sure I can budget properly. But there are other ways of budgeting, like making parties 'bring-your-own' events. Friends do the same too so we never have to fork out loads of money for a good time!

If I didn't have my friends I think I would be lonely and bored. I think that lots of people who have learning disabilities are lonely and bored. With nowhere to go and nothing to do, they can get bored very quickly. Sometimes they are close to their parents or their sisters and brothers. But they don't have any friends outside the family and finally their parents are no longer there and their brothers and sisters have moved away. I'd be very lonely and depressed if it had not been for all the friends I have because my mother passed away and my sisters have their own lives to lead. If you are lonely, bored and depressed you have fewer things to do and no reason to keep healthy. That really is so important. The thing is that everyone needs someone who loves and cares for them as a friend. Friends are also very important when you are ill and I will tell you about that a bit later.

I think special friends are important as well. I have had a few boyfriends and have one at present. There is nothing more important to me than knowing there is someone there who loves and cares for me like no other person, someone I can rely upon for the rest of my life. But having a boyfriend leads me on to other things to do with my health.

Knowing about health and illness is important to my health

Lots of people who have learning disabilities want to have close relationships and some to have children when they are ready. I think it really is important that like any other children, young people who have learning disabilities learn about sexual health. I worked with a People First group who put together a book on sex and sex education. The book talked about some of the dangers of sex such as sexually transmitted diseases. It also talked about contraception.

I was very angry to find out about these things so late on in life. It could have been too late! I was lucky, but I don't think people who have learning disabilities should be treated differently from anybody else. They have a right to know about their bodies and about how best to make decisions about what they do with them. There seems to be the idea that because we have a learning disability that all of us should, and will, have decisions made for us by others. That's not right. It's true that we cannot be responsible for what we do not know or have not been told about. But the answer to that is to pass on the right information, for example in relation to healthy lifestyles or safe sex. And it's also true that we have minds of our own and that if we need help with making a decision we can ask the right person.

This means that people who have learning disabilities have the right to be educated in all areas which may affect their health. They should also be shown how they can make the best of their bodies and how to recognize any worrying signs. I think women should be informed about matters that concern women. I have an example from having put together this very article. When Paul asked me about cervical screening I told him I did not want that because I was a bit shy, not only about having the screening but about talking to others about it. So there are things about education that can help people to make the right decisions about themselves and to recognize any worrying signs like lumps, slight pains in the chest, aching feet and so forth. But sometimes things happen and you do not know what's wrong. I had a friend who was like Peggy in Eastenders. She had breast cancer. The thing is, if they had kept a regular check of her health she could have been fine. So a regular health check would really make a lot of difference. It would also make people feel confident doing all the things they have to do.

But there are other times when you can't ignore that you're not well. For example, recently I had nasal problems and from that seemed to become allergic to damp, dustmites and cats. The doctors found this out by putting a long strip of substances onto my arm to see if any of them irritated my skin. They found out I was particularly allergic to cats and that I should not put my face near them or kiss them.

There are also other things that keep people healthy. For example, personal hygiene and having a bath daily is very important. But then again, all these things would not be any use if you were not living in a clean and healthy environment. For example, I tried for a long time to get the council to come and look at my window surrounds because they are letting in the damp. That really was no good for my health. How can I keep healthy if I'm freezing in my house and it is damp? The thing is that preventing illness and staying healthy are not only our responsibility but the responsibility of others too sometimes. People who have learning disabilities should have somewhere to live that is clean, safe and warm.

Summary

Being healthy and staying healthy happens when you have a meaning to your life. It is no good asking people to look after themselves if they have no reason to do so. Having meaning to your life means having a reason to keep fit and healthy such as going to work, participating in leisure and seeing friends. Friends help you to care for yourself and care if you are not feeling well. But to stop being ill you need good housing and living conditions. You also need to know how to look after yourself. If that is not possible, because it isn't for everybody, whether they have a learning disability or not, you need people around you who do know and who do care enough about you to keep an eye on your health. Finally, a lot of illness could be prevented if everyone had a regular health check.

ILLNESS AND GETTING WELL

When I think of being ill I usually think about getting a headache or having a cold or the flu or a tummy upset. I also think about how rotten I felt when I had chicken pox or when I had my accident. I always feel totally grotty when I get ill. I remember when I was a little girl and had to stay home from school, mum was always there to fuss around me when I got ill. I really used to love that. If I didn't have people around me to look after and care for me and sympathize with me I think I'd feel a lot worse. I think it was like that when my mum was dying and I was looking after her. I tried my hardest to give her all the love and attention she had given me when I was growing up. I was 28 and I couldn't be with her when she died. I was stunned and had counselling. They talked to me about mum and what we had together and it really helped me through.

Sometimes you do need to call out the doctors. I called the doctor once with a bad dose of flu. The doctor came and examined me and made out a prescription. Later on Paul, who was visiting at the time, told me that the doctor had pulled him aside to have a private word about how I should look after myself (lots of liquid and rest and so on). The doctor just assumed that somebody else would have responsibility for me and Paul had to tell the doctor he should tell me about this and not him. The other thing about the doctor talking to Paul was that he didn't even ask who Paul was and yet told him *my* health problems! I think this is what they must mean when they say people should be treated with dignity and respect and be treated like individuals. Despite his best intentions, the doctor who saw me didn't treat me in this way and unless he has some training he may not ever know he is doing anything that infringes people's rights.

A particularly bad time for me was after my accident, when I had been hit by a motorbike. It was not my fault but I was very badly injured. A woman bystander said out loud, 'What is this person with Down's syndrome doing walking on her own?'. I was in so much pain but that really made it worse and I was so angry with her. Would she like me to be shut up in a room all day without the right to move about freely? Anyway, I was rushed to the hospital and had an operation and stitches all down my leg. I had nine broken ribs, my femur and tibia were broken and leg bent in half, I had a broken shoulder, a collapsed lung and badly cut arms and legs. I had staples and a metal plate put in my leg and stitches on my shoulder. When they did the stitches they did not put me under anaesthetic and I was sick everywhere. I think they could have done that for the pain.

My mum stayed in the nurses' home to be with me. I also remember June coming in and seeing me with all these bandages and a cast and stitches. I bet she could hardly have seen any of me through all that stuff. I said, 'Hiya June' and she said, 'how are you then?' and I said, 'I'm all right'. It was a stupid question but it made us laugh through the pain. Having mum and June there showed me there were people who really cared for me.

My friends also visited me and that was really uplifting. I was in hospital for 2 months including my 27th birthday and we had a party on the ward. The nurses were really wonderful and really looked after me well, giving me lots of attention. They always listened to what I said and we could have a good laugh sometimes. I sometimes felt that the hospital could have been kept a little cleaner though.

The problems really started when I was discharged from the hospital. I really wanted to get home. My mum was a bit worried about me using the stairs and the staff said to me, 'If you can't cope at home then do come back in'. I said, 'I'm only just getting out!'. I had a walking stick and a zimmer frame and my flat is two flights of stairs up. It was one of the worst experiences of my life getting up those stairs. They should have provided someone to help. Instead they sent someone over to suggest I went back into hospital.

Once at home I was stuck in the sitting room for about one and a half years. I started to get visitors and that was really great. But getting better was one of the most lonely and boring experiences of my life. I was very isolated, especially when my mum went out. I could not get around on my own and needed others to help me. But I did get about very slowly and improved bit by bit. I know lots of people who have learning disabilities who use wheelchairs and who cannot do things for themselves. They can get very very bored because there are often not people there who they can ask to take them out. And they get fed up asking or other people get fed up of them asking to be taken out.

So, when you have friends who you can rely on it helps, especially when you are ill and unable to do things for yourself. But I have to say this. I think you can only expect so much of your friends. Especially when my mum was out, it would really have been useful to have had some sort of extra help like home-help who could clean and cook when necessary. As it was, I often had to really struggle around to get myself even a sandwich. If mum wasn't there I couldn't even answer the door and I really had to fight for an entry phone to be put in. Looking back, these experiences were really not good enough and they should have been planned before I left hospital.

It took ages to be able to start my life where I had left off. But the accident has left some problems. I cannot do as much walking as I used to do and cannot run or jump either. There's nothing I can do with the damage to my arm, leg and the scars and they will stay with me forever, but I have to live with that and move on. That raises another question about the health of people with Down's syndrome that I feel strongly about.

Before talking about this it would be useful to say that when you are ill you need friends and family as well as doctors and other health people. The doctors and nurses and others need to treat you as an adult, to tell you everything so that you can understand. They should be very friendly and seem to have the time for you. When you are very ill or getting better you may need extra help and people should be asked whether they require this help. Friends provide you with company and keep your spirits up. They do things for you and make you feel wanted at a time when you are likely to be feeling very low. In some cases it might be an idea for family, friends and a person who has a learning disability to meet with doctors and others where there are lots of things that need to be done to help the person get better.

WHEN IS HEALTH NOT HEALTH AND ILLNESS NOT ILLNESS?

I went to Barcelona for a conference some years ago now. The doctors and researchers there were talking about doing testing for Down's syndrome in babies and I stood up and told them to stop treating us like guinea pigs. I asked them if they would prefer it for me not to be there and not to have been born. I asked them if I had not got a valuable life and did not have lots to offer the world. I really do wonder how much money is spent on trying to prevent people like me being born. I think I have made a good life for myself and for the people I know.

I don't think testing for Down's syndrome is about health. It is about how much people think they can love and value people like me and it makes me really sad to think how much time and money are spent trying to stop people like me being born. Are we worthless or is it other people who think we are?

The same question can be asked about plastic surgery on people with Down's syndrome to get rid of their lovely features. It doesn't change the person inside (except by scarring them for life). Plastic surgery is therefore a cosmetic change. It is not about health or at least not the health of people with Down's syndrome. It is more about the health of a society. If people cannot accept and value us as we are then we need to change them and not change us. Why should we have to undergo the scalpel and bear the scars so we *look* different?

That is what I was saying at the beginning of this chapter. When people tell me that I am overweight, I ask 'overweight for what reason?' Am I overweight because some people just cannot stand looking at someone who has a few extra pounds on them? Or am I overweight because it stops me feeling good in myself? Or am I overweight because I can't do the things I really want to do? Or is it that because I'm overweight, my friends are expressing fears about my long-term health, that I may have illnesses that are to do with my weight?

What I would never think about doing is losing weight because people think I look better. I am me and I am proud of what I am. I do not go around saying things like 'I don't like that person over there because of the way they look' or because they have a particular label. I would prefer to get to know them first and then choose if they should be my friends on the basis of who they are.

There are things that are using up public money as if it will get individual people better. For Down's syndrome testing they are really saying it will be better for you as parents not to have a child like me. With plastic surgery they are really saying that they can cure the ills of society by getting rid of our lovely features instead of saying they should work to get rid of prejudice. These are not issues of health and illness. They are about how much a society can value all of its people.

In summary, it is vital to understand that people who have learning disabilities are not ill because they have learning disabilities. Trying to 'put right' a learning disability or to cover it up or to prevent it is not about health or illness.

It is about prejudice and about people's lack of knowledge. Each person, whether they have a learning disability or not, brings their own unique gifts to society and to our world.

CONCLUSION

I have had to learn a lot through my life by fighting and by other people fighting for my rights. I think I have a right to be looked after when I am ill and to information that will keep me healthy and will act as a warning sign that I may be ill. I think I should have a right to a check-up every so often to ensure I am healthy. I also think I have the right to be myself whatever others may think of me as a person.

But for these rights to be meaningful to me, I need to have a meaning to my life. I need something to live for. I need friends. I need respect. I need love from others. Without any of these, having rights doesn't seem as important. Whilst I have made a life for myself and am very happy with who I am and what I'm doing, a lot of people who have learning disabilities need support to find themselves and the meaning to their lives. This is why I chose the title for this chapter – 'Being well and my well-being'. The simple fact of the matter is that you cannot have one without the other.

REFERENCES

Souza A, Ramcharan P 1997 Everything you ever wanted to know about Down's syndrome ... but never bothered to ask. In: Ramcharan P, Roberts G, Grant G, Borland J (eds) Empowerment in everyday life: learning disability. Jessica Kingsley, London

10 Self-concept and people who have learning disabilities

Mark Statham and Diane Timblick

KEY ISSUES

- Exploring the meaning of self-concept
- Perceptions of the physical body
- Relationship between perceptions of the body and the development of self-concept
- The importance of relationships to self-concept
- The impact of disability on the development of self-concept

INTRODUCTION

This chapter will explore the relationship between self-concept and health. This interrelationship will be placed in the context of social constructions of disability and an inclusion versus assimilation approach to service delivery. Within this, health is recognized in its broadest context and includes dimensions of physiological, psychological and sociological well-being (WHO 1986, cited in Gates 1997). Although there has been an increased emphasis upon the medical needs of individuals who have learning disabilities (DoH 1995, 1997), there is a need to address the more subtle and perhaps insidious effects of self-concept on overall well-being, quality of life and subsequently upon health.

Within this chapter it will be asserted that there exists a disparity between a national agenda of inclusion and partnership and a service philosophy based upon assimilation and conformity. In doing this, the chapter will utilize findings from a small-scale research study undertaken by the authors. In addition, this chapter invites you to consider your perception of the work you undertake, to explore the way in which you practise and the impact it can and does have upon those you support.

The research provided evidence of underlying themes identified within the literature which impact on the development of self-concept. These themes provide a basis from which it will be argued that there is a need to reevaluate the philosophies upon which contemporary models of support are based. This can lead to the need to review the nature of relationships we have with people who have learning disabilities, challenging accepted practice throughout services and the community at large. Throughout the text you will be encouraged to draw upon personal experience and reflect upon the relationships you presently have with people who have learning disabilities.

RESEARCH FINDINGS

In an attempt to gain a clearer understanding of the perceptions that people who have learning disabilities have about the importance of body size, a research project was undertaken. Its aim was threefold.

1. To identify the importance that body size has in forming initial perceptions in context with other factors such as gender, clothing, ethnicity and disability.
2. To gain a further insight into the factors that influence the ideas of people who have a learning disability.
3. To gain a further understanding of the levels of control that people who have learning disabilities have in maintaining the body size of their choice.

Full details of the research process will not be explored in detail here but key themes from the findings will be discussed. Although the research was not aimed at exploring the concepts of the self in terms of value and worth per se, some of the findings have particular relevance to issues being discussed in this chapter.

In total, 14 people took part and only one of these individuals could be considered as being overweight. Participants were encouraged to discuss where they got their ideas from in relation to things such as exercise, food, clothing and disability. As a result the perceptions of this sample group may contrast with those who may have direct experience of a weight difficulty. Due to the small sample size, there is no attempt to generalize the findings of this research to a larger population.

THE IMPLICATION OF LEGISLATION

Philosophies such as normalization (Wolfensberger 1972), social role valorization (Wolfensberger 1983) and services accomplishments (O'Brien 1987) have shaped the transition from segregation to inclusion with choice, advocacy and empowerment now being themes considered central to the development of person-centred services. The important question, however, is to what extent these services are truly person centred.

In the Mental Health Foundation report *Building expectations* (1996) the need to feel valued was identified as a key principle of importance to people who have a learning disability. Likewise, shared values are considered to be fundamental to ensuring good practice in services for people who have a learning disability. The goal to 'create a seamless service based entirely around the needs and wishes of users of care and their carers' as stated by Virginia Bottomley, the then Minister of Health (DoH press release 1991, cited in Philpot & Ward 1995), was in theory central to the provisions of the NHS and Community Care Act 1990. In reality, promises of wider access to services, consumer choice and user-centred assessment and packages of care were in direct conflict with the creation of an internal market which was governed by increasing demands on limited resources. In such a context genuine choice and real person centredness can become rhetoric rather than reality (Philpot & Ward 1995).

The failings of the NHS and Community Care Act 1990 in ensuring equal access to services are not specific to people who have learning disabilities. However, their problems may have been more acute. People who have learning disabilities are more likely to become a low priority, not on the basis of need but due to limited specialist provision from health services (Gates & Beacock 1997).

Not only are services limited but the policies that drive their provision are in direct conflict with the philosophies that underpin care for people who have a learning disability (Gates & Beacock 1997).

The new Labour government's agenda for reversing the fragmentation of the NHS was set out in *The new NHS: modern, dependable* (DoH 1997). This initiative replaced the internal market with integrated care built on principles of a 'genuinely national' service which depends on 'local responsibility' for the delivery of healthcare, with a key focus upon 'partnership', 'efficiency' and 'excellence' in order to rebuild 'public confidence'. The clear message is that efficiency and excellence are driven by quality in service delivery and performance, with all NHS trusts being held accountable through clinical governance frameworks for the quality of care delivery (DoH 1998a).

Within this agenda consumer representation has been identified as crucial in monitoring service development and care delivery. However, for people who have a learning disability to truly participate in the development of services they need to be more effectively involved in the development of policies and associated legislation. Initiatives such as the advisory group informing ministers of the agenda that is important to people who have a learning disability need to be positively supported in order to challenge the concept that consumers are simply expected to ascribe to the beliefs of those in power. Crucial within this consideration is the meaning of words such as 'efficiency' and 'excellence' for people who have a learning disability. Other questions relate to issues of genuine partnerships between service users and service providers as well as equality of access.

Although *Modern, dependable* (DoH 1997) and *First class service* (DoH 1998a) do not include direct reference to people who have a learning disability, this need not be viewed negatively. In essence, it can be seen as a crucial re-inforcement of the move to access ordinary community facilities in the same way as any other member of the public. This scenario positively reinforces the fact that people do not automatically require specialist health service input simply because they have a learning disability (DoH 1998b). However, a difficulty often experienced by people who have a learning disability when accessing these services is the skill and expertise of the professionals they come into contact with. This can lead to some very negative experiences which in turn will impact upon a person's self-concept and self-worth. In keeping with this, suggestions have been made to both the NHS and the Health Education Authority that a national public information exercise to correct the false images associated with people who have a learning disability could be a valuable strategy (Mental Health Foundation 1996). This challenge has not yet been addressed.

ISSUES OF SELF-CONCEPT

The relationships that make up our daily lives provide references from which we establish our identities within the world in which we live. It is these day-to-day interactions that lay the foundations from which a concept of self is constructed (Brechin & Walmsley 1989, Jenkins 1996).

Individuals do not develop an identity divorced from the environment within which they exist. Self-concept is a social construct, one that is mediated by a number of external elements that form one's own presentation of self.

ACTIVITY 10.1   Consider the image you have of yourself. What are the key elements of this perception? Ask a friend how they would describe your image. Compare notes and consider the similarities and differences. How does the way in which others perceive you make you feel?

If you spent some time considering this question you may have come up with a list of factors that includes your physical appearance in terms of dress or size. You may consider your personality, the roles you fulfil or cultural interests. The feelings you identify in relation to how others perceive you are also important, particularly as these may contribute to feelings about yourself that can challenge your self-concept.

Image

The concept of self arises from two factors: self-image and self-esteem. The image we have of ourselves is affected by the way in which we value the image we believe we present. Moreover, we all aspire to an ideal image of ourselves and the distance we perceive ourselves to be from it determines the value we place upon ourselves (Rogers 1959, cited in Atkinson et al 1993). Although we make choices based upon what we would like to be, this is heavily influenced by a society which places heavy emphasis upon the 'ideal person'. Personal experience raises awareness of this and through such experience there is a tendency to evaluate oneself against such ideals. Inherent within these discussions is the recognition of the individual as unique and it is within this context that the experiences of people who have learning disabilities will be explored.

In modern society an increasing emphasis is put on the importance of the body. We are surrounded by idealized images of what our bodies should look like, with emphasis continually being placed on the desire to combat any signs of deterioration and decay. We are told that creams and lotions will help prevent the effects of ageing while diets and surgery can alter our shape, creating a body looking youthful and beautiful.

It could be argued that in a democratic society we should have the right and freedom to choose how we express our own individuality in terms of character, appearance and lifestyle. Indeed, many people do. Body piercing, tattoos, alternative fashions are a few examples of how some individuals may mark their own identity. Although these all carry a risk of social disapproval they are nonetheless part of a consumer culture built around body image and perceptions of physical attraction. However, when chosen lifestyles are seen to have a negative impact on health, those choices may also carry moral sanctions that have a significant impact on the individual's value in society. Therefore your right to choose a particular lifestyle is balanced with the need to look good and be healthy. Our bodies provide a basis on which we can be judged by others and subsequently have a significant impact on the way we feel about ourselves and our sense of self-worth.

It has already been suggested through the work of McCarthy (1998) that people who have a learning disability are not immune to pressures to conform. In her exploration of how women who have learning disabilities feel about their bodies, the sample group found it difficult to identify anything positive about their bodies. McCarthy highlights her uncertainty in determining whether this resulted from a lack of belief that there was anything good about their bodies or a more general difficulty in saying positive things. However, her own conclusions lean towards the former, equating a negative body image to a form of oppression that is shared by women who have learning disabilities. High levels of dissatisfaction that women who have learning disabilities have with their own weight reflect a wider trend in society. This is understandable when the consumer market is built upon the assumption that people want to change their bodies and appearance in search of not only what is deemed to be physically attractive but also what is considered by society as acceptable.

Films, TV, magazines, high street shops and advertising all contribute to the creation of the 'body beautiful', filtering expectations of what is considered attractive into our daily lives. No matter how much some people may try to convince themselves that they are not going to buy into the consumer culture that perpetuates the desire for physical attractiveness, it is hard to escape from the pressures it imposes, with many people, both male and female, aspiring to the classic body shape as presented by the media. Therefore an important question for service providers is the extent to which such expectations impact upon the way in which people who have a learning disability perceive themselves and how they are perceived by others.

Overweight and obesity: the national agenda

The maintenance of healthier bodies and a healthier lifestyle has received increased focus on a national level. Overweight and obesity have received particular attention and somewhat ambitious targets have been set to reduce the number of men who are obese by 25% and the number of women who are obese by over a third, by the year 2005 (George 1996).

Cardiovascular disease, stroke, cancer, gallstones, hypertension, diabetes (Perry 1996), gout, decreased lung function, osteoarthritis (Bell & Bhate 1992), hypercholesterolaemia, degenerative joint disease and obstructive sleep apnoea (O'Meara & Glenny 1997) all are more likely to occur in a person who is overweight or obese. Yet despite being recognized as avoidable risk factors, the prevalence of overweight and obesity continues to increase. The experience of people who have a learning disability is no exception (Perry 1996), with evidence suggesting that the prevalence of overweight and obesity is higher amongst this group than among the general population (Bell & Bhate 1992, Prasher 1995, Wood 1994). Dietary intake and low activity levels may be compounded in some cases by additional physical factors specific to a diagnosed syndrome, e.g. abnormalities in appetite control in Prader–Willi, hypothyroidism in Down's syndrome and prescription of some medications such as antiepileptics and antipsychotics. Causes of obesity in people who have a learning disability have, however, generally been found to be the same as in the general population.

Although a greater emphasis is now placed on the need for weight loss in order to reduce health risks rather than the need to achieve an ideal weight, what is deemed to be successful weight loss may be hard to achieve by those who are defined as obese and consideration may need to be given to the impact of unrealistic goals, particularly in relation to an individual's feelings of self-worth. The awareness of the need to lose weight, whether imposed by self or others, places an immediate pressure on individuals to enter into a regulated dietary regime. While some may thrive on diets, gaining confidence through investing in and glorifying the body, for others the need for a diet may engender feelings of failure and inadequacy. Even if weight loss occurs a sense of failure may still arise if what is considered as an 'ideal' weight has not been achieved. If people feel good about themselves they are more likely to be successful in achieving their goal (Vines 1995).

Perceptions of the body

Vines (1995) suggests that obesity is 'the last socially acceptable form of prejudice'. Literature on sociological theorizing of the body suggests that fatness has come to signify a lack of control (Lupton 1995). Overweight and obesity are visible stigmas and the penalties of neglecting the body are seen in the 'lowering of one's acceptability as a person as well as an indication of laziness, low self-esteem and even moral failure' (Featherstone 1982). In contrast, being slim is associated not only with physical attractiveness but also with success, discipline and achievement. It is interesting to note, however, that within the authors' research, perceptions of being slim do not reflect trends in wider society with a greater importance being attached to health.

RESEARCH FINDINGS

Comments relating to the need to lose weight were evenly divided between participants who felt that people represented in the pictures would definitely 'want' to lose weight and those who 'ought' to lose weight. From these comments it would not be possible to suggest what the motivation for weight loss would be.

It is evident from the focus groups that images of large people were associated with activities that reflect undesirable attributes symbolized through 'blemishes of character' (Goffman 1963), which discredit the individual in the eyes of the public. Particular associations were drawn between people who were large and drinking alcohol, drink driving which could cause an accident and an aggressive personality. In addition to ascribing attributes, there was a general feeling amongst participants that being large would also be accompanied by feelings of sadness, depression and being upset.

In contrast, attributes of people who were 'small' or 'average' were ascribed on the basis of their clothing rather than size and were generally positive. Comments related to descriptive accounts of what each person was wearing, making some associations with the type of activities they may be involved in, such as working hard and going to the pub. In this context, the consumption of alcohol was not seen negatively.

Self-concept is influenced by society. The negative stereotypes and generalizations ascribed to people who have learning disabilities have a profound effect upon individual perceptions of themselves and the way in which others view and relate to them (Harris 1995, Susman 1994). The perception of disability in Western culture is particularly strong and associated with abnormality. Positive self-image is difficult to achieve if one is continually represented as a distinctly 'separate species' (Oliver & Barnes 1998). The work of Goffman (1968) explores the internalization of this separation and the development of a self-deprecating or 'spoilt identity'.

<table>
<tr><td>

RESEARCH FINDINGS

</td><td>

One participant drew some associations between fashion and physical attractiveness, expressing the view that some young girls may be at risk of becoming depressed through being unable to achieve the looks and lifestyle of fashion models. Clothes were evidently important to the rest of the research participants but for very different reasons. A more dominant theme that arose during focus groups and interviews related to the need to look clean, tidy and smart. Participants were unanimous in the belief that cleanliness was of central importance in how you are viewed by others but also to avoid being the subject of ridicule.

</td></tr>
</table>

Oliver (1996), as an advocate of a social constructionist approach, sees disability as arising from the barriers of prejudice and discrimination rather than the physical or learning disability. Disability has been socially constructed through the meanings attached to physical and learning disabilities and defined in terms of personal disadvantage. Impairment is therefore equated with a deficit, which is at the root of negative images held by the able-bodied and should not be a point of reference within a disabled identity. However, the difficulty a social model faces is the creation of what has been referred to as an 'untenable separation between the body and culture, impairment and disability' (Hughes & Paterson 1997). Therefore by removing impairment from disability discourse and locating it within a purely medical focus of attention, some would argue that a central part of their identity has been removed from the public arena. Coming to terms with impairment is essential for some individuals before they can address the social barriers it may construct. Being able to understand and acknowledge the loss experienced through impairment is necessary in being able to identify the things you want to change (Szivos & Griffiths 1990).

<table>
<tr><td>

RESEARCH FINDINGS

</td><td>

From focus group and interview data, it is apparent that the possession of a physical disability has far greater consequences in terms of social acceptability. From the responses made, five distinct themes were highlighted.

1. The perception that some members of the general public feel that people who have disabilities should not be accepted into society.
2. Having a disability implies the notion of dependence, being unable to do anything for oneself.
3. The desire to be like the able-bodied – to be normal.
4. Having a disability was a source of humiliation.
5. Having a disability was a source of sympathy and pity.

Participants were asked to list the disabilities they were aware of. Responses were dominated by references to physical disabilities involving 'strokes, epilepsy, poor legs, bad eyes, cripples, limping and wheelchairs'. This reinforces the 'personal tragedy' model of disability (Oliver 1996) in which disability is located within the individual.

</td></tr>
</table>

Prejudice and discrimination would appear to be central to the stigmatized disability identity. Being disabled has been strongly associated with notions of dependence. The visibility of a disability may legitimate the inability to undertake certain tasks of daily living. Such views perpetuate traditional assumptions that people who have disabilities are unable to take control of their own lives, a characteristic that has been considered a failing in modern society. In response to this, research participants identified the perceived desire of those who are disabled to be like able-bodied people.

In general discourse, the able-bodied are used as a reference point of normality to which it is assumed disabled people aspire. However, emphasis upon rehabilitation has not been welcomed universally, being viewed as a mechanism of power shaped by the ideology of normality (Oliver 1996). The images portrayed of disability are in stark contrast to those of non-disabled people with the focus of attention drawn immediately to what are considered as deficits in terms of their impairment. When the history of prejudice and discrimination against disability has been based upon notions of individual difference, it is difficult to provide any basis for suggesting that having a learning disability in some way excludes you from the pressures of having to conform to idealized images of what is accepted as beautiful. People who have learning disabilities may face an additional barrier in their attempts to develop a mark of individuality within society's expectations of acceptable appearance. Choices to adopt alternative fashions may be viewed as inappropriate, bringing unnecessary attention to themselves. Subsequently the chance to explore and experiment with one's appearance may be reduced by the opportunities and choices made available to individuals who have a learning disability by families and carers who play a key role in informing their ideas. The visibility of a disability has significant repercussions on how individuals are viewed during social interactions, bringing into conflict virtual and actual identity (Goffman 1963). Research participants clearly identified the possession of a disability as being the subject of ridicule and embarrassment.

Goffman (1963) suggests that stigma is associated with acceptance. Although disability is prone to victimization it is not an inevitable consequence. The stigmatized must reduce the tensions surrounding their acceptance in a social occasion, helping them to act more appropriately. This is built on the premise that difficulties are encountered as a result of societal responses to disability rather than their functional limitations (Susman 1994). This view can be criticized for placing responsibility on the disabled individual to break the barriers created by wider social processes forcing them into a position of having to justify their own existence and mediating their own acceptance. Ultimately, the possession of a disability signifies difference and mixed contacts between the stigmatized and 'normals' may lead to uncertainty over how to interact (Goffman 1963).

Relationships

The value that we place upon the opinions and judgements of others can have a profound effect upon us. This becomes increasingly important when we are seeking inclusion as part of a group or activity (Argyle 1994). Various factors can contribute to the nature of relationships that we have. The interaction with those around us and the way in which we respond to them differs over time as certain individuals or groups wax or wane in importance to us. Our perception of ourselves and indeed others is a dynamic one.

ACTIVITY 10.2

Consider the relationships you have in your daily life. What role do these relationships play and what importance do you attach to them?

The relationships you may have considered are that of brother, sister, lover, mother, father, student, friend, etc. The role relationships have may not be unique to you in themselves but are unique in both their nature and quality as experienced by you. It is this experience together with body image that enables you to develop a concept of yourself.

ACTIVITY 10.3

Imagine that you have just been told by your doctor that you need to lose weight. Think about the following points and write down your responses.
- How do you think you would feel about the advice given to you?
- How did you reach a decision on what action to take?
- What factors would influence your decision?
- How much control did you have over the decision?
- What support would be available from others to help you if you chose to lose weight?

In making a decision about one's own health and lifestyle behaviour, it would be necessary to weigh up the pros and cons of different options. This may involve a range of different approaches in accessing more factual information in relation to weight loss to find the most effective way to manage it. What may be of greater importance and value is the individual's attitude towards the importance of losing weight. External factors that may influence those attitudes, such as media images and consumerism and the perceived costs and benefits that particular actions may have, may relate not only to health but also to the practicality of making significant changes in one's lifestyle, the responses of others around us and support that would be required from family, friends and colleagues to make those changes.

ACTIVITY 10.4

Having considered your own responses in Activity 10.3, consider some health advice that you have recently given someone who has a learning disability. Ask the person the same questions and compare responses.

It is evident from the research that carers and professionals play a dominant part not only in the role of information giver and educator but also as friend and confidant. The research below indicates additional responses of importance from the perspective of people who have a learning disability.

RESEARCH FINDINGS

It was evident that the research participants had a fairly extensive knowledge of what were considered to be 'good' and 'bad' foods. The association of greasy, fatty and sugary food as being 'bad' and fruit, vegetables and non-fatty food being 'good' reflects findings of other research (Lupton 1996). During the focus groups, a significant number of responses were made associating food with being large, with particular reference to having too many chocolates, crisps, fatty foods and 'ginormous' meals. However, when exploring ideas of what may happen to the body if individuals consumed too many 'bad' foods, responses focused primarily on issues relating to health difficulties such as heart problems and strokes, rather than on issues of actual size. (Although the words 'good' and 'bad' may appear to be immediately value laden, they are terms that participants generally seemed to relate to more clearly than 'healthy' and 'unhealthy'.)

Only two participants referred to factors other than food that may lead to people putting on weight. These were medication and glands. There appeared to be some awareness of the importance of exercise, with five participants being able to articulate the link between losing weight and keeping fit. Interestingly, however, one of these participants felt that the need to build up strength was important not only for health reasons but also to stop being bullied. While acknowledging the importance of exercise, more comments were made in relation to the potential harmful effects of exercise than to its benefits and enjoyment factor.

It would appear from this information that very clear messages about the potential health risks related to excessive eating of unhealthy foods are being learnt by participants in this research sample. Yet to what extent does this new knowledge influence actual health behaviour? Without social supports in place to enable individuals to develop a healthier lifestyle, the use of this information may be inconsistent and on occasions inappropriate. The challenge for professionals, in this instance, is to facilitate people who have a learning disability to take personal control to achieve and maintain a body size and shape that is meaningful to them.

Service providers play a vital role in delivering knowledge that is up to date and based on sound evidence and in a manner in which the recipient can understand it. The relevance of that information may vary, however, according to the personal, social, environmental and emotional context in which it is given and how it can be acted on.

This raises two particular issues. First, carers and professionals are in a position to dominate and control the information given about a range of issues in relation to content and access. Research participants found it quite difficult to articulate where their ideas came from but there was a very limited number of responses that referred to television, magazines and other media images. Research participants were more likely to talk to family, carers and nurses about ideas than to friends and social networks.

Second, as a professional it is often difficult to draw the line between where a personal and professional relationship begins and ends. Subsequently, there may be a conflict of interests in the advice and support that is given in providing a balance between meeting specific health needs and enabling individuals to take greater control in determining their own desires, wishes and choices. It is not unusual for different members of one family unit to have different likes and dislikes. For people within this research, however, it is evident that staff have a greater control in determining many decisions. In addition to providing relevant health-related information and supporting decision-making processes about essential issues such as diet, it is evident that nurses and carers are playing a dominant role in supporting decisions about personal image.

RESEARCH FINDINGS

When exploring where people got their ideas about clothes, participants identified magazines, TV and catalogues. In relation to their own lives, however, carers were cited as the dominant source for helping to make decisions. This was generally done by looking at clothes in shops with the majority of participants referring to Marks and Spencers, Littlewoods, John Reins and Debenhams.

ACTIVITY 10.5

Cast your mind back to the last time you purchased an item of clothing. What influenced your ideas of what you were looking for and what you purchased?

In answer to this question it is likely that you will consider price, colour or size. It is perhaps unlikely that at the time of purchase you will consider the influences within the wider context of a consumer culture, which may operate at a more subconscious level. As previously stated, advertising, TV, magazines and books were all cited by participants as sources of learning and ideas. Difficulties in relating the significance of these factors to daily lifestyle choices is perhaps not surprising. For people within this research, influences on choice of purchase or lifestyle were more obvious and immediate, relating to the support given by family and carers. Evidence of strong reliance on their support was not necessarily viewed negatively by the research participants as they clearly valued the support received. However, it does question the extent to which choices are shaped by the beliefs and expectations of others, however innocent their intentions.

Staff need to consider how they negotiate their role in enabling individuals to develop their own sense of control and self-determination. In doing so, it is important to consider the variety of functions that relationships have.

ACTIVITY 10.6

Think of an individual who has learning disabilities with whom you have spent some time. How does the extent and nature of your relationships with them differ from relationships you have with non-disabled people?

Although you may have been able to describe the extent of these various relationships and experiences, how would you interpret their impact upon the person you thought about? What is your reply based upon – assumption or empathy? As carers, friends, acquaintances and relatives, it is essential that we recognize the value individuals place on different aspects of their lives.

In recognizing the importance of relationships that individuals have with carers, it is important to consider what individuals who have learning disabilities get out of the relationships that they have. Nunkoosing & John (1997) explored the relationships of a group of people who have learning disabilities and identified a number of key themes that arose. These were acceptance and mutuality as characteristics of friendship, the experience of and dealing with rejection, the experience of and dealing with loneliness, 'accepting relationships' between individuals who have learning disabilities and their non-disabled friends and the constraints on the development of relationships. Within the study, relationships based upon acceptance and mutuality were identified. Individuals participated in exchanges concerning emotional support, practical assistance, companionship and acceptance. Mutualism can be regarded as a fundamental component of meaningful relationships and from an eclectic social psychological perspective is seen as irrefutable evidence of the interdependence of human beings (Jenkins 1996). It is surprising that we need to prove that people who have learning disabilities are able to engage in the type of recipro-cal relationships that non-disabled people have. Interestingly, the themes that emerge from this study are not necessarily different from those experienced by us all. The fear of rejection and loneliness and how we deal with these are part of the equation which develops our self-concept.

Within these relationships we develop a perception of ourselves, our abilities, status and roles together with how people view and evaluate us. Hopes and aspi-rations and our perception of our ideal self combine to make up what we are. However, there remains a fundamental contradiction in the relationships supporters often have with people who have learning disabilities, particularly as the locus of control often remains with supporters and service providers (Brown & Smith 1992) whilst a positive and enduring self-concept can only arise from individuals taking control over their own destiny.

CONSTRUCTION OF GROUP IDENTITIES

The stigma associated with having a disability appears to have a significant impact on social acceptability and often those who are stigmatized in one respect express all the normal prejudices towards those stigmatized in another (Goffman 1963). The interesting issue here is the extent to which people who have a disability identify themselves as being disabled.

RESEARCH FINDINGS

Participants were asked to list the disabilities they were aware of. Responses were dominated by references to physical disabilities involving strokes, epilepsy, poor legs, bad eyes, cripples, limping and wheelchairs. While associations were drawn between people in the sample group and the possession of a physical disability, only one indi-vidual openly identified themselves as having a learning disability. It is interesting to note, however, that all participants, who are themselves members of a disadvantaged stigmatized group, shared the same stigmatizing perceptions of disability that are commonly attributed to the general population. It is not clear from this sample, however, whether the views expressed in focus groups and interviews were a projec-tion of participants' own lived experiences or a reflection of dominant discourses promoted through the medical professions, carers, families and media images. Doctors, nurses and healthcare professionals were again identified as key sources of knowledge about disabilities although it was recognized that not enough was known.

Within the sample groups there was a degree of sympathy expressed towards friends who had a disability. It is possible that participants share an affiliation with the stigmatized through their own experiences, but the main emotions expressed related to a fear that they too could become disabled. This view reflects the dominant culture that disability is something to be avoided as much as possible (Stone 1995). The research participants' perceptions about the importance of having a disability appear to reflect attitudes and beliefs held by the general population.

Normalization and social role valorization (Wolfensberger 1972, 1983) fail to respect the value individuals may place upon the groups to which they belong. Individuals are expected to not only act like but also look like perfect citizens. The work of Todd & Shearn (1995, 1997, cited in Rapley et al 1998) attempts to provide an argument that individuals become 'invisible to themselves'. That is, the label of learning disabilities is so tarnished that they do not recognize it as relating to themselves. Moreover, the issue of 'invisibility' suggests that individuals do not recognize the part disability plays in their lives. Studies, however, demonstrate that people are often acutely aware of the impact it has on them and others (Booth & Simons 1989, Harris 1995, Sinason 1992, Stone 1995, Szivos-Bach 1993). A more significant issue that needs consideration is not whether individuals wish to acknowledge the impact of a particular label but how they deal with the circumstances in which they find themselves. Denial of a label or membership of a group should not automatically be seen as abnormal; in reality the rejection of group membership with negative associations is a common part of everyday life (Tajfel 1979, cited in Finlay & Lyons 1998).

A re-evaluation of the work of Todd & Shearn by Rapley et al (1998) provides a positive review by recognizing that people who have learning disabilities are essentially managing issues of identity construction by acknowledging and contesting their membership of a construct of disability they do not accept. They are in effect being ordinary.

Wolfensberger (1972) reflects upon the social expectations of marginalized groups and postulates that such groups are under considerable pressure to conform to the expectations associated with the role they are identified with. In relation to people who have learning disabilities, these were subhuman, holy innocent, eternal child, object of ridicule, object of pity, burden of charity, menace and an object of dread (Gates 1997). The risk for professionals in this situation is that they will interact with the learning disability and the social constructions around this rather than the *person* who has a learning disability. This distinction is important as it lays the foundations of the way in which we perceive and relate to people who have learning disabilities and the way in which they may perceive themselves and us. The social construct of disability and the labels and the imagery which it portrays provide further arguments to suggest that they assist in reducing the impact of disability by creating low expectations of individuals to conform by society (McCarthy 1998).

By placing an emphasis upon conformity to social norms and expectations, individuals or particular groups are denied the opportunities to explore mutual concerns and experiences from which to enhance or construct an identity of belonging that promotes self-identity and from it autonomy and self-determination. It is pertinent to note that knowledge about disabilities comes predominantly from those without them, rather than those who have experience of disability themselves. The assimilation approach advocated by adherents of normalization 'theory' reinforces society's negative attitude towards disability by accepting social norms and promoting conformity and integration based on terms that are not in partnership and certainly not equitable. Support is unilaterally perceived in the context of partnership and collaboration in a professional–client relationship not from a recognition and acceptance of meaningful relationships between disadvantaged individuals and/or groups.

Collective action and support are still universally identified with 'deviancy' (Wolfensberger 1972). Conceptual frameworks based upon service outcomes of community participation, community presence, choice, dignity and respect (O'Brien 1987) can only prove meaningful in an environment of mutuality and personal continuity and can be prejudiced by access to opportunities and an unchallenged assumption about the underlying concepts which inform professional practice (O'Brien & O'Brien 1998). As we have explored, the development of self-concept is influenced by personal experience. Active disassociation of individuals from the means to develop their identities based upon their own valued relationships, both formal and informal, actively denies choice and the possibility of collective support and action based upon common histories and life experiences. Indeed, the power of 'self-validation' and the recognition of 'communities of choice' (Campling 1981) provide a strong challenge to the universally accepted philosophy which underpins many services today.

CONCLUSION

As members of society and professional groups, we remain somewhat impotent in dealing with the fundamental challenges that personal constructs of disability pose to us. Our research has clearly highlighted that people who have a learning disability share the same perceptions and stereotypes as the general population and will be affected equally by the consequences of them. It is also evident that professionals and carers are not only a dominant source of knowledge and information but also influence ideas that have a direct impact on the construction of individuals' appearance and identity. This chapter has sought to address the idea of power in relationships that influence the construction of self-concept. Self-concept cannot be disengaged from its social context and active devaluing of individuals' choice of partnership within groups that celebrate commonalities rather than differences denies personal growth.

While national agendas are clearly linked to improving health and the greater inclusion of people who have learning disabilities in mainstream services, greater attention needs to be paid to the philosophies that govern our approaches to practice and the understanding of having a learning disability. Such approaches should not depend on the need to conform to societal norms and expectations. The stripping away of individual identity weakens the foundations from which people develop a sense of belonging and source of strength to challenge the concepts people have of them and the groups which they inhabit. Communities have much to learn from people who have disabilities and an adherence to principles of assimilation has proved detrimental to people who have learning disabilities in perpetuating disability as stigmatized and devalued.

FURTHER READING

Heyman B, Swain J, Gillman M, Handyside E C, Newman W 1997 Alone in a crowd: how adults with learning difficulties cope with social network problems. Social Sci Med 44(1):41–53
This qualitative research article explores the negative impact that social contexts may have on the development of valued identities and the coping strategies adopted by six adults who have learning disabilities in response to a stigmatizing world. The implications of this study on service provision in Britain have also been considered in brief.

Opie A 1998 'Nobody's asked me for my view': users' empowerment by multidisciplinary health teams. Qualitat Health Res 8(2):188–206
This article raises some key issues relating to the power relations that exist between healthcare professionals and service users. Based on work undertaken in New Zealand, this research explores the practices of multiprofessional teams in promoting the empowerment of service users on an individual and structural level. Although this work does not focus particularly on issues of self-concept it addresses the importance of developing partnerships between policies and practices.

Pearpoint J, O'Brien J, Forest M 1998 Path: a workbook for planning positive possible futures. Inclusion Press, Toronto
An informative guide for the use of one kind of person-centred strategy. A powerful tool that can be used for individual or group development.

Sanderson H, Kennedy J, Ritchie P, Goodwin G 1999 People, plans and possibilities. Developing person centred planning. SHS Ltd, Edinburgh
An inspirational text that challenges traditional support frameworks and reinstates the person at the centre of care.

Shilling C 1993 The body and social theory. Sage Publications, London
This book provides a comprehensive introduction to key social theories that contribute to our understanding of the relationship between the body and self-identity. It is an accessible read for anyone interested in exploring the increasing importance that is attached to the body within consumer culture, raising some important questions relating to the presence and experience of disability within society.

Wertheimer A 1995 Circles of support: building inclusive communities. Available from Circles Network, Bristol
An essential read for those wishing to explore the development of inclusive communities and to challenge how services traditionally support individuals with learning disabilities.

REFERENCES

Argyle M 1994 The psychology of interpersonal behaviour, 5th edn. Penguin Books, London

Atkinson R L, Atkinson R C, Smith E E, Ben D J 1993 Introduction to psychology, 11th edn. Harcourt Brace, London

Bell A J, Bhate M S 1992 Prevalence of overweight and obesity in Down's syndrome and other mentally handicapped adults living in the community. J Intellect Disabil Res 36:359–364

Booth T, Simons K 1989 Whose terms? Commun Care October: 19–22

Brechin A, Walmsley J 1989 Making connections. Hodder and Stoughton, London

Brown H, Smith H 1992 Normalisation. The reader for the 90s. Routledge, London

Campling J 1981 Images of ourselves – women with disabilities talking. Routledge and Kegan Paul, London

Department of Health 1995 The health of the nation: a strategy for people with learning disabilities. HMSO, London

Department of Health 1997 The new NHS: modern, dependable. The Stationery Office, London

Department of Health 1998a First class service. The Stationery Office, London

Department of Health 1998b Signposts for success. The Stationery Office, London

Featherstone M 1982 The body in consumer culture. Theory Culture Society 1:18–33

Finlay M, Lyons E 1998 Social identity and people with learning difficulties: implications for self advocacy groups. Disability Society 13(1):37–51

Gates B 1997 Learning disabilities. Churchill Livingstone, London

Gates B, Beacock C 1997 Dimensions of learning disability. Baillière Tindall, London

George M 1996 Missing the target. Nursing Standard 11(6):26–28

Goffman E 1963 Stigma. Simon and Schuster, New York

Goffman E 1968 Asylums: essays on the social situations of mental patients and other inmates. Penguin, Harmondsworth

Harris P 1995 Who am I? Concepts of disability and their implications for people with learning difficulties. Disability Society 10(3):341–351

Hughes B, Paterson K 1997 The social model of disability and the disappearing body: towards a sociology of impairment. Disability Society 12(3):325–340

Jenkins R 1996 Social identity. Routledge, London

Lupton D 1995 The imperative of health: public health and the regulated body. Sage Publications, London

Lupton D 1996 Food, the body and the self. Sage Publications, London

McCarthy M 1998 Whose body is it anyway? Pressures and control for women with learning disabilities. Disability Society 13(4):557–574

Mental Health Foundation 1996 Building expectations: opportunities and services for people with a learning disability. Mental Health Foundation, London

Nunkoosing K, John M 1997 Friendships, relationships and the management of

rejection and loneliness by people with learning disabilities. J Learning Disabil Nursing Health Social Care 1(1):10–18

O'Brien J 1987 A guide to life-style planning. In: Wilcox B, Bellamy G T (eds) A comprehensive guide to the activities catalogue. An alternative curriculum for youth and adults with severe disabilities. Paul Brookes, London

O'Brien J, O'Brien C L 1998 Members of each other. Building community in company with people with developmental disabilities. Inclusion Press, Toronto

Oliver M 1996 Understanding disability: from theory to practice. Macmillan Press, London

Oliver M, Barnes C 1998 Disabled people and social policy: from exclusion to inclusion. Longman, London

O'Meara S, Glenny A M 1997 What are the best ways of tackling obesity? Nursing Times 93(22):50–51

Perry M 1996 Treating obesity in people with learning disabilities. Nursing Times 92(35):36–38

Philpot T, Ward L 1995 Values and visions. Butterworth Heinemann, Oxford

Prasher V P 1995 Overweight and obesity amongst Down's syndrome adults. J Intellect Disabil Res 35(5):437–441

Rapley M, Kiernan P, Antaki C 1998 Invisible to themselves or negotiating identity? The interaction management of 'being intellectually disabled'. Disability Society 13(5):807–827

Sinason V 1992 Mental handicap: the human condition. Free Association Books, London

Stone S S 1995 The myth of bodily perfection. Disability Society 10(4):413–424

Susman J 1994 Disability, stigma and deviance. Social Sci Med 38(1):15–22

Szivos S, Griffiths E 1990 Group processes involved in coming to terms with a mentally retarded identity. Mental Retardation 28:333–341

Szivos-Bach S E 1993 Social comparisons, stigma and mainstreaming: the self esteem of young adults with a mild mental handicap. Mental Handicap Res 6(3):217–236

Vines G 1995 Fighting fat with feeling. New Scientist 1987:14–15

Wolfensberger W 1972 The principle of normalisation in human services. National Institute on Mental Retardation, Toronto

Wolfensberger W 1983 Social role valorisation: a proposed new term for the principle of normalisation. National Institute on Mental Retardation, Toronto

Wood T 1994 Weight status of a group of adults with learning disabilities. Br J Learning Disabil 22:97–99

11 Valued occupation for people who have a learning disability

Caroline Heason, Lynne Stracey and Dommie Rey

KEY ISSUES

- Valued occupation is a lifestyle issue, not a label
- The importance of person-centred approaches
- Cultural specificity in occupation
- Ethical dilemmas and risk taking
- Social inclusion
- Continuity of opportunity and flow routines

INTRODUCTION

This chapter will take the reader through a journey of aspirations, hopes, dreams and the fulfilment of those dreams. This passage of life planning applies to us all and our journey is continuous, starting when we are very young, through the middle years and into old age. It is a process through which we explore and find out about what we enjoy and what we want to do with our lives. Through exploration, we develop skills and attitudes that lead us to become better at those activities or tasks that are important to successful achievement in the life choices that we make. We find out about those activities pleasurable or necessary for us; the task, the people, environment and time of day. We also discover ways of adapting occupations to make them easier and more to our taste. We go through a process of elimination, sometimes making mistakes and at times with a complete change of direction. This applies to all aspects of our social and occupational lives. We are then able to establish what we want to do, how we are going to do it and with whom.

Although some aspects of our lives may take on greater significance according to our life stage and assumed responsibilities, this process is not singular in nature. It applies to all aspects of our lives, bringing together the many strands to form an integral whole. In this way our individual lifestyle is created.

Since this journey of life planning applies to all of us we are not going to write a chapter about disability. There are no formulaic ideas here about how to

ACTIVITY 11.1

- Consider and list your current roles.
- What experiences throughout your life have shaped and influenced these roles?
- What makes these roles yours as opposed to a series of timetabled events that could be performed by anybody?
- Consider previous roles you have had. Write them down in a path format to illustrate how you have arrived at your current roles (Fig. 11.1).

Think about the following.

- Have you ever changed life course?
- When you changed course was this based on a lot of experience or no experience?
- Did you consider the risks involved?
- Are you satisfied with the choices you made?
- Do you envisage changing life course again?

FIGURE 11.1

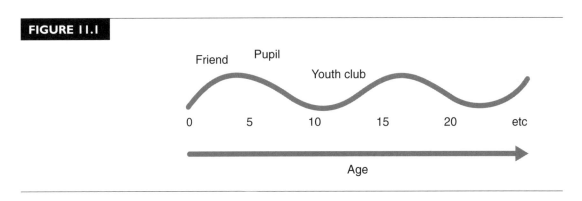

organize valued occupation with a person who has a learning disability, how to set it up, how to conduct an initial interview; we hope to provide helpful hints and strategies that may be useful. However, the difference for people who have a learning disability is that the aspirations, the expectations afforded to them by others mean that they do not often have the same sorts of opportunities as people without a learning disability.

We would also like you to consider the thought that there are no simple answers within life. Having accepted this, it is important to acknowledge that everything in our lives is connected to something or someone else. It is this interconnectedness that makes things more complex. It is therefore impossible to think of supporting someone to develop opportunities in their life in isolation from other aspects or roles the person may have. For example, work can be connected with leisure if I meet my colleagues for a drink; with running my home if I share childcare organization; and with education if I go on a course from work. Friendships, relationships, families' emotional well-being creep into this and blur the boundaries. These things help to make my life and my job easier, more fulfilling and more enjoyable.

It is impossible to separate opportunities and occupation into a 'block of flats' model, where everything is facilitated separately, ensuring that a person is a passenger rather than someone who is empowered to have a go, make mistakes, try again and to find their dream.

We hope you enjoy this chapter. We have aimed to make it 'interactive'. By that we mean we have posed questions and given scenarios throughout prompting reflection on your own experience and those you know.

ACTIVITY 11.2

Think about all the experiences, play, thoughts, discussions and arguments you have had; films and TV programmes you watched; people you respected, both current and historical, in order to help you decide what you value in connection with work, leisure, education and running a home.

When you have done this consider how these experiences have shaped your life and how they have informed your decisions about your own roles. You may have thought about why you chose to do the work that you do and what influenced that decision. You may have thought about your family life and how this may have coloured your life choices.

HISTORICAL PERSPECTIVES

The concept of occupation seems to have become increasingly person centred over the last century. Wolfensberger (1975) describes occupation in the 19th and 20th centuries in the USA where it was centred around the independence of the institution rather than the individual or the family. He describes farms, laundries, kitchens where people had very clear tasks, the process of promotions and the hierarchical status placed upon certain jobs but not preparing the person for valued occupation in their own neighbourhood for themselves (Wolfensberger 1975).

> Pear picking was one activity pursued in this so-called farm colony. It was the hope that with sufficient farm land able-bodied imbeciles of both sexes could be kept in our state at a weekly cost of not more than $1 per capita in addition to what the farm would produce.
> (Wolfensberger 1975, p 32)

This use of a segregated workforce to provide the economization and enlargement of the institutions had not always been the case. Again, Wolfensberger (1975) describes in the middle 19th century how Howe (1852), Seguin (1870) and Johnson (1898), all in the *Journal of Insanity*, noted that the institutions they were involved with were not intended to be dumping grounds. They were viewed as schools and had a habilitative and training function to them. The schools were viewed as being within and not segregated from society. For example, the first such institution in the USA was built in Boston, Massachusetts, in 1848 in the middle of a highly populated residential area.

Barton (1959) describes recreating work environments, social clubs, social events and shops within the hospital setting in a strictly chaperoned environment. Again, this did not address supporting people to develop their confidence, capabilities and choice in enhancing their opportunities away from the hospital. Mental health and learning disability services have all gone through a habilitation or rehabilitation model. Moya Wilson (1983) discusses the use of challenging schools of thought such as humanism and Goffman's work on socialization activities with people who have enduring mental health problems. However, she doesn't seem to address the difficulties of supporting a person as a fellow human being to develop capabilities to fulfil their aspirations and dreams within their neighbourhood and community in a supported rather than sheltered setting.

The person-centred approach inherent in person-centred planning and in Circles Networks started with Wolfensberger's work first on normalization and then more recently on social role Valorization. Laudably, these works advocated the inherent value and individualism of people who have a learning disability. However, his work was misinterpreted by many. Valued opportunities were not individualized and little account seemed to be taken of people's ethnic and cultural background which meant that services were based on white middle-class stereotypes.

Adult training centres could also be criticized in the same way as the large institutions of the 19th and early 20th century. This is because a lot of their work promoted the independence of the organization. It was not person centred and relied on the readiness model, in which people had to be trained and ready for 'outside employment' before being supported to find a job. Supported employment schemes such as the Shaw Trust, Right Employment in Oxford and VISION have gone a long way to change this. They look at both the capabilities and support needed to enable the person to pursue the opportunities they want to based on earning a real wage in a real work setting.

DEFINING VALUED OCCUPATION

Before considering the meaning of valued occupation for people who have learning disabilities, it is necessary to define the meaning of 'occupation' if we are to provide informed and focused support. The term 'valued occupation' has no single universal definition. It may be considered to be a cultural concept, in that the culture in which occupation takes place will define the meaning or value that is attached to it.

In our efforts to define occupation we often attach words to it such as 'meaningful' or 'purposeful'. This enables us to distinguish activities that are not occupational in nature in that they are arbitrary, involuntary or purposeless. Inherent to this concept is the meaning and value that occupation conveys for the individual personally. However, 'meaning' and 'purpose' are not necessarily synonymous. An occupation may be purposeful without being meaningful to the individual just as it may be individually meaningful without having an identifiable purpose. The purpose will be found in the context within which the occupational activity takes place. We do not always do the things we enjoy well; neither are they always necessary nor vital to the overall responsibilities of our lives. Though we may strive to achieve competency and this may be necessary to some tasks in our lives (for example in our employment) of equal importance is our drive to participate. It does not necessarily follow that lacking the capacity for expertise should preclude participation in activities that are meaningful to the individual. There is sometimes a tendency for services to people who have learning disabilities to overemphasize the importance of some aspects of occupational activity, such as self-care and leisure, whilst ignoring the overall productive potential that is unique to the person's particular lifestyle.

> It is through valued occupation that an individual gains expression of self-identity, social connection and productive management of time. Increasingly occupation is being regarded as the day-to-day basis of quality of life, wellness, empowerment and social equity.
>
> (Townsend et al 1997)

Societal values and perceptions will determine whether or not particular occupational activities or roles receive positive validation. Wolfensberger argues that human perceptual processes are inherently evaluative. What is perceived, either consciously or subconsciously, is evaluated by an individual, or a culture, as positive or negative. He argues that there is no such thing as value-free perception (Wolfensberger 1988). The place we take in society, the things we do and the opportunities we have to do them will be greatly influenced by the perceptions of others and in this way occupational forms are profoundly affected. The opportunities we have to engage in specific activities and the way in which we approach them will be defined by cultural values and practices.

When considering whether occupation is valued, it is first necessary to consider what it means to be devalued. In general, this occurs when a place, object, task, person or group is invested with low or negative value by the perceiver. This often leads to being considered of lesser worth. When this happens to people or social groups, they are often afforded fewer or poorer quality opportunities. It is possible to identify what a specific culture devalues by examining what it values positively. The people who characterize the opposite of what a society values will be cast into devalued status and consequently denied access to valued roles and opportunities. In this way, historically, people who have learning disabilities have been marginalized and excluded from access to or full participation in valued occupational roles.

As services have become increasingly person centred, focused attempts have been made to support people who have learning disabilities to develop valued lifestyles. Central to this theme is the need to support people to access the same culturally sensitive opportunities for valued, meaningful occupations as are enjoyed by society at large. In building inclusive opportunities, it is important to consider the need for a person to feel a sense of flow and connectedness in their lives. This means that they are supported to develop patterns and routines that link chunks of activity taking place in their day into an integral whole. Without this (and all too often) the lives of people who have learning disabilities become a series of inflexible, timetabled events that the person has access to, whilst remaining passive and dependent on others. In this way, they are inhibited from seizing control over their lives.

ACTIVITY 11.3

- Consider your day. What routines connect and facilitate flow in order to link the main activities that take place?
- Who else is important in enabling these routines to happen?
- What would happen if these 'flow routines' changed or were interrupted?
- Could you sustain the important things in your day/life without them?

Valued occupation provides a means of organizing one's life into patterns, habits and roles. It may be conceptualized as doing culturally meaningful work, play or daily living tasks in the stream of time and in the context of one's physical and social world (Kielhofner 1995).

Peter has worked for many years assembling and labelling boxes for a small company producing health foods. Despite being fully independent in these work tasks, he continued to be dependent on full support to enable him to work. Peter was rarely ready to leave for work in the morning as he was often still caught up in the routines of the staff-supported household in which he lived. At work, Peter was unable to locate his locker without support and therefore did not engage in the link behaviours which facilitated the initiation of work activity, i.e. taking off his coat on arrival at work, putting on his overall and making his way to the bay in which he worked. He relied on his supporter to initiate these routines. Throughout his day at work Peter did not easily interact with other employees. As a result of these things, despite being able to carry out the tasks required to do his job, Peter lacked contentedness in his work role.

ACTIVITY 11.4

- Consider what constitutes your work role.
- At what point in your day does this role begin and end?
- What link routines would enable Peter to successfully take control of his work role?
- What factors does the service provider need to consider in supporting Peter effectively at work?

CONCEPTS OF HEALTH AND OCCUPATION

The impact of occupation on health and well-being is well recognized. The concept of wellness is increasingly being challenged as being more than the absence of disease. It could be argued that positive health status may in part 'depend on people having access to meaningful occupations that provide them with housing, employment, community and enjoyment' (Townsend et al 1997).

> People know from their own experience that their health is strongly influenced by what they do in working, playing and generally living – this common knowledge is gaining support from research which indicates that health improves when people are empowered to direct what they do each day.
>
> (McKnight 1989)

Within any culture, health beliefs can be broadly separated into two groups: theoretical perspectives presented by professionals and lay beliefs and ideas expressed by members of society.

In the context of occupation and people who have learning disability, throughout this chapter we are exploring how these beliefs may influence lifestyle and therefore occupational behaviour.

FIGURE 11.2   *Personhood.*

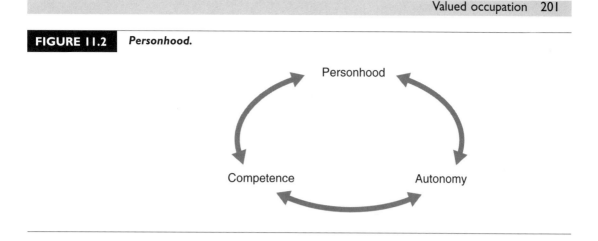

ETHICAL DILEMMAS

Being aware of one's own values and beliefs is a prerequisite for coping with ethical dilemmas.

A multitude of issues in the care and support of people who have learning disabilities have strong ethical implications. Many of these are underpinned by one or more major issues: the concepts of personhood, autonomy versus paternalism and competence.

Personhood

The concept of personhood invites us to explore what we mean by a 'person' and what criteria we can use to define a person, when personhood might begin and end.

Part of the basis of the move away from institutional care for people who have learning disabilities to a client-centred individual approach is founded upon our desire to recognize and encourage personhood and individuality. One of the prime objectives of support is to encourage, assist and enable the individual to function as independently as possible; that is, to exercise as much autonomy as possible (Hessler & Key, in Shanley & Starrs 1993).

Later in the chapter we will discuss the depersonalizing nature of the institutional patterns of care which characterized the provision of services to people who have learning disabilities throughout the first half of the 20th century.

Autonomy and paternalism

In this context autonomy is defined as the right to or state of self-government and the freedom (and ability) of an individual to determine his or her actions and behaviour.

In contrast, paternalism is a system in which care is apt to pass into (unwelcome) interference or where the freedom of the individual is subject to well-meaning regulations.

This approach is clearly undesirable in the context of preventing either the development or exercising of autonomy in those individuals who have both the desire and the potential ability to do so.

The principles of normalization emphasize the importance of individuals being able to exercise informed choice and being enabled or empowered to make decisions about their own lives. The concept of risk taking has to be considered in this context (Hessler & Kay, in Shanley & Starrs 1993).

Competence

In relation to competence we are exploring an individual's ability to undertake a course of action or even to decide whether to embark upon a course of action.

We need to explore the criteria upon which we decide whether a person is competent and to consider the effects of declaring someone incompetent. To link these three key issues to occupation, consider these questions.

ACTIVITY 11.5

You are considering two jobs. One is in a restaurant in a busy out-of-town shopping centre, the other one is in a quieter café in a suburb. Someone decides on your behalf that you are not competent to work in either. What are the issues that arise regarding personhood?

■ *Personhood* – this decision is depersonalizing as it does not allow you to identify your desired position yourself and assumes that you would not cope.

■ *Autonomy and paternalism* – it is paternalistic as you are not allowed the freedom to try a job to see if it is right or not.

■ *Competence* – you are firstly not considered competent to decide or make a choice and secondly, you are not competent to do the job.

Think how you would wish to be supported to spend time in both environments to see if they are right for you and to carefully consider your choice and to identify your own areas of competence and areas for development.

RISK IN VALUED OCCUPATION

Concepts of risk and risk taking are not new. Saunders (1998) suggests that by defining the term 'risk taking' we can put it in context. Risk taking can be defined as pursuing a course of action in order to realize a beneficial outcome in the knowledge that there are consequences that would be perceived as negative or harmful in nature should they occur.

Carson (1988) identified that a risk has two significant aspects:

■ *likelihood* – the probability that a particular event will occur
■ *consequence* – the nature of the outcome.

The challenge for us is how people who have a learning disability can be enabled and supported to access valued occupation, taking into account that a certain degree of risk may be inherent in many aspects of daily life. Risk is present for us all in many of the roles and responsibilities we take on. The element of risk in occupation should not in itself automatically inhibit access. We all take risks in our occupational lives, both in an emotional and physical sense. Despite this, there is an overwhelming tendency in services to protect people who have a learning disability from potential harm by reducing exposure to risk. Behind the fear of risk taking often lies an assumption such as 'What if I can't handle the consequences if things go wrong?'. Professional responsibility can also act as a deterrent: 'What if I am blamed if things go wrong?'.

PSYCHOSOCIAL ASPECTS OF HEALTH AND OCCUPATION FOR PEOPLE WHO HAVE LEARNING DISABILITIES

Blaxter (1990) suggests that there are three states of health:

- freedom from illness
- ability to function
- fitness.

In this tripartite definition she identifies health as function and defines this as being 'able to do things'. This theme can be extended by considering functional occupation to be the way in which a person creates balance and finds purpose in life. It provides a means of participating and interfacing in the world in a purposeful way. As suggested in the introduction, it is through purposeful occupation that an individual is able to adapt to, transform and progress within their environment to find personal meaning, empowerment and growth throughout the life stages. Adaptive human occupation is not static, it is a fluid concept that, whilst suggesting constancy, supports the capacity for change and rejuvenation.

Occupations therefore provide continuity in a person's life, what have been termed 'flow experiences' (Csikszentmihalyi 1991, cited in Townsend et al 1997). A sense of flow is achieved when the demands of occupation are in harmony with the person's values and skills. Anecdotally, most of us can confirm that the balance of our occupational roles significantly affects our mental, emotional and physical well-being.

Generally speaking, a person who has a learning disability will not differ in their basic needs, wishes, wants and desires from the non-learning disabled population (O'Brien 1999). Services may be overly cautious in assuming that people who have a learning disability may be unrealistic or extraordinary when making occupational choices. This can lead to the assumption that a certain degree of control or restriction is necessary. In actuality this is rarely the case since on the whole all people of all societies want access to ordinary culturally valued things.

CULTURAL DIVERSITY AND VALUED OCCUPATION

We have already briefly explored the concept of occupation being given meaning by the culture in which a person lives. It is through cultural construction that 'valued occupations are generated which are given shape and significance' (Kielhofner 1995). What we choose to do, the way in which we do it and the setting we choose will be to some extent determined by our cultural attitudes and beliefs.

In a multicultural and multiracial society it is vital that services should be able to appropriately meet the occupational needs of people who have learning disabilities from minority ethnic groups.

Some writers have noted that the thrust towards personal autonomy currently reflected in person-centred planning might not take account of the person's place in the dynamics of the family, which in some communities may be more highly prized than individualism. This may sometimes alienate ethnic minority people who have learning disabilities and their families from services. An example of this is given by Baxter (1998) as 'training for independence'; she cites this as an example of how Western values may conflict with the traditional values of the extended family.

When assisting someone who has learning disabilities from a minority ethnic group to develop meaningful occupational roles, it is important to consider the specific values within the culture from which they derive validation. There may be important gender considerations, for example, with regard to appropriateness of occupations and the place in which they take place. Similarly, there may be significant cultural differences in the way in which tasks are approached.

Occupations must be considered within this context and should be fashioned to meet the cultural needs of the individual where this is relevant or meaningful to the person. This will require providers to be informed about the person's cultural background. However, whilst being culturally competent and sensitive practitioners, we should avoid the trap of stereotyping and cultural preoccupation (Baxter 1998). There is a diversity of attitudes and behaviour in any group (Khamisha 1997a,b). Generalizations about specific racial groups should be avoided, as should formulaic solutions where all decisions are based on cultural differences alone.

ACTIVITY 11.6

Return to your reflections in the introduction and imagine yourself in each of the following scenarios.

1. The only options you have are:
   - working in your hostel's laundry
   - sorting plastic nuts and bolts in the training unit.

2. You have lived at home with your family, your elder brother has gone to university, your younger sister is a mechanic and loves rally driving and you have a passion for working with animals. You meet with your care manager and the only options available to you are:
   - a sheltered training centre offering a mixture of work, education and leisure-type opportunities
   - staying at college part time – no opportunity for working with animals and it is a course specifically for people with special needs.

3. You desperately want to work in a library. You are introduced by your care manager to a supported employment agency, a leisure agency and adult education. You work with these agencies together so how can you fulfil your dream and pursue a GNVQ qualification at the same time?

Which option is preferable? And why? Which option is closest to your own experience? Discuss the options available to a person who has a learning disability: now; 10 years ago; 20 years ago.

SERVICE OPTIONS AND PARTNERSHIPS IN ACTION

There are two aspects to each scenario: first, the number of service options available and second, the development of partnership in action.

The NHS and Community Care Act 1990 heralded the first of those service options. Before this the majority of service options were led by the NHS, Social Services and, to a lesser extent, Mencap, the Shaw Trust, etc. In the last 10–11 years the market became more 'pluralistic', i.e. increasing numbers of agencies offering services, e.g. MacIntyre, Home Farm Trust, SCOPE and Advance. This was helpful and useful in that it reduced the monopoly held by the NHS and Social Services and more creative options have been established.

Short-term breaks	■ in your home, for a day or other period of time
	■ in a short break centre
	■ with a family in their home
Work	■ sheltered environment offering retail experience in a high street
	■ supported employment in a supermarket, department store, factory or library
Leisure	■ art class with other people who have a learning disability also interested in art and design
	■ evening class with a supporter
	■ fishing with a supporter

This has been an important social change in that what may have been 'Cinderella' services have increased 'in-house' options and also support to enable people who have a learning disability to access 'open' options. Options moved from limited and second best to creating a person-centered service.

The last aspect of this has been Partnership in Action which is a recent innovation by the Labour administration. The NHS and Community Care Act advocated pluralism but also a market economy. This set up services to 'compete', in an informal market, with each other for work. This led to an atmosphere of not sharing innovations, mistrust and a lack of knowledge of available options. Partnership in Action has heralded joint projects and communication. For example, a community team recently invited a group of women who had a learning disability to meet for 12 weeks to discuss issues of sexual health and relationships. The women have identified that they would like to pursue personal safety courses; after discussions with the women, joint commissioning, the community team and the employment agency, the employment agency are going to lead this opportunity.

These recent developments, in conjunction with developments in social inclusion, service options and partnership, mean that for a person supported by their circle (at all stages of their life) planning becomes a much more natural (not necessarily easier or less challenging) process with commitment from the person and their circle of support. The Circles Network is a powerful instrument of change; the organisation was started in Bristol in 1993 and now spans the whole of the UK. The facilitator helps the person to identify important relationships and then supports the person and their circle to plan and bring to fruition the person's dreams and aspirations. A circle is made up

| FIGURE 11.3 | *Building inclusive communities (from Wertheimer 1995, with permission)* |

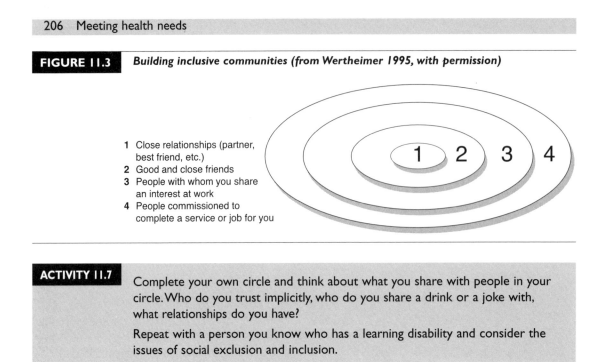

1 Close relationships (partner, best friend, etc.)
2 Good and close friends
3 People with whom you share an interest at work
4 People commissioned to complete a service or job for you

ACTIVITY 11.7

Complete your own circle and think about what you share with people in your circle. Who do you trust implicitly, who do you share a drink or a joke with, what relationships do you have?

Repeat with a person you know who has a learning disability and consider the issues of social exclusion and inclusion.

---

of people who love, care for and know the person well, friends, colleagues, employees, etc. (see Fig. 11.3).

DISCUSSION

It has become clear that in order for occupation to be meaningful, it cannot relate to a series of isolated events that will simply happen to the person, with the provision of well-intentioned support. It is a process of exploration and learning where competency and sometimes mastery in the task or role are developed. We have discussed the importance of flow routines that link the tasks and activities in an individual's life into an integral whole.

When considering the roles we occupy, it is important to be mindful of the components of the role, where it begins and ends. If people who have learning disabilities are to experience true role occupation, it is important to identify the meaningfulness of the role for the individual. It could be argued that unless a person can conceptualize the role that they occupy, it is not possible to fully engage in it. It is therefore not a true role. In these circumstances it is essential that aspects of a role be broken down into achievable and individually meaningful tasks that will support the person to develop an overall understanding of the role being considered. A final consideration on this point is that we do not have to understand something intricately to enjoy and value it, for it to become meaningful to us and for others to recognize it as such.

In order for service providers to support people who have learning disabilities to form meaningful lifestyles, a considerable and focused shift in thinking is required. They must be considered as individuals, with particular needs, wishes, wants and talents. Without careful and intentional planning the person may experience a series of activities that fill chunks of their day, the remainder being 'desert time', where the person is lacking meaningful engagement. Mansell et al

(1987) state this is particularly true where a person may have a series of thera-peutic plans that are programmed to take place throughout the day, the times in between being ignored by services. This becomes particularly relevant where people who have learning disabilities may be living in supported accommoda-tion in small groups. In these kinds of settings there is a risk of the needs of the organization overwhelming the needs of the individual service user. Services should therefore ensure that plans are not service led but truly reflect the needs and desires of the individual. A suggested example of a planning method can be found below.

TOWARDS ENABLING VALUED OCCUPATION FOR PEOPLE WHO HAVE LEARNING DISABILITY

Using a person-centred process, identify how the person would like and needs to spend their time. This typically begins by forming a vision and asking questions of the person.

Consider

- What are their personal values and beliefs?
- What are their dreams and aspirations?
- What are their responsibilities?
- What are they good at?

A story-telling approach may be useful. The person is encouraged to talk about the things they have done in the past, things they do now and what they would like to do. Were/are these of personal value to the person? Are there aspects of the person's life that they would like to change?

The individual and/or people who are closest to them may spend time considering a typical day. What makes a good day? What makes a bad day?

Then think about

- What are the obstacles to the person achieving the things they would like or need to do?
- What are the options available to the person? What opportunities already exist and what needs to be developed?
- What support does the person require to fulfil these roles and responsibilities:
  - direct support?
  - new skills that may be needed?
- Who needs to provide support?
- What physical and social resources does the person need to be available to them? For example:
  - a culturally appropriate environment
  - financial considerations
  - time

- people
- specialist requirements that facilitate and enhance participation.

■ What does the organization need to do to provide optimum support? How does it need to change?

Finally (and only if relevant) consider

■ Are there any negative associations inherent in the person's occupational choices that may inhibit or hinder access to valued occupation?
■ Is the person burdened with a negative reputation that may impact on fulfilment of their occupational desires? (This may already have been highlighted when considering the obstacles to meaningful occupation.)
■ Are there any risks involved in the person's occupational choice?
■ How can we best support them?

Then, support the person to develop their plan for the future

■ Identify timescales and responsibilities
■ Remember that planning is an ongoing process, since a person's life changes and evolves

It is important that people with limited life experience have the opportunity for exploration before making choices and decisions.

In order for plans to be successful, careful monitoring is required. Additionally, it is important to check that they are translated into action, as all too often admirable plans are written but the person's life changes little. Ironically, the more familiar services become with systems of support, such as person-centred planning, the more they may combine them into their routine so that eventually they go by unnoticed and may be eventually seen as unnecessary and even intrusive.

In order to avoid service lethargy, O'Brien (1999) has suggested that whilst planning, providers should ask themselves regularly 'What do I/we need to do?'. Self-reflection and questioning in this way throughout the planning stages will automatically result in steps being taken to ensure that the person will be afforded actual opportunity. This process takes considerable commitment on the part of supporters and an enduring sense of personal responsibility for the part that we play in assisting someone with a learning disability to effect change.

Some exponents of social role valorization have recommended the use of individual activity planning or timetabling in order to ensure that regular and consistent opportunities are available. This method is a focused way of planning the support that services will need to provide in order to ensure that opportunities are in place. They should define the time of day the activity needs to happen and the resources (including staff) that will be required. Activity plans should reflect the individuality of the person, following on from the essential lifestyle plan, and as such are a further way of ensuring action after planning. They are not intended to be inflexible timetables that the individual must adhere to or that reflect the only opportunities that will be available to the individual. A further consideration when planning in this way is the importance of taking into account 'flow routines', discussed previously, that link the chunks of activity into an integral and personalized whole. This part of planning will take account of the actual task, the preparation needed and the components or requirements needed to ensure that opportunities exist for positive engagement as well as the individual's particular style and habits around a task.

Services are increasingly demanded to support people who have learning disabilities creatively and with an enthusiasm for ensuring that human rights are considered as paramount. This requires services to develop a culture of continual improvement and to invest heavily in the training of staff to enable them to support people in an informed and focused manner. Training cannot therefore be considered to be a short-term activity; it is an integral part of service management, making certain that staff attain a level of competence that will secure the quality of the service and support they provide. This should not, however, take place within a 'culture of blame', where there is no room for mistakes. Reflective thinking should be encouraged, alongside positive monitoring of staff. This will involve shadowing staff occasionally and reflecting with them on their thinking and performance in a non-judgemental manner.

When supporting people who have learning disabilities to develop meaningful lifestyles in a resourceful and imaginative way, risk taking and ethical dilemma may be inherent aspects of planning. Services must therefore ensure that solutions are sought that reflect the needs of the person at hand and not the unwillingness of the service provider to put itself in perceived jeopardy. Service providers may feel vulnerable during this aspect of planning and professional courage may be necessary to enable us to support people who have learning disabilities to divert from the perceived norms and take emotional and physical risks occasionally as they arise. That is not to indicate, however, that potential risks should be approached negligently. Careful planning, including potential benefits and harms, should be considered and there are many tools available that can assist in this process.

CONCLUSION

In this chapter the authors set out to take the reader on a reflective journey. The chapter examined and defined the concept of meaningful occupation and introduced the prerequisites, thinking and reflection needed in order to approach the subject in a person-centred manner. The main debate explored:

- definitions of meaningful occupation
- concepts of physical and emotional health and occupation
- the history of occupation in learning disability
- social isolation versus inclusion
- career and life planning
- the importance of debating issues from a legal and ethical perspective
- the importance of respecting and recognizing an individual's culture and ethnicity when supporting them to make plans
- service implications and partnerships in action.

Through a series of activities, the reader has been encouraged to consider their own life and occupational choices alongside those of people who have learning disabilities and the processes involved in establishing 'meaningful occupation'.

It is hoped that through reflection, the reader will be able to identify the steps, thinking and supports necessary to enable a person who has a learning disability to experience, fully take on and maintain a meaningful lifestyle. In addition to this, to be able to identify support strategies and structures that facilitate and respect the right for individuality in the occupational choices that people who have learning disabilities make.

FURTHER READING

Blaxter M 1990 Health and lifestyles. Routledge, London
This book is based on a national survey of 90 000 individuals carried out by an interdisciplinary team at the University of Cambridge Clinical School, investigating issues related to health, health-related behaviour, attitudes and beliefs.

Ewles L, Simnett I 1996 Promoting health, 3rd edn. Baillière Tindall, London
This book sets out to provide a comprehensive, practical guide for all practitioners involved in health promotion. It can be used as a self-teaching guide yet it also provides ideas for group teaching.

Gates B 1997 Learning disabilities, 3rd edn. Churchill Livingstone, London
This is an essential core text for preregistration nursing students and is an excellent reference book for those involved in supporting people who have a learning disability.

REFERENCES

Barton R 1959 Institutional neurosis. John Wright, Bristol

Baxter C 1998 Learning difficulties. In: Rowaff S, Bahl V (eds) Assessing health needs of people from minority ethnic groups. RCP, London

Blaxter M 1990 Health and lifestyles. Routledge, London

Carson D 1988 Taking risks with patients: your assessment strategy. Prof Nurse April: 247–250

Khamisha C 1997a Cultural diversity in Glasgow Part 1: how do we meet the challenge? Br J Occup Ther 60(1):17–22

Khamisha C 1997b Cultural diversity in Glasgow Part 2: are we meeting the challenge? Br J Occup Ther 60(2):73–76

Kielhofner G 1995 A model of human occupation: theory and application, 2nd edn. Williams and Wilkins, Baltimore

Mansell J, Felce D, Jerkins J et al 1987 Developing staffed housing for people with mental handicaps. Costello, Tunbridge Wells

McKnight 1989 In: Finkelstein V Disabling barriers, enabling environment. Open University Press, Milton Keynes

O'Brien J 1999 Lecture at Oxford Learning Disability NHS Trust

Saunders M 1998 Management of risk. In: Pickering S, Thompson J (eds) Promoting positive practice in nursing older people. Baillière Tindall, London

Shanley E, Starrs T 1993 Learning disabilities. A handbook of care. Churchill Livingstone, London

Townsend E, Stanton S, Law M et al 1997 Enabling occupation: an occupational therapy perspective. Canadian Association of Occupational Therapists, Ottawa

Wertheimer A 1995 Building inclusive communities. Circles Network, Bristol

Wilson M 1983 Occupational therapy in long term psychiatry. Churchill Livingstone, London

Wolfensberger W 1975 The origin and nature of our institutions. Human Policy Press, New York

Wolfensberger W 1988 A brief introduction to social role valorization: a high-order concept for addressing the plight of societally devalued people, and for structuring human services, 3rd (revised) edn. Training Institute for Human Service Planning, Leadership & Change Agentry (Syracuse University), Syracuse, New York

12 Sexual health

Damian Dunn

KEY ISSUES

- Sexuality and sexual expression
- Sexual expression as a right
- Needs assessment
- Facilitating healthy lives
- Service accessibility
- Evaluation
- Ethics

INTRODUCTION

In recent years sexual health has been a priority area for those with a health promotion or public health role. In Britain, as in many other affected countries, this has largely been due to fears aroused by the HIV/AIDS pandemic which came to light in the late 1970s. Public health policy in Britain has reflected these concerns (DoH 1987, 1992) and recent statements about the need for a national sexual health strategy demonstrate the importance of this area of work (Jowell 1999).

Much of the response to the HIV/AIDS pandemic has been fuelled by bigotry. Negative attitudes in society such as homophobia, sexism and racism, mingled with an ambivalence towards sex and sexual expression, have made sexual health a difficult area in which to work. Discussion of sexual health issues is something that many people find difficult even in ideal circumstances, so when we contemplate relating these issues to a group of people often stigmatized by their learning disabilities and who are often viewed by many in society as either undesirable or asexual (Anderson 1982), the size of the task can seem quite daunting.

At this point it is important to remind ourselves that people who have learning disabilities have rights which must be acknowledged and realized. Any health promotion work geared to the needs of those who have a learning disability should have a sexual health component if we are taking the kind of holistic approach to health commonly advocated by many writers in the area of health (Maslow 1954, Seedhouse 1986).

WHAT IS SEXUAL HEALTH?

In its strategy document *The health of the nation* (DoH 1992), the Department of Health set out six general sexual health objectives.

- To reduce the incidence of HIV infection

- To reduce the incidence of other sexually transmitted infections
- To develop further and strengthen monitoring and surveillance
- To provide effective services for diagnosis of HIV and other STDs
- To reduce the number of unwanted pregnancies
- To ensure the provision of effective family planning services for those people who want them

A quick glance at these objectives reveals their rather limited scope. This is a view of sexual health which suffers from being oriented towards very narrow, largely medical preoccupations. They also reflect something of an obsession with what can be measured, as this can transferred into numbers and percentages, which has a certain appeal to the scientific mind. How meaningful they are is, however, open to debate (Porter 1992). It could be argued, quite justifiably, that sexual health has as much to do with having a fulfilling sex life, which allows sexual expression, as it has to do with absence of infection or unwanted pregnancy.

A more comprehensive view of sexual health is provided by the World Health Organization (1986a). It defines the three essential components of sexual health as:

- a capacity to enjoy and control sexual and reproductive behaviour in accordance with a social and personal ethic
- freedom from fear, shame, guilt, false beliefs and other psychological factors inhibiting sexual response and impairing sexual relationships
- freedom from organic disorders, diseases and deficiencies that interfere with sexual and reproductive functions.

If the appropriateness of the DoH sexual health targets can be criticized in relation to the population at large, how much more inappropriate are they for those people who have learning disabilities? Before concerns about gonorrhoea and unwanted pregnancy are considered, more basic issues concerning the right to recognition as a sexual being must often be addressed. For an individual who has a learning disability, being allowed to masturbate without fear of censure may be a much more important issue than having an understanding of the routes of HIV infection.

Sexuality in its fullest sense incorporates such things as sensuality, personal relationships, political affiliations, physical activity (i.e. sport), social and cultural oppression and sexual orientation. It involves a good deal more than sexual attraction and sexual practice. This more comprehensive view of sexuality is represented in Figure 12.1 (Adams & Painter, unpublished, 1998) and is much more in keeping with the holistic approaches now advocated in understanding health issues, whether they be personal or social. It recognizes that human beings are complex organisms inseparable from their environment and that psychological and social factors play as central a role in a person's well-being as their physical state (Hinchliff et al 1993).

It follows from this that sexual health problems or frustrated expression of sexuality are likely to have a negative effect on the totality of an individual's health experience, which can adversely affect their quality of life. An understanding of sexuality is therefore central to understanding sexual health.

We express our sexuality in a variety of ways from our infancy through to old age (Dixon 1992). This is as true for those who have a learning disability as

FIGURE 12.1   *The sexuality flower (from Adams & Painter 1998, unpublished, with permission).*

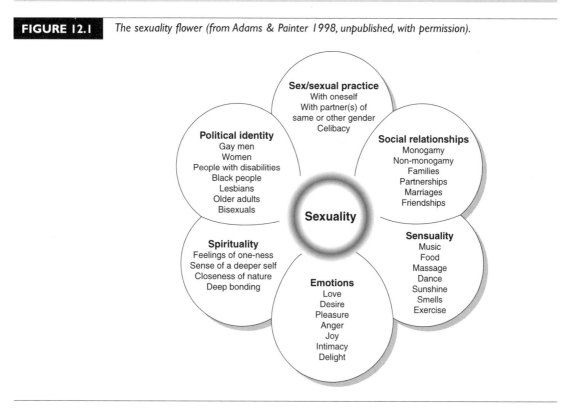

it is for others. How we support the sexual expression of those who have learning disabilities will form a significant part of this chapter.

SEXUAL HEALTH AND RIGHTS

In 1975 the United Nations defined the rights of disabled people in the following way.

> Disabled persons have the inherent right to respect for human dignity. Disabled persons, whatever the origin, nature and seriousness of their handicaps and disabilities, have the same fundamental rights as their fellow citizens of the same age, which implies first and foremost the right to enjoy a decent life, as normal and as full as possible.
>
> (UN 1975)

The right to express one's sexuality and meet one's sexual needs is implicit in this statement. However, as with many rights acknowledged in UN declarations, the gap between theory and practice is immense. This can be clearly seen if we look at what this right is supposed to mean in more detail.

Organizations working with those who have learning disabilities have formulated more specific rights due to their clients. Mencap incorporates the following charter into its staff induction pack.

> People with a disability have a right …

- to be informed of, advised about and supported in making choices in daily living
- to be treated with dignity and respect
- to be accepted as an individual with feelings and emotions
- to be accepted as a person with a past, present and future
- to have cultural, religious and social values respected
- to have sexuality and personal relationships respected
- to be consulted about important decisions and have personal opinions respected
- to be protected from exploitation and neglect
- to have access to all medical and professional services according to individual needs, e.g. dental, chiropody, speech therapy, physiotherapy, etc.
- to have training, support and opportunities to be helped towards independence.

(Gillett & Greenwood 1995)

Realizing these very laudable ideals is fraught with problems, most of which relate to the level of ability and autonomy of those who have a learning disability. This can vary tremendously. It is fair assumption that most people who have mild to moderate learning disabilities will find it easier to realize these ideals than those who have severe or profound levels of disability. How we determine an individual's level of ability is the next point to consider.

WHO ARE WE TALKING ABOUT?

If we take a broad definition of the term, individuals who have a 'learning disability' can be affected by anything from a hearing impairment to cerebral palsy. For the purposes of this chapter we will be focusing on those people who are affected by intellectual impairment or, more precisely, those people who are in a 'state of arrested or incomplete development of mind which includes severe impairment of intelligence and social functioning' (DoH 1982).

Other authors in the field of sexual health education have described the general characteristics of those affected by learning disability as:

... likely to include a decreased ability to make use of informal, unstructured social and sexual learning opportunities. They do not pick up cues, ask questions or acquire information from friends in the same way that other youngsters do. This is often compounded by the often very sheltered lives that students lead outside of school hours.

(Craft et al 1996, p 11)

Although the above statement was made specifically in relation to young people who have learning disabilities attending full-time education, similar problems of awareness and autonomy exist for adults with similar issues. Clearly, sexual health needs, and approaches to meeting those needs, can be influenced by an individual's level of ability. This means that the needs of each individual must be carefully assessed before any useful interventions can be undertaken.

HOW DO WE ASSESS NEED?

Before any meaningful health promotion work can be undertaken, it is advisable to assess the needs of the group or individual at whom it is aimed. There is a potential problem here, in that needs can vary depending on the perspective of those assessing them. Typically, health need can be viewed from four conceptual standpoints (Bradshaw, cited by Ewles & Simnett 1996): normative, felt, expressed and comparative need.

Normative need

Normative need refers to need as defined by a professional or an expert in a particular field of work, determined by their profession's ethos and value system. Problems can exist when these professionally defined needs conflict with those of the service user. There is an assumption within society as a whole that people who have a learning disability are asexual and therefore do not have the right to a fulfilling sex life. For many individuals who live with their parents or within residential services, this can result in a form of oppression, whereby people do not develop expectations that they will engage in intimate relationships. In addition, they do not experience opportunities in which this can take place and as such do not always learn the skills that support developing intimate relationships and fulfilling sex.

An additional issue for professionals working with people who have a learning disability is the understandable desire to protect clients from potential harm or exploitation. This may be reinforced by professional codes which identify the need to protect individuals in the care of the professional from any harm, either as the result of an act of commission or omission. A family planning nurse, for example, may believe that an injectable form of contraception (or even sterilization) is desirable for a young woman with a learning disability because of the perceived problems associated with a pregnancy. The client, on the other hand, may find the idea of pregnancy leading to parenthood very appealing and may want to choose other contraceptive options that allow her more immediate control over her fertility. The normative values of the practitioner, combined with his or her power in relation to the client, could in these circumstances lead to a very unsatisfactory outcome for the client.

Further problems can arise when different organizations working with a particular individual or group have different priorities resulting from their different professional ideologies. Nurses, for example, have a set of guidelines which should inform their work with clients who have a learning disability (UKCC 1998) as do social workers (BASW 1996). Slight differences of emphasis may exist between these two sets of professionals and this can cause problems. In the case of parents who have a learning disability, conflicting objectives may occur between those professionals working on a community team for people who have a learning disability, the health visitor and the child's social worker. The essence of this conflict would be based around the person at the focus of care delivery with the health visitor and the child's social worker primarily concerned, responsible and accountable for the child's well-being. The learning disability professionals are likely to be primarily concerned with the needs of the parent.

Felt need

This type of need is felt by an individual or group and often leads to them wanting something to meet it. Awareness of what is available can affect felt needs so that, for example, a woman who has learning disabilities who masturbates using the neck of a shampoo bottle may suddenly feel the need for a vibrator following an education session in which sex toys and their use are discussed. Of course, in this instance she may encounter the negative attitudes and values of significant others, whether carers or professionals, who may find the idea of using sex toys quite distasteful. The challenge for all practitioners working with people who have a learning disability is to develop strategies or processes that enable people to communicate their felt needs, thus translating them into expressed need.

Expressed need

An expressed need is a need (often a felt need) that has been given a voice in the form of a demand or request. So, if the woman cited in the example above was to ask for a vibrator, this would become an expressed need. Of course, not all felt needs are expressed as many people are unable to express their needs in any way other than in services that they are familiar with or believe are available to them. For example, this woman may well have expressed the need for a vibrator because she perceived that this would be a way in which services would be able to assist her. Further exploration with her may identify her felt need to be the need for a partner and an intimate and fulfilling sex life.

Additional difficulties that may be experienced by people who have a learning disability are those of communication and perceived power bases. The woman in our example may not have the assertiveness or communication skills to be able to give expression to her felt need, nor feel that she is in a position to do so. This problem may be compounded if organic damage has affected her ability to communicate effectively. In a situation like this it may be appropriate for an advocate to speak on her behalf. An advocate who has a long-standing relationship with a client is likely to have a good understanding of the client's needs and may be able to support the service user in expressing their needs and wants.

As we have already seen, it is not uncommon for the expressed needs of an individual or group to be in conflict with the normative needs of professionals.

Comparative need

This need is ascertained by comparing two or more similar groups. Essentially this means that if one group receives a service and a similar group does not then a comparative need exists. An example of this can be clearly seen when considering access to antenatal services. This service is made available to all women and therefore any woman who does not receive this would be seen as having a comparative need. A further example can be seen within the area of cervical smears, as this is also a service available to all women. However, for women who have a learning disability, this service is not easily accessible. Whilst acknowledging the complexity of gaining informed consent for such a complex and invasive procedure, it has to be noted that the failure to provide this service to women who have a learning disability identifies a very clear comparative need.

Matching personal and professional perspectives of need

Looking now at how these various types of need can interact, we can see that there is potential for the development of a dialectical relationship between professionals and clients who have a learning disability and/or professionals and carers. A dialectical relationship between the feelings that carers have for those who have a learning disability and the social roles they are cast into also often exists (Wolfensberger 1984). Educational materials dealing with these conflicting sets of interests are available and can be useful as discussion starters when working with carers and clients (West Lambeth HPS 1992).

Crucially, when assessing health needs professionals often need to remind themselves of the rights of clients as cited above. Failure to do this can result in an apparently thorough and systematic assessment of need from the perspective of the professional or service provider that bears no real relevance to the needs and wants of the service user. Collaboration and partnership with clients whereby they are supported to lead the agendas in relation to assessment, planning and all subsequent stages of care delivery is essential. Achieving this can be a significant challenge when working with service users who do not have intentional verbal communication, particularly in relation to sexual health. However, it is important that the needs of this group of people are not negated on the basis of communication difficulties.

Some useful needs assessment materials do exist in the area of sexual health. One training pack produced for work with clients has a checklist of topics, from differentiation between male and female bodies to assessing a person's ability to use a condom correctly (O'Sullivan & Gillies 1993). However, this particular pack was designed for use with clients who have moderate learning disabilities and may need to be adapted for use with those who have a more severe disability.

A client who has multiple and profound learning disability is likely to find it extremely difficult to express their felt needs. This sets a considerable challenge to any person assessing the sexual health need of this group of people. The use of Makaton signs is problematic, as the available vocabulary is not adequate and British Sign Language is also of very limited use. A close examination of the *Dictionary of British Sign Language* will in fact reveal that there are no signs given for sexual organs and hardly any for sexual activities (Brien 1992). In order to explore needs relating to sex and sexual expression, a specialist collection of signs should be used – for example those in *Signs of a sexual nature* (Coleville 1985).

In situations like this, normative attitudes and beliefs of both professionals and carers become even more significant. If the attitudes of those people supporting the client in this situation are that sexual health needs are not a priority, then the client may find it extremely difficult to get their needs acknowledged and acted upon. Indeed, they may well find themselves in a state of enforced asexuality.

Good practice, then, should involve practitioners and carers making every possible effort to discover the views and feelings of the client and putting those before their own reservations. This is one of those situations where practitioners need to remind themselves of the bill of rights presented at the beginning of this chapter and those that other organizations have developed.

However, it seems likely that any thorough needs assessment will comprise elements of all of the above. A triangulation of felt/expressed needs, normative and comparative needs will provide a good baseline on which to plan work.

WHAT HELPS PEOPLE STAY SEXUALLY HEALTHY?

Most theoretical models of health promotion have been developed over time and can be justifiably applied to any aspect of health. They do, however, have a normative outlook and assume a certain level of intellectual development. This can pose problems for people who have learning disabilities and a brief examination and critique of these models is appropriate at this point.

There are many factors that interact to produce a healthy person. Some factors are genetic, some environmental, some relate to the beliefs held by individuals and some are to do with attitudes and values they possess. The possession of life skills and wealth is also very significant in determining a person's health experiences.

The health action model as developed by Tones (Tones & Tilford 1994) has been a very influential conceptualization of the factors leading to actions conducive to health. It identifies three behavioural responses – routines, quasiroutines and discrete single-time choices – which are influenced by three systems – those of beliefs, of motivation and the normative system – and mediated by facilitating or inhibiting factors (Fig. 12.2).

A routine behaviour is one that has become habitualized, often as a result of socialization (Tones & Tilford 1994). A good deal of health promotion activity is geared towards encouraging healthy habitualized behaviours. From a professional carer's point of view it may be desirable for a client to use a condom every time they have vaginal/anal sex. This could be considered healthy habitualized behaviour.

Some older clients who have spent many years in institutionalized care may have been subject to normative experiences which are considered undesirable in other situations. Same-sex relationships may have been commonplace in institutional settings. Same-sex activity of this sort could be described as quasiroutine in the context of the health action model described above. This is because quasiroutine '... describes a situation in which a particular practice (healthy or unhealthy) is so pervasive that the individual is unaware that a choice is really possible' (Tones & Tilford 1994). People who have learning disabilities who have experienced institutional care may provide particularly good examples of this mechanism at work. This could have implications for the likelihood of adopting safer sex practices in the future, particularly in relation to anal intercourse. The client's normative system may allow for anal intercourse. Their belief system may be telling them that this is how sex is for everyone and their motivation system may be influenced by the pleasure they

FIGURE 12.2   *The health action model (from Tones & Tilford 1994 with permision).*

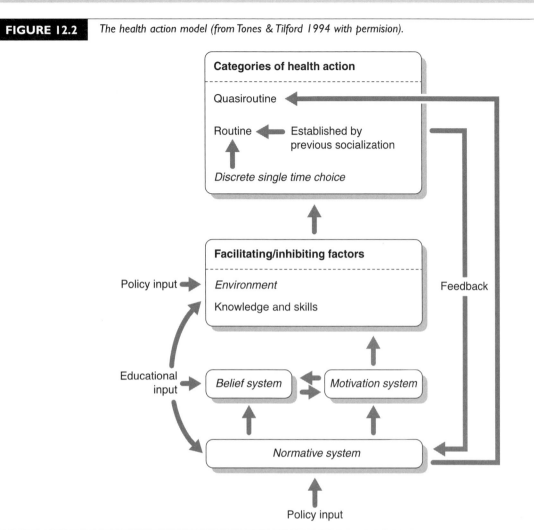

experience. This might be a very uncomfortable thing for professionals to acknowledge but it may be true nonetheless.

Clearly, from the sexual health perspective of a professional, it may be desirable to bring about changes to this behaviour but from the point of view of the client, there may be no need to alter behaviours that he or she finds quite acceptable. The normative needs of the health professional may clash with the normative quasiroutine of the client in this instance.

The last type of health behaviour to be considered in relation to the health action model is the discrete single-time choice. This refers to '... a single specific decision' (Tones & Tilford 1994, p 92). An example of this in relation to sexual health may be that a woman who has learning disabilities attends her GP practice for a cervical smear test. Her experience of attending the surgery may then affect her future actions. If the experience is a good one and she is treated well, there is a greater likelihood that she will attend again. If, however, her experience is unpleasant or frightening, she may decide never to repeat it.

FACTORS WHICH INFLUENCE DECISIONS ABOUT HEALTH

So much, then, for the potential health actions of an individual client. Let us now examine the factors which influence these decisions by starting with the systems which underlie them.

The normative system incorporates the prevailing cultural, power and socioeconomic deadwood of the past and has a significant effect on the sexual health experiences of all people in any given society. Some feminists might, and do, argue that patriarchy, which views women as chattels to be used or disposed of as men see fit, has a negative influence on the normative system in relation to the sexual health of women. If women are possessions then they can be justifiably used for sexual gratification by male partners, including fathers or brothers.

Cultural influences are particularly important in understanding the development of beliefs and normative elements of social life. These influences can be 'big' ones, which can be generalized throughout society, or 'small' more specific influences relating to subgroups within society. Religious beliefs, for example, can have a very strong bearing on moral judgements relating to sexual expression. Judeo-Christian culture may have a different perspective to Islamic or Buddhist orthodoxy.

The culture of professional groups can have secondary socialization influences on individuals who join them. The attitudes and values of individuals who become nurses or social workers are likely to be influenced by the normative cultural outlook of that particular group. These influences on big and small culture are very significant factors affecting sexuality and sexual expression.

Policy inputs to protect women and girls, such as laws prohibiting sexual abuse, are offset by long-established social mores which devalue women in relation to men and a general acceptance that it is normal and right for men to be in positions of power. Sexist attitudes of this type have remained remarkably resilient in the face of the much-vaunted 'girl power' of our times.

Policy factors such as equal opportunities legislation can have a positive effect on the self-esteem of marginalized groups. This in turn can have a positive effect on the normative system and could enhance the quality of life of those who are disadvantaged largely as a result of socially constructed concepts of disability. Having access to good-quality sex education and life skills training in special schools (where many people who have learning disabilities are educated) is initially a policy issue, which then needs to be translated into good practice by caring or teaching staff. In this way normative values can be changed positively and the right of those who have learning disabilities to have access to this type of information is taken for granted rather than seeming inappropriate.

Moving on now to look more closely at the belief system, it is possible to observe the effects it has on health behaviour. It has been argued (Tones & Tilford 1994) that the most important set of beliefs influencing health behaviours are the beliefs individuals hold about themselves. These beliefs collectively form an individual's self-concept. In particular, an individual's perceived susceptibility is of great significance because this affects their judgement of risk.

Throughout the 1980s and 1990s many sexually active people made few if any changes to their sexual behaviour (HEA 1997) despite the gloomy predictions of the WHO (1992) and widely disseminated information on HIV transmission, which showed quite clearly that sexual activity was by far the most significant route for HIV transmission between individuals, most of whom, if looked at in a global context, are heterosexual.

This information was offset by a widely held belief that only homosexual men were at risk of HIV infection. This led to a situation in which many people did not believe that they were susceptible to the HIV virus because of their sexual orientation. Even after almost 20 years of HIV/AIDS awareness education, there still remain many sexually active, non-monogamous heterosexuals who will not acknowledge their susceptibility to this condition. Consequently the adoption of safer sex techniques by the general population has been very slow.

If we now try to relate this fact to people who have a learning disability, the problems are obvious. For many such people it will be even more difficult to undo or unlearn inaccurate information about susceptibility due to their level of intellectual impairment. If, as seems likely, they have never been given the opportunity to discuss the variety of sexual expression open to human beings and weigh up the relative risks associated with different sexual activities, they are much more prone to misunderstanding and consequently may be unable to grasp their potential susceptibility to infection or pregnancy. The critical ability to treat information with justifiable scepticism is often underdeveloped in clients who have learning disabilities, with soap operas and tabloid newspapers being invested with an inordinate amount of credibility.

Another important element of the belief system concerns the concept of self-efficacy. This relates to an individual's belief in how much personal control they have over factors which affect their lives. An individual with an external *locus of control* (Rotter 1966) will perceive themselves as being at the mercy of outside factors and individuals over which they have no control or influence. This is likely to have a disempowering effect and can lead to them being resigned to what they see as their fate. They believe that their self-efficacy is minimal and that they are at the mercy of forces which are beyond their control.

Once again, if we think of the number of agencies and individuals who are likely to have a say in how people who have learning disabilities conduct their lives, we see that there is a considerable risk that such negative beliefs relating to self-efficacy will be commonplace. This is one reason why promoting and encouraging the empowerment of clients is so important and why it should be the *leit motif* of all relationships between professionals, carers and clients. Only through encouraging a sense of autonomy and self-reliance can self-efficacy be fostered. Any group of staff working in this field should understand this and make serious efforts to place this approach at the centre of their relationship with clients. For this reason, Mencap are careful to spell out its importance in their staff training manual, which is worth quoting in detail.

To help others to become empowered we need to ...

- teach decision-making and action-taking skills
- encourage people to explore their own ideas and feelings about their life and lifestyles
- accept that we cannot protect people from all of the risks and consequences that arise from informed choices

- stand back from controlling people who have a learning disability
- encourage people to think about the risks and consequences of their decisions and actions.

(Gillett & Greenwood 1995)

The authors of the above principles go on to point out some of the dilemmas intrinsic to this approach, most importantly the temptation to protect people from the consequences of what professionals may perceive to be bad choices. This has to be balanced with the desire to promote independence and encourage growth in the client. These dilemmas are difficult to resolve and will be discussed further when we examine ethical issues later in the chapter.

The third system, already mentioned in passing but worth further elaboration as part of the health action model, is that of motivation, which has been described as '... a complex of affective elements which ultimately determines an individual's attitude to the specific action and his or her intention of adopting it' (Tones & Tilford 1994).

This complex includes values, attitudes and drives. Values are sets of beliefs with an affective character acquired as a result of socialization. They refer to particular aspects of experience. Strong religious values could, for example, influence sexual behaviour. A person who has a learning disability could become involved in an exploitative sexual relationship because of the value they place on the relationship with their exploiter.

Attitudes have been defined in the following way: 'An attitude represents a person's general feeling of favourableness or unfavourableness towards some stimulus object ...' (Fishbein & Ajzen 1985). Values can spawn a whole host of attitudes. If, for example, a person who has a learning disability places a negative value on monogamy this is likely to affect their attitude to having multiple sexual partners. This obviously has implications for their sexual health. If this same person places a high value on penetrative sex, it is unlikely that they will be open to safer sex techniques which place emphasis on oral sex or mutual masturbation.

It follows from this that positively influencing values from an early age is key to creating the base on which the superstructure of a healthy individual is built. The most significant individuals influencing person's values are those with most contact with the developing child, usually the parents. Policy inputs at this stage could include parenting skills training and providing good respite and counselling support services for parents/carers.

The training of professionals working closely with such families should place due emphasis on helping carers to understand the importance of their attitudes in shaping the attitudes of the developing child and how these attitudes, once acquired, can either positively or negatively affect the sexual health experiences of the child for the rest of their lives.

The third set of factors to consider as part of the motivation system are drives. These have been described as being for the most part inherent and species specific and include such things as hunger, pain and, more importantly for our discussion, sex (Tones & Tilford 1994). The strength of these drives is often underestimated by those with a health-promoting role. Even those with strong moral beliefs, values and attitudes can be overwhelmed by the drive for sexual gratification. The most pious of individuals, of whatever religious persuasion, is likely at some stage of their life to wrangle with sexual drives which could lead them into fornication or adultery!

All of the above factors are intrinsic to the individual. They are components of consciousness or awareness but they are not static and can be influenced by external factors. In psychodynamic terms, the *superego* represents the more acceptable, civilized, altruistic elements of the human psyche, with the *id* represented by drives, passions and hedonistic self-gratification. Most human beings are subject to this moral/drive dialectic as part of their conscious life. It could be argued that people who have a learning disability, particularly those who have multiple and/or profound disabilities, are less likely to have the same constraints on drive-initiated behaviour. This may be as a result of organic damage to the higher centres of the cerebral cortex, the areas of the brain with which we associate 'personality' aspects of our being. They are, moreover, the areas of the brain which we associate with intellect and moral/ethical judgements.

The point here is that the drive element of motivation may be unconstrained by the counterbalancing values and beliefs acquired through the processes of socialization. This could lead in some circumstances to the types of behaviour which cause embarrassment, for example starting to masturbate in a public place or inappropriate touching. The drive to spontaneously express sexual need is acted upon without thought for the appropriateness of the behaviour. This is not only embarrassing for carers but can bring the client into conflict with the law or potentially dangerous conflict with members of the public. A good deal of sexual health work with people who have learning disabilities is about appropriateness of behaviour, for this reason. This can be achieved by appropriate educational interventions and policy inputs.

So far much of our discussion has focused on the individual client and factors which are internal to them, such as beliefs and motivation, though the point has been made that these systems are influenced strongly by the normative system, which is a social construct. We will now consider the effects of facilitating/ inhibiting factors as part of the health action model (Tones & Tilford 1994).

It is an educational and developmental truism that the environment, with which we interact on a daily basis, will influence the type of person we are and the way in which we behave. This assumption has been intrinsic to health promotion since the Alma Ata declaration (WHO 1978) and was reaffirmed as part of the Ottawa Charter (WHO 1986b).

Creating environments that are conducive to health is as important a task for those with a health-promoting role as positively influencing beliefs, attitudes and values. We have touched on the importance of environment in creating a positive healthy environment when we examined the normative system but it is worth pursuing this further. Public policies, such as equal opportunities legislation, help to create an environment which is more fair and equitable for all. This has benefits for everyone but particularly for those who may have previously been subject to either covert or overt discrimination. They help to create more positive and inclusive 'normative' values.

Creating an environment in which sexuality and sexual issues are discussed openly and freely is likely to facilitate better sexual health. Educational and residential settings serving those who have learning disabilities need to appreciate this and incorporate it into their ethos. The home environment too can be affected positively, by ensuring that parents/carers are given adequate support on sexual health issues.

Statutory and voluntary services have a responsibility to make themselves accessible to those who have a learning disability. Cervical cytology services, family planning services and genitourinary medicine (GUM) services need to ask themselves how easy it would be for someone who has a learning disability to get the most out of what they have to offer. What aspects of these particular environments could be improved to increase uptake of the services they provide?

Of course, in order to access a GUM service and get the maximum benefit from it a client would need certain levels of knowledge and possibly quite highly developed life skills. A lack of communication skills, for example, could lead to difficulties when trying to find out the session times for the service. An even greater obstacle would be a lack of awareness that such a service exists. Knowledge and skills therefore are essential and can be influenced positively by providing good educational inputs for clients.

The clinic environment can also facilitate good sexual health by treating clients who have a learning disability on an equal footing with those who do not. A disapproving attitude on the part of staff members is unlikely to be helpful from the client's point of view. Training and education of frontline staff is the issue here.

Service providers should also create a physical environment which is conducive to use by those who have a learning disability. Those clients who have mobility problems as well as learning disabilities need to be catered for. Badly designed buildings can present an insurmountable barrier to some of those wishing to access the service.

THE HEALTH ACTION MODEL

If we now attempt to tie all of the above points together by looking at a particular example we can see how all of these factors relate to, and influence each other.

CASE STUDY 12.1

Let us imagine a young woman who has a learning disability who has been sexually active from her very early teens and who has never had a cervical smear test. This is not unlikely, since we know from recent research that people who have a learning disability are less likely to visit their GP and that very few of them have regular cancer screening checks (Mencap 1998).

The young woman in question may have been neglected by primary care staff because of incorrect assumptions about the level of her sexual activity. This may be compounded by the fact that she does not see the necessity for a smear test because she is not used to visiting her GP (*normative system*). In addition, her previous experiences of treatment at the hands of her GP may have been quite negative, affecting her willingness to attend (*motivation system*).

A lack of educational input regarding cervical cancer may mean that she does not see herself as being susceptible to cancer because she does not smoke and that smoking causes cancer (*belief system*). This scenario does not augur well for the sexual health of our client.

However, even if we assume that she is able to overcome the systems impediments she is confronted with, she may then encounter a service which is difficult for her to access because of the attitudes of her GP and practice nurse (*environmental factors*) and her inability to express her felt need due to a lack of confidence in the face of professionals who may be playing down her concerns (*assertiveness skill*). Therefore her discrete single-time choice, to have a cervical smear test, is unattainable.

It could be argued that all the inhibiting factors in the above example could be overcome if carers and professionals took their health-promoting role seriously and made a sustained effort to equip this young woman with the skills, attitudes and knowledge necessary to facilitate a more positive outcome.

EFFECTIVE HEALTH PROMOTION INTERVENTIONS

Most people reading this chapter will have a desire to work more effectively with clients in an effort to improve the sexual health aspects of their lives. Individual workers are most likely to be interested in aspects of health education and skills acquisition of relevance to individual clients or to small groups of clients. They may also have an interest in how to influence, in a positive way, the relevant policies of the organizations or institutions in which they work. It is worth considering these interventions at this point.

The Ottawa Charter (WHO 1986b) has already been mentioned in passing. However, we will take a closer look at the main points of the charter, as many would say they form the basic principles on which good health promotion practice is built. The charter identifies five key elements which, in theory at least, should be synergistic.

- Healthy public policy
- Supportive environments
- Community action
- Individual skills
- Reorientate health services

Healthy public policy should help to create a climate wherein sexual health issues are given the priority they deserve. As we have already seen in our discussion of the health action model (Tones & Tilford 1994), public policy influences the normative system and the environment in which discussion and practice concerning sexual health take place. A good deal of this policy is formed by institutions outside the health sector in the fields of economics and politics (Katz & Peberdy 1997).

The campaign to being down the age of consent for homosexual sex is a good example of public policy and its implications for sexual health. It is obviously absurd to have an age of consent for heterosexuals which is different from that for homosexuals. This discrimination helps to foster a set of values and attitudes in society at large which can have a damaging effect on the self-esteem of those who are sexually attracted to members of the same sex. It is also likely to give tacit approval to homophobic attitudes and create a climate of fear and shame for anyone outside the 'normative' heterosexual majority. This is hardly conducive to good sexual health.

A normative climate of this kind can lead to certain homosexual activities becoming furtive and hurried. The classic activities of this sort are cottaging and cruising which are often conducted without a great deal of negotiation and are often unsafe in sexual health terms (Aggleton et al 1991). It could be argued that a more tolerant or broader normative set of values concerning sexual expression would help obviate the need for risky sexual encounters in public environments. However, the same authors also point out that one of the attractions of sex in public environments is the element of risk involved which adds a certain *frisson* to the activity.

Sexual health policies may be desirable for organizations and institutions working with clients and carers. Their ethos could, and some might argue must, be based on the principles enshrined in the United Nations *Declaration of the Rights of Disabled Persons* (UN 1975) already cited. These rights are spelled out in more specific terms in the staff training induction manual developed by Mencap (Gillett & Greenwood 1995).

As well as making sexual issues acceptable things to talk about, policy should make services more accessible and equitable. This should be an aim for all primary and secondary services (NHSE 1998). For those people who have learning disabilites who often spend a certain amount of their time in the 'care of professionals', policies should exist on such things as intimate care, to minimize the chances of sexual exploitation of clients. Such policies exist in many organizations but not all.

Sexuality policies that recognize the right of an individual to form relationships of their choosing can be of use in some settings. This is an empowerment issue. There may be occasions when carers are tempted to discourage relationships that they believe are not in clients' interests, particularly a same-sex relationship. It may be that the carer is being influenced by their own disapproval of such relationships rather than thinking of the client's best interests, though that may be the rationale given by the carer. Training, which involves an element of values clarification, can be the starting point for policy development in relation to sexuality.

Moving on now to consider knowledge and skills requirements, certain points need to be made. Having conducted an appropriate needs assessment of the individual client or group of clients, we can plan a package of interventions to meet these needs. Depending on the disability a client has or their level of confidence, they may be able to express their own sexual health needs, using one of the needs assessment questionnaires already mentioned (O'Sullivan & Gillies 1993) or one tailored to the particular needs of a client or group of clients.

It is clearly very difficult to use this approach with clients who have multiple and/or profound levels of disability, for reasons we discussed in the section on needs assessment, and in these instances the level of need may be determined (rightly or wrongly) by carers who have a close daily relationship with the client and who may have observed behaviour which they believe may be the result of frustrated sexual expression. The classic observed behaviour in many situations is that of masturbation or inappropriate touching of others.

There are materials available in relation to these issues for working with clients who are profoundly disabled. They can offer suggestions and give guidance (Craft 1992, Downs & Craft 1998, McCarthy & Thompson 1996).

Caring staff may base their judgement of need on comparison, as previously discussed in the section dealing with needs assessment. They may have worked in other settings where sexual health issues and sexual expression are higher up the agenda than in their current situation. This may lead to them wanting to extend good practices brought from their previous working environments. Such staff are also likely to be influenced by their own attitudes, values and beliefs and the normative aspects of needs assessment discussed earlier.

So, what are the important issues likely to be? Many of the needs likely to surface from a good needs assessment will relate to gaps in knowledge, including such basic issues as body awareness, relationships and how to form them, gender differences, sexual awareness and exploration. At a slightly more sophisticated level issues such as contraception, sexually transmitted diseases, safer sex practices, how to use sexual health services, etc. will also be of importance.

The importance of skills acquisition cannot be overestimated in this work. Knowledge of the importance of contraception is of little use if the skills to access it from provider services are absent. In this particular case it may be lack of communication skills which is the problem. To give another example, if a man who has learning disabilities wants to use a condom for penetrative sex due to his anxieties about HIV, but his sexual partner does not, then there is an assertiveness issue here. Any lack of assertiveness skills on the part of the client could lead him into unsafe sexual activities, which could have negative consequences for him.

Other useful social skills training looks at issues relating to appropriateness of behaviour and how to approach and form relationships with people. Those interested in how to conduct this education can now quite easily find resources to help them. Many of the resources cited above will provide ideas to take this work forward but there are many others and catalogues of useful resources are available.

How carers approach this work will very often be determined by the issues arising in a particular environment. In some situations it may be thought unnecessary to plan a comprehensive sexual health education programme, very often due to lack of time. More often, both formal and informal carers find they are reacting to a particular problem.

Another aspect of the Ottawa Charter worthy of discussion is that of community action. The term 'community' in this context refers to a body of people with a set of common characteristics, in this case their shared learning disabilities, rather than a geographical location. Supporting self-help groups is a valid health promotion activity for carers. Political and lobbying activities to demand equity of service provision or access to information are very empowering experiences for those involved and are likely to enhance self-esteem and a sense of self-efficacy. As has already been argued, these are significant factors in accessing health services.

The idea of 'supporting' a self-help group may seem like an oxymoron but encouraging the establishment of such groups, and encouraging client participation in them, is a valid health promotion activity. Carers and professional staff do need to curb any tendencies to take charge or impose their own agenda but can offer advice when asked for it. The crucial element in this approach is the sense of empowerment engendered within the group. This can lead to very useful outcomes.

The first UK-produced video/training pack dealing with sexual health issues for people who have learning disabilities came about due to the establishment of such a group (West Lambeth HPS 1992). The characters in the video are all adults who have learning disabilities and the issues explored are very true to life. This is an excellent example of what can be achieved by people who have learning disabilities who take up an issue of importance to them and then tackle it in their own way. This is in keeping with the ethos outlined in the Mencap staff induction manual referred to above (Gillett & Greenwood 1995).

The reorientation of health services is the final aspect of the Ottawa Charter to be considered. In practice this means that services should develop a more health-promoting ethos and be less curatively focused. The medical model of health should be seen as it is, with its emphasis on curative rather than preventive services.

To achieve this reorientation of health services means challenging the power of the medical profession. It could be argued that they have a vested interest in keeping things as they are and find it difficult to overcome the medical model prejudices they picked up in medical school. Health promotion is often quite low on the agenda of the medical profession and their understanding of what it entails can be quite woeful, though examples obviously exist which disprove this, as illustrated in *Signposts for success* (NHSE 1998).

The accessibility of services is another important aspect of their reorientation. One of the findings of Mencap's research *The NHS – health for all?* (Mencap 1998) was that people who have learning disabilities do not access services as readily as members of the general population. This may in part be due to the physical difficulties of accessing some services and partly due to the attitudes of staff encountered when a client gets through the door and their sensitivity or lack of it (NHSE 1998). Education and training on disability issues and communication/interpersonal skills are important aspects of increasing accessibility.

Of course, all the above measures require the commitment of adequate levels of funding. The NHS now consists of a series of businesses, often competing with one another for increasingly scarce financial resources. In an environment like this, those who shout the loudest and make the most fuss are more likely to have their needs met than those who do not assert their rights so forcefully and yet often have greater needs. This phenomenon, known as the inverse care law (Tudor-Hart 1988), is certainly not a new one but its existence is an affront to any notion of equity.

Carers of those who have a learning disability have a role in all these elements of the Ottawa Charter, whether it be helping to develop life skills with clients, developing relevant policies, providing education or supporting self-help groups. The key word in relation to all this work is empowerment.

EVALUATING HEALTH PROMOTION

The extension of good practice is one of the aims of health promotion. It follows from this that health promotion activity of any sort should be evaluated to see if it met the criteria for success determined at the outset. The evaluation of health promotion activities should be discussed at the planning stage and not tagged on to the end as an afterthought, as so often happens.

There are two main categories of evaluation: outcome or summative evaluation and process or formative evaluation (Aggleton et al 1992). Outcome evaluation relates to outcomes or outputs of particular pieces of health promotion activity. This type of evaluation is a measure of how effective activities have been. So, for example, if a particular health promotion activity was to ensure that men attending a day centre were given educational input relating to testicular self-examination and their knowledge at the end of the session was greater than it had been at the beginning, then the activity could be said to have been successful in terms of outcomes.

Process evaluation, on the other hand, is more concerned with how things were done. This could relate to the techniques employed as part of the activity. This in turn will often reflect the ethos of the group involved. If, for example, a group of health professionals decide to carry out a sexual health needs assessment on a group of people who have learning disabilities but do not take account of the expressed needs of the group or involve them in any way, then it could be argued that this is a flawed piece of work and that the process was flawed.

Evaluation is important for several reasons. Outcome evaluation is often important in sustaining a piece of work over a period of time. Those providing the funds or staff time necessary for a particular piece of work will usually want some evidence that it is being effective before committing themselves to further involvement. Process evaluation may be needed to assess how well particular inputs or approaches have done in achieving a particular outcome.

Most evaluations of health promotion activity should have both. Even the evaluation of a training workshop should take into account the methods used to convey information, such as group work, didactic methods, etc., as well as assessing any gains in knowledge or changes in attitudes.

So when embarking on any health promotion activity, decide what the desirable outcomes are and then think about the most appropriate process for achieving them. Remember, of course, that monitoring the process throughout is useful (Downs & Craft 1998) because then if something does not appear to be working other methods can be employed.

LEGAL AND ETHICAL ISSUES

Many professional carers are reluctant to tackle their clients' sexual health issues. In some situations this is due to genuine fears and concerns relating to the legality of certain activities (Gunn 1996). On other occasions, raising concerns about the legality of such work is a convenient smokescreen behind which to hide, particularly if staff are reluctant to tackle a subject with which they are not comfortable.

Clear policies relating to sexual health issues in formal settings are very useful in creating a secure environment in which clients can develop and staff can work effectively. As we have already discussed, the development and constant review of policy is an essential part of sexual health promotion.

Philosophical and moral issues often arise in any area of health promotion activity but work which involves sex and sexual expression raises particularly visceral concerns. It goes without saying, then, that guidance on how to resolve ethical dilemmas is useful in finding a safe way through what can be something of a minefield. In this respect the 'ethical grid' devised by Seedhouse (1988), and illustrated in Figure 12.3, is very helpful.

In Seedhouse's view several questions need to be asked in relation to any proposed health promotion activity.

- Does it safeguard equity and respect and further the creation of autonomy?
- Will the activity do good and avoid harm?
- Are the consequences of the action likely to be good and if so, for whom?
- How does the activity measure up to external considerations, such as weight of evidence, legal responsibilities or risks?

The grid can be used to assist carers in answering these questions. If we now try to illustrate the application of the grid to a realistic situation we can see how it might work in practice.

| FIGURE 12.3 | Seedhouse's (1988) ethical grip (reproduced from Seedhouse 1988 with permission of John Wiley publishers). |

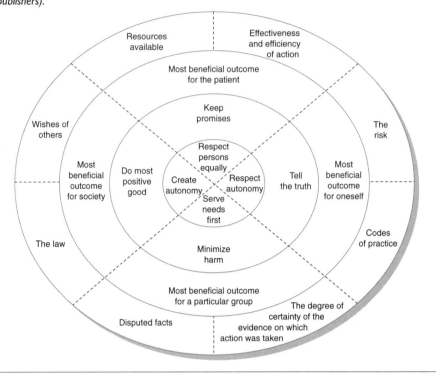

| CASE STUDY 12.2 | **A practical test for the ethical grid** |

A group of young people who have a range of learning disabilities are invited to take part in a discussion which will examine issues around mutuality and exploitation within personal relationships.

After the preliminary introductions, the group are shown a series of line drawings which show people in a range of intimate encounters and are asked to comment on the amount of mutuality or exploitation revealed by the body language and facial expressions of those represented.

One of the drawings shows a young woman in an intimate embrace with an older man and it is evident from the expression on her face that she is not happy with the situation. In fact, the drawing shows quite clearly that she is frightened and considerably distressed by the experience.

Halfway through the session a coffee break is taken and one of the young women in the group takes the opportunity to disclose to a group leader that her father has been forcing her to have sex with him for some time. She is obviously quite distressed.

As a result of her disclosure Social Services become involved and investigate the validity of her claims. This takes some weeks of difficult interviews with parents and various agencies, the outcome of which is that her claims are found to have been true in all probability.

However, her parents are very angry with the workers who set up the original workshop and the Social Services department, and refuse to let her attend any more sessions or take part in any other social activities which the group have arranged, causing more distress to the young woman involved. The police and Crown Prosecution Service become involved and charges may be brought against the young woman's father.

The question to be asked is whether or not this piece of work can be justified from an ethical standpoint. After all, the young woman obviously has feelings for her father and clearly loves him. She is also very confused by her present situation and is very sad to be unable to go back to the group, as many of the members are her friends.

Did this health promotion activity safeguard equity and respect and further the creation of autonomy?

It could be argued that dealing with this subject matter ensured that the group were allowed access to information which they had previously found difficulty in obtaining. This information is useful and is the sort of information which people who do not have learning difficulties take for granted. As part of the process of normalization, then, it is a sound piece of work and was allowing a certain amount of equity with the population at large.

It is also empowering in that it emphasizes that relationships and behaviours which individuals find distressing or unpleasant do not have to be tolerated and they can take measures to stop them. By emphasizing the self-efficacy elements of assertiveness, the group members are encouraged to take more control of their own destinies.

Will the activity do good and avoid harm?

This is far from straightforward. The young woman in our example has asserted her right to choose who she has sexual relations with and it is hoped that any further exploitation of her will be more difficult. However, the trauma of her disclosure and the effect it will have on her relationships with both of her parents are certainly negative consequences. Where the balance falls between harm and good in this respect is likely to be a subjective judgement.

Are the consequences of the action likely to be good and if so, for whom?

The consequences of this particular activity are a mixture of negatives and positives. The young woman in question is likely to have her relationship with her father damaged, certainly in the short term and possibly in the longer term. She is also likely to suffer as a result of her parents' unwillingness to let her attend any more sessions of a group which she had quite clearly enjoyed. On top of this her father may be prosecuted at some point which may be highly stigmatizing for the family.

On the positive side of the equation, she has been able to take a very difficult step by disclosing her abuse. This, it could be argued, came about because of the supportive environment created by the workers organizing the group. She has now taken a certain amount of control over her situation and has therefore been empowered to a certain degree. This is in accordance with the principles of good practice set out at the beginning of the chapter.

On the whole, it could be argued that the long-term consequences of the health promotion activity are likely to be good. The young woman may have learned something about exploitation and mutuality which will stand her in good stead for her future life.

One possible negative consequence, however, may be that the staff involved in the initial session may be frightened off further activities due to fears of uncovering more unpleasant issues which they find personally challenging.

How does the activity measure up to external considerations, such as weight of evidence, legal responsibilities or risks?

In terms of the activity itself, evidence exists which testifies to its validity. Many of the available resources for work with people who have learning disabilities use line drawings and photographs as ways to start discussion on a range of sexual health issues (Craft 1992, Downs & Craft 1998, McCarthy & Thompson 1996, O'Sullivan & Gillies 1993).

The activity is not in breach of any law and does not infringe the rights of anyone involved. However, it could be argued that there is a certain amount of risk associated with this approach. Whenever work of this kind is undertaken there is a risk that uncomfortable or difficult feelings will emerge. In most circumstances this is a justifiable risk when set against the benefit which will ensue. In this particular case, then, it would seem that the work undertaken passes the ethical criteria set out in the ethical grid.

CONCLUSION

The promotion of sexual health for this group of clients is fraught with difficulties but the existing body of theoretical knowledge can help those interested in this field of work to be effective in their interventions.

The central themes of rights and empowerment should provide the ethical framework for any work undertaken. Equity of service provision is an issue for policy makers and for those who have a learning disability. Service providers must ensure that their services are accessible and those who have a learning disability have a responsibility to lobby for improvements where these are deemed necessary:

- Carers should be supportive of those who have a learning disability but should not be controlling, however difficult this may be.
- Knowledge issues concerning such things as body awareness, sexual awareness, relationships, sexual relationships, service availability, HIV/AIDS, sexually transmitted diseases and contraception need to be addressed.
- Skills such as assertiveness, communication, decision making and how to use a condom must be part of any programme of activities.
- Both professional and home carers can have a positive effect on the long-term sexual health of those they care for but they too will have training needs that have to be met.

Above all, a sense of respect for people who have learning disabilities is essential. Altering our perspective and seeing human beings with needs but also with positive qualities and things to offer society is crucial. Only in this way can we help to improve the sexual health experiences of clients and be able to offer them the quality of life which others, not similarly disabled, very often take for granted.

FURTHER READING

Ewles L, Simnett I 1996 Promoting health: a practical guide. Baillière Tindall, London
This is an excellent book for anyone working in a practical setting who wishes to begin approaching health promotion with clients or other colleagues. Nurses and social workers who have regular contact with people who are learning disabled will find it particularly useful.

Gunn M J 1996 Sex and the law. Family Planning Association, London
This book is a very useful guide through the minefield existing around the legal culpability and responsibility of people who have learning disability and their carers, in relation to sexual expression and sexual behaviour. It is very accessible and is an ideal reference source for anyone wishing to engage in sexual health promotion.

Seedhouse D 1988 Ethics: the heart of healthcare. John Wiley, Chichester
An understanding of ethical considerations is essential to all healthcare practitioners. This book provides a framework to help people unravel some of the difficult ethical dilemmas with which they can be confronted. The ethical grid is a useful tool which can be used to this end.

Tones K, Tilford S 1994 Health education: effectiveness, efficiency and equity. Chapman and Hall, London
Anyone wanting to understand the theoretical assumptions and perspectives that underlie health promotion practice is well advised to read this book. It provides a vital presentation of the need for synergy in different areas of health promotion work.

REFERENCES

Aggleton P, Jordan S, Stoakes P, Wilton T (eds) 1991 Outreach work with men who have sex with men. Southmead Health Authority, Bristol

Aggleton P, Moody D, Young A 1992 Evaluating HIV/AIDS health promotion. Health Education Authority, London

Anderson C 1982 Teaching people with mental retardation about sexual abuse prevention. CA Network Publications, Santa Cruz

Brien D (ed) 1992 Dictionary of British Sign Language/English. Faber and Faber, London

British Association of Social Workers 1996 The code of ethics for social work. BASW, Birmingham

Coleville M 1985 Signs of a sexual nature. Cheshire Deaf Society

Craft A 1992 Nottinghamshire SLD sex education project. Living your life. Learning Development Aids, Cambridge

Craft A, Stewart D, Mallet A, Martin D, Tomlinson S 1996 Sex education for students with severe learning difficulties. Health Education

Department of Health 1982 Mental Health (Amendment) Act 1982. HMSO, London

Department of Health 1987 AIDS Control Act. Department of Health, London

Department of Health 1992 Health of the nation. Department of Health, London

Dixon H 1992 Chance to choose. Sexuality and relationships education for people with learning difficulties. Brook Advisory Centre, London

Downs C, Craft A 1998 Sex in context. Pavillion Publishing, Brighton

Ewles L, Simnett I 1996 Promoting health: a practical guide. Baillière Tindall, London

Fishbein M, Ajzen I 1985 Belief attitude, intention and behaviour: an introduction to theory and research. Addison-Wesley, Reading, Mass

Gillett E, Greenwood C 1995 Making the most of life. Royal Society for Mentally Handicapped Children and Adults, London

Gunn M J 1996 Sex and the law. Family Planning Association, London

Health Education Authority 1997 Health update – sexual health. Health Education Authority, London

Hinchliff S M, Norman S E, Schober J E 1993 Nursing practice and healthcare. Edward Arnold, London

Jowell T 1999 First ever government strategy on sexual health launched. Proceedings of the Family Planning Association Annual Conference, 23 March, London

Katz J, Peberdy A (eds) 1997 Promoting health: knowledge and practice. Open University Press, Milton Keynes

Maslow A 1954 Motivation and personality. Harper and Row, New York

McCarthy M, Thompson D 1996 Sex and the 3 R's: rights, responsibilities and risks. Pavillion Publishing, Brighton

Mencap 1998 The NHS – health for all? People with learning disabilities and healthcare. Royal Society for Mentally Handicapped Children and Adults, London

National Health Service Executive 1998 Signposts for success. Department of Health, London

O'Sullivan A, Gillies P 1993 You me and HIV. Daniels Publishing, Cambridge

Porter M 1992 Promoting sexual well-being. Family Planning Today, first quarter.

Rotter J B 1966 Generalized expectancies for internal versus external control of reinforcement. Psychological Monographs – General and Applied 80(609):1–28

Seedhouse D 1986 Health: the foundations for achievement. John Wiley, Chichester

Seedhouse D 1988 Ethics: the heart of health care. John Wiley, Chichester

Tones K, Tilford S 1994 Health education: effectiveness, efficiency and equity. Chapman and Hall, London

Tudor-Hart J 1988 A new kind of doctor. Merlin Press, London

UKCC 1998 Guidelines for professional practice. UKCC, London

United Nations 1975 Human rights: a compilation of international instruments. UN, New York

West Lambeth Health Promotion Service 1992 My choice, my own choice. South East London Health Promotion Service, London

Wolfensberger W 1984 A reconceptualization of normalization as social role valorization. Mental Retardation 34(2):22–26

World Health Organization 1978 Alma Ata declaration. WHO, Geneva

World Health Organization 1986a Concepts for sexual health. EUR/ICP/MCH 521. WHO, Copenhagen

World Health Organization 1986b Ottawa charter for health promotion. World Health Organization, Health and Welfare Canada, Canadian Public Health Association, Ottawa

World Health Organization 1992 Current and future dimensions of the HIV/AIDS pandemic: a capsule summary. WHO Global Program on AIDS, Geneva

13 Mental health

Steve Moss and Pauline Lee

KEY ISSUES

- How do we define mental illness in a person who has learning disabilities?
- Are the risk factors for mental illness greater than for the general population?
- What is the true prevalence of mental health problems in this population?
- The relationship between psychiatric disorders and challenging behaviours
- Obstacles to assessment and practical steps to overcoming them
- Identifying mental health problems in the community
- Mental health problems across the lifespan
- Appropriate treatments

INTRODUCTION

The mental health of people who have learning disabilities is a topic which has come to increasing prominence over the last 15 years. There is now a growing recognition of the need to respond more adequately to mental health problems in this population, with a number of countries developing specialist training and clinical services, as well as devoting significant resources to research in this field. While considerable effort is now being put into the development of better mental health services for people who have learning disabilities, there are still major obstacles to overcome. Indeed, the problems of recognizing, diagnosing and treating mental health problems in people who have learning disabilities, many of whom cannot give a clear account of their subjective experiences, challenge our fundamental concepts of mental illness.

DEFINING MENTAL ILLNESS

Although most of us have a concept of mental illness, we are likely to disagree about those individuals who are mentally ill. This reflects the fact that psychiatric conditions are to a large extent socially defined and hence highly interactive with the context in which the person lives. Certain social situations seem more able to contain or deal with the psychiatric symptoms than others, while other social situations may actually produce or exacerbate such symptoms. Most of us have had the experience of 'things getting on top of us', although in most cases we manage to cope with the help of our support networks. Goldberg & Huxley (1980) have discussed the factors which determine whether someone with a neurotic disorder becomes a psychiatric 'case'. They point out that the severity of symptoms is not necessarily directly related to degree of incapacity or interference with day-to-day life. Both interpersonal factors and external social factors may determine whether a given set of symptoms results in presentation to a doctor.

Most mental disorders, even the very severe disorders such as schizophrenia, do not have clearcut biological bases for their origin. True, schizophrenia tends to run in families, so we know there is some genetic component, but genetic predisposition does not seem to be enough to ensure that a specific individual contracts the illness. Also, schizophrenia can have so many different symptoms that a non-expert could easily assume that two cases had completely different disorders. The same goes for depression and anxiety. Some people suffer panic attacks, others lose their self-confidence and others lose their ability to do things they once enjoyed. Frequently, people suffer from a wide range of symptoms relating to a variety of these disorders.

Defining mental illness in people who have learning disabilities is further complicated by the issue of challenging behaviour. Problem behaviours are common in the population of people who have learning disabilities and are frequently the subject of psychiatric referrals. Although it is clear that there is an association between challenging behaviours and psychiatric problems, there are many cases of challenging behaviour which have nothing to do with mental illness. Indeed, one of the major issues facing the field of learning disability psychiatry is to develop a better understanding of the true association between these different types of disorders. This particular issue will be discussed more fully in a later section.

For the purposes of focusing the discussion in this chapter, the definition of a mental disorder furnished by the American Psychiatric Association is probably a good starting point.

> A clinically significant behavioural or psychological syndrome or pattern that occurs in an individual and that is associated with present distress (e.g. painful symptom) or disability (i.e. impairment in one or more important areas of functioning) or with a significantly increased risk of suffering death, pain, disability or an important loss of freedom ... Whatever its original cause, it must currently be considered a manifestation of a behavioural, psychological or biological dysfunction in the individual. Neither deviant behaviour (e.g. political, religious or sexual), nor conflicts that are primarily between the individual and society are mental disorders, unless the deviance or conflict is a symptom of a dysfunction in the individual, as described above.
>
> (American Psychiatric Association 1994, p xxi)

RISK FACTORS FOR MENTAL ILLNESS

Mental health is inextricably bound up with quality of life issues. A good quality of life tends to protect us from mental illness and minimize the severity of illness when it does occur. Indeed, most of us have so many supportive elements contributing to the overall quality of our lives that we are probably unaware of their influence, unless circumstances remove them from us. The strength of these supports is such that the vast majority of mental illness in the community can be dealt with by the individuals themselves and their carers and in most cases does not come to the attention of mental health services. Obviously, the more severe and debilitating the condition, the more likely that medical help will be sought. However, there are many factors apart from severity of the condition which determine whether outside help is sought. Broadly speaking, these are the same factors which contribute to our quality of life in the absence of mental illness, e.g. the amount and quality of social support which is available to the person, the amount of stress in the person's life, the presence or absence of additional physical illness, and the effectiveness of the person's coping mechanisms.

Most of us are in the fortunate position of being able to take for granted our basic life quality, perhaps only questioning it at times when stress or major negative life events affect us. However, this is not true for all persons. Many people who have learning disabilities, even if they have a good quality of life now, continue to suffer from the effects of their past life. Others may continue to live in adverse circumstances, having little integration with the wider society, perhaps having few friends, and no contact with their family.

Apart from these social risk factors, the development of behavioural and psychiatric disorders in people who have learning disabilities also reflects the interactions between complex genetic, chromosomal, perinatal and environmental factors. These may all have a significant impact on brain development and thus on the pattern of intellectual and social development shown by the person. In addition, they may have direct and indirect influences on the person's vulnerability to develop psychiatric disorders and/or challenging behaviour. Obvious examples include high rates of Alzheimer's disease in people with Down's syndrome (Dalton 1995, Dalton & Wisniewski 1990); severe self-injurious behaviour in people with Lesch–Nyhan syndrome (Oliver & Head 1990); overactivity in people with fragile X syndrome (Murphy 1994); and overeating and severe obesity in people with Prader–Willi syndrome (Holland 1991).

It is important to remember that the *level* of learning disability can be an important factor when considering the individual's mental health needs. In people who have severe or profound learning disabilities, mental health problems are likely to relate primarily to complex neurological, genetic and other biological abnormalities. People who have mild or moderate learning disabilities, on the other hand, are likely to demonstrate to a greater extent the impact of social risk factors, e.g. parental rejection, long-term institutionalization, impoverished social networks, lack of self-esteem, etc. Eaton & Menolascino (1982) and Reiss (1982) reported that people who have learning disabilities are subject to a wide range of emotional disturbances and that depression has been shown to be associated with a low level of social support (Meins 1993) and a high level of stigmatization (Reiss & Benson 1985). Moss (1999a) has discussed the importance of the person's wider ecology in supporting and maintaining their mental health, and drawn attention to the impoverished ecosystem of many individuals who have learning disabilities. It is quite clear that many people, not just those who have disabilities, have life circumstances which are far from ideal. Boredom, monotony, lack of a sense of autonomy, the stress of increasing job insecurity, family breakdown – these are all factors contributing to mental health problems in the community. The crucial difference from most people who have learning disabilities, however, is that most of us have compensating aspects which make up for our problems. Thus, one might have an unfulfilling job but a rewarding and supportive home life. One's job may be stressful but may afford good status, high self-esteem and an income which can help make the rest of life more comfortable. When compensating factors are absent we are at greatest risk.

Specific life events can also have an impact on mental health, people who have learning disabilities being particularly vulnerable because of their reduced ability to conceptualize and to express their feelings. For instance, the inability to share and express grief has been reported as leading to the development of an affective psychosis (McLoughlin & Bhate 1987). There is also a risk of exploitation and abuse, which can result in mental health problems. Varley (1984) presents the cases of three young women who developed schizophreniform psychoses following sexual assault.

PREVALENCE OF MENTAL HEALTH PROBLEMS

Review articles have noted a wide variation in reported prevalence rates in people who have learning disabilities, Campbell & Malone (1991), for instance, reporting that prevalence rates varied from 14.3% to 67.3%. There are two main reasons for this lack of consistency. First, different methodologies lead to markedly different results. In particular, studies relying on routine clinical assessment techniques tend to produce much higher estimates than studies employing standardized methods of data collection using rigorously applied diagnostic criteria. The second reason is the uncertain status of challenging behaviour. Since behaviour problems are so prevalent in people who have learning disabilities, the criteria for their inclusion or exclusion as mental health problems can have a large effect on measured prevalence. Generally speaking, prevalence studies that have only included symptom patterns which meet clear diagnostic criteria for psychiatric conditions tend to produce much lower estimates of morbidity compared with those studies which include challenging behaviours. Unfortunately, many studies have not clarified their criteria to a degree sufficient to make comparisons with other estimates.

Across the spectrum of mental disorder, evidence from large-scale studies of morbidity does suggest that the pattern of prevalence is somewhat different from the general population. Table 13.1 gives a comparison between two extensive studies of morbidity, one relating to the general population (Bland et al 1988) and the other specifically to people who have learning disabilities (Lund 1985). It can be seen that the general population shows a much higher prevalence of substance abuse disorders, affective disorders and neuroses. People who have learning disabilities are reported as showing higher rates for psychoses and autism and a very high rate for behaviour disorders.

PSYCHIATRIC DISORDERS AND CHALLENGING BEHAVIOUR

In the UK, challenging behaviours are the most common reason for which people who have learning disabilities are referred to a psychiatrist, accounting

TABLE 13.1	Comparison of prevalence figures (excluding dementia) for persons who have/do not have learning disability

General population*		Associated DSM IV codes	Mentally retarded**	
Diagnostic category	Prev. %		Prev. %	Diagnostic category
Alcohol abuse	5.4	F10.0–10.9	0.0	Substance abuse
Drug abuse	1.7	F11.0–19.9		
Schizophrenia/ schizophreniform	0.3	F20.0–29	6.3	Schizophrenia/ psychosis of uncertain type
Austism†	0.04	F84.0–F84.12	3.6	Autism
Manic episode	0.1	F30, F31, F34		
Major depression	3.2	F32, F33	1.7	Affective disorder
Dysthymia	3.7	F34.1		
Phobia	5.1	F40.1, F40.2		
Panic	0.7	F40.0, F41.0	2.0	Neuroses
Obsessive/compulsive	1.6	F42.0		
Antisocial personality	1.8	Not comparable	10.9	Behaviour disorders

* Bland et al 1988
** Lund 1985
† Ritvo et al 1989

for a third of the admissions from the community (Day 1985). A similar trend has been noted in the USA (Jacobson 1998). There is, however, considerable uncertainty regarding the relationship between challenging behaviours and psychiatric disorders. This uncertainty arises partly because of the lack of clarity surrounding the definition of these various constellations of behaviours and symptoms and partly because of the lack of basic research into the topic. Understanding the possible links between these defined constellations is important, not just from a theoretical perspective but also because a greater understanding may lead to the subsequent development of more effective treatment approaches (Emerson et al 1999).

Behaviours which come to be regarded as 'challenging' are, by definition, behaviours which transgress social rules. Whether a particular behaviour will be 'challenging' will be based on complex interactions between what the person does, the setting in which they do it and how their behaviour is interpreted or given meaning. Given this complexity of factors, challenging behaviours are likely to range widely in their form and in the psychological and/or biological processes which underlie them. The determinants of challenging behaviour are poorly understood and are in many cases likely to be highly complex – a combination of factors relating to: history of learned behaviour, biological, environmental, social and psychological factors. As such, they often do not fit the established criteria for diagnosable psychiatric conditions (Corbett 1979). Indeed, it is probable that behaviours often have multiple causation (e.g. a challenging behaviour exacerbated by a coexisting psychiatric disorder or a psychiatric disorder expressing itself partly in terms of a challenging behaviour). In order to understand the complexity of factors it is thus crucial to distinguish true psychiatric disorders from problems arising from other causes, e.g. due to an environment which is poorly matched to the person's level of adaptive skills. At present, the majority of diagnostic instruments for mental health problems do not make it possible to tease out these various factors (Edelbrock Costello 1988). It is to be hoped that more sophisticated assessment models, with the power to make these complex analyses of behaviour, are developed in the future.

Regarding the nature of possible links between challenging behaviour and psychiatric conditions, there is some evidence that psychiatric disorders may in some cases underlie or exacerbate problematic behaviour.* Thus, for example, recent evidence suggests that some forms of self-injurious behaviour may be associated with obsessive–compulsive disorder (Bodfish et al 1995, King 1993) and that fluctuations in mood state associated with affective disorders may provide the motivational basis for other forms of self-injury (Sovner et al 1993). A number of studies have also suggested that challenging behaviours may sometimes be symptoms of affective disorders. Reid (1982), for example, suggests a variety of clinical features which may be indicative of depression among people whose level of disability makes it difficult to verbalize their feelings. These features include somatic symptoms (e.g. headache and abdominal ache), hysterical fits, agitation and disturbances of physiological functions such as sleep, appetite and bowel movements. More recently, Meins (1995) showed that, in people who have more severe disability, the severity of existing behaviour problems was higher in the presence of depression as defined by DSMIIIR criteria. He points specifically to the diagnostic significance of aggressive and self-injurious behaviour, stereotypies, screaming and spontaneous crying. Similarly, Reiss & Rojahn (1993) found levels of depression to be evident in four times as many aggressive as non-aggressive subjects. Jawed et al (1993) describe the case of a man who has severe learning disabilities whose pica became uncontrollable during episodes of depressive illness.

ASSESSMENT OF MENTAL HEALTH PROBLEMS

The diagnosis of mental disorders, whether in the general population or in people who have learning disabilities, depends on the interaction of a variety of factors: what the person states they are experiencing, what others say about them, how they are seen to behave and the history of their complaint. For many people who have learning disabilities the first of these factors is usually limited because of reduced linguistic ability and is often totally absent. As a result, the diagnostic process becomes reliant on third-party reports and observations. The consequence of this is that the validity of diagnosis for non-verbal people is most uncertain (Moss 1995, Moss et al 1996).**

---

* For a more extensive discussion of the relationships between challenging behaviours and psychiatric disorders, see Emerson et al (1999).

** Lack of space precludes detailed description of the theoretical issues relating to diagnosis. For a detailed discussion of issues relating to assessment, see Moss (1999b).

Practical approaches to assessment

In order to facilitate a thorough diagnostic and treatment formulation, clinical mental health assessments of individuals who have learning disabilities should seek to integrate information from a wide range of relevant sources (Reiss 1982, Szymanski 1988). A multidisciplinary assessment may include clinical opinions from a psychiatrist, other specialist medical professionals (e.g. neurologist, geneticist), psychologist, social worker, nurse, behaviour therapist, speech/language pathologist, staff and family members. The main areas that are typically covered in a mental health assessment of an individual who has learning disabilities include: a thorough review of the individual's history (e.g. medical, psychological, behavioural, ecological, social and psychiatric details), psychiatric interview with individual (mental status examination, physical examination), interview with carers and at least a 2-week period of data collection (e.g. observations, mood charting, behavioural charting, etc.). The following outline is drawn from an assessment model used by a specialist learning disabilities mental health team in Vancouver, Canada. It shows the steps involved in a multidisciplinary assessment leading up to the formulation of the diagnosis.

Referral

Typically, individuals who have learning disabilities are referred for a mental health assessment by a carer or family member. It is rare for an individual who has learning disabilities to self-refer him or herself for an assessment. Usually, the reason for referral is some deterioration or change in the individual's behaviour which has caused some distress. Given that usually the referral has been made by a third party, the team needs to ensure that the individual is in agreement with the referral. Similarly with children, where referrals to mental health professionals are often made by parents, it is impractical to expect the individuals themselves to seek treatment or to recognize a problem in themselves.

First meeting

The purpose of the first meeting is to allow the individual who has learning disabilities and their carers to meet with the core team of professionals (e.g. psychiatrist, nurse, psychologist, behaviour therapist, social worker) who will likely be involved in the assessment. Before this meeting, a package of forms will have been sent out to the individual and carers, asking for details on demographics, reason for referral, brief history, and current situation (e.g. residence and employment). The meeting provides an opportunity for the individual and their carers to describe in detail the nature of the referral problem and their expectations from the outcome of the assessment. This particular discussion usually allows the assessment team to evaluate the relative significance of the referral problem to the individual compared to the carers. At this meeting the assessment team also has the opportunity to describe and explain the process of the assessment, detail the information to be collected and discuss consent issues.

FIGURE 13.1   *Stages in the assessment process described in the text.*

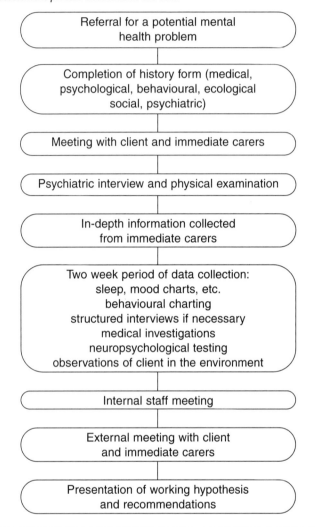

Assessment phase

With so many potential sources of information, it is beneficial to have a primary therapist assigned to the case who can be responsible for coordinating all the information. The primary therapist is also a key person who can summarize and present all the information to the assessment team. It is important that the collection of data follows a structured format (such as Gardner's (1996) multimodal model).

History review

The value of a thorough history review cannot be overestimated. Many individuals who have learning disabilities have difficulty recalling their personal histories, yet crucial information such as hospitalizations, family history of psychiatric illnesses, changes in patterns of behaviour, changes in living situations, specific educational difficulties, etc. are important in providing a full clinical picture. Such information is often sought by retrieving past records from institutions, hospitals, schools and day centres and by interviewing families and carers. It is important to obtain longitudinal information on behavioural and mental health symptoms. (This particular assessment team had developed specific history forms for this purpose.)

Interview and examination

Given the difficulties of assessing and diagnosing mental health problems in people who have learning disabilities it is not surprising that considerable attention has been devoted to the development of assessment schedules. In terms of instruments designed to detect a broad spectrum of disorders, the Psychopathology Instrument for Mentally Retarded Adults (Matson et al 1984) was one of the first to achieve recognition. The Diagnostic Assessment for the Severely Handicapped (DASH) scale (Matson et al 1991) provides, as its name suggests, a schedule which is specifically designed for use with people functioning in the lower end of the ability spectrum. A somewhat different approach is taken by the Psychiatric Assessment Schedule for Adults with a Developmental Disability (PAS-ADD) (Moss et al 1993, 1997) which is a semi-structured interview using operationally defined diagnostic criteria (Spitzer et al 1978), based on the Schedules for Clinical Assessment in Neuropsychiatry. The instrument produces research diagnoses and involves present-state interviewing of the patient, followed by a similar interview with a key informant. Either interview can detect symptoms and produce diagnoses, so the PAS-ADD can also be used for the assessment of individuals whose linguistic ability does not permit a clinical interview.

In terms of initial case and symptom identification the Reiss screen (Reiss 1987) has achieved widespread use, particularly in North America. The scale includes not only psychiatric symptoms but also items on aggressive and self-injurious challenging behaviour and items relating to dependency and assertiveness. In the UK, the Mini PAS-ADD (Prosser et al 1998) and the PAS-ADD Checklist (Moss et al 1998) have been designed with the specific aim of improving case recognition through a two-level filtering system.*

A number of broad-spectrum diagnostic instruments have also been developed for children and adolescents who have learning disabilities. The Adolescent Behavior Checklist (Demb et al 1994) is a self-report scale for use by adolescents who have mild or borderline learning disabilities. The Child Behaviour Rating Form (Aman et al 1996, Tasse et al 1996) is an informant rating scale for use by parents and teachers.

In addition to these broad-spectrum instruments, schedules have been specifically designed to diagnose depression. The Beck Depression Inventory (Beck et al 1961) and the Zung Self-Rating Depression Scale (Zung 1965) have been simplified and adapted for use with learning-disabled individuals by Kazdin et al (1983). The Hamilton Rating Scale for Depression (Hamilton 1960) has also

---

* For information about the PAS-ADD instruments contact Dr Steve Moss

been used with members of this population. More recently, a number of researchers have reported successful use of the informant version of the Children's Depression Inventory with adults who have learning disabilities (Benavidez & Matson 1993, Meins 1993).

Despite the availability of these tools, it is common practice for clinicians not to use any structured interview schedule. The main reason is probably because these instruments have mainly been devised for non-psychiatrists. Rather, they can be valuable in collecting detailed information on day-to-day behaviour, information which can only be known by the people who live and work alongside the individuals who have learning disabilities.

In general, it is important for the clinician to gain enough information about the individual to get an idea of their past and current life situation and previous mental health and behavioural difficulties. It is helpful if the interview follows a clear structure and to be aware that the pace of an interview with an individual who has learning disabilities tends to be slower than normal. It is important for the clinician not to readily accept answers to questions but to make further inquiries to ensure that the individual has fully understood the questions being asked. To help make the individual feel relaxed and at ease, the clinician may begin by asking questions about their interests, what they enjoy doing and what they consider are their strengths. Usually after this stage the clinician is more able to access information about mental health symptoms and behavioural difficulties from the individual (Russell & Tanguay 1996).

In situations where the individual is non-verbal or severely impaired, an interview can still be conducted. Communication can be facilitated with the use of pictures, drawing, play materials and gesturing. While it may be difficult, and at times impossible, to access detailed information about the individual's feelings, through the process of interaction the clinician will gain insight about the individual's mental status and ability to relate to others.

A physical examination of the individual also plays an important role in identifying the presence of key symptoms such as dysmorphic features, abnormal thyroid, signs of self-injurious behaviour and presence of tardive dyskinesia and extrapyramidal side effects.

Interviewing staff and carers

It is essential to interview staff and/or carers about their knowledge and observations of the individual's mental health symptoms and behavioural difficulties. Such investigations provide additional information about the individual interacting with different people in different settings. The interviews also provide another opportunity for the assessment team to evaluate staff and carers' attitudes and tolerance to the individual and their difficulties.

First internal meeting

Once the history review, interview and examination of the individual and interviews with staff and carers have been completed, an internal meeting with the members of the multidisciplinary team is held to examine all the information. Following an established structure to review the information in all the domains (e.g. psychiatric, psychological, medical, ecological, behavioural and social) the team can begin to formulate hypotheses about the cause and nature of the individual's problems. At this time, requests for further information are made before the final conclusions and treatment recommendations are made and presented.

Behavioural observations

It is beneficial to allow at least a 2-week period of data collection for gathering additional information to substantiate hypotheses regarding the significance of symptomatology. The type of data collection may include behavioural observation (on-site observations of the individual), video-recording, and behaviour charting (frequency, severity, duration, and antecedent–behaviour–consequence). For example, if there is a suggestion that the individual suffers from highs and lows in mood, then a mood chart completed over a 2-week period may provide further evidence of a potential bipolar affective disorder. The 2-week period is also useful to gather other information such as a neuropsychological evaluation, a structured interview (e.g. autism diagnostic interview) and medical investigations (e.g. thyroid tests, genetic testing, etc.).

Second internal meeting

By this stage in the assessment process, all the information needed to complete the assessment has been collected. The primary therapist for the case presents all the information to the multidisciplinary team. It is more effective if the presentation follows a structured format. For example, feedback is provided on the following areas as it relates to the individual: medical, psychological, psychiatric, behavioural, ecological and social domains. Members from the various disciplines are asked to provide verbal reports on their findings during the assessment (e.g. psychological and psychiatric reports). Based on all the information presented, the team formulates a number of conclusions one of which will include a diagnosis. The diagnosis is seen as only part of the case formulation and its prominence in the overall feedback will vary. At this time recommendations for treatment are also made. If the team is unable confidently to formulate a diagnosis then a diagnostic hypothesis is usually put forward and further data collection and follow-up is recommended to clarify the picture.

Case conference

The case formulation is presented and explained in detail to the individual and their carers in a manner that is understandable to all. It is important that adequate time is taken to explain carefully what information was collected, how it was pulled together to formulate the conclusions and how they specifically relate to the individual. While it is not necessary for all members of the multidisciplinary team to present their findings, key findings from specific members of the team facilitate further understanding of the case formulation process. It is only after the case formulation has been presented and explained that treatment recommendations are presented.

CASE STUDY 13.1   ## The importance of in-depth multidisciplinary assessment

Mary was a 45-year-old woman who had moderate learning disabilities and cerebral palsy and who was confined to a wheelchair. She was referred to a mental health team for an assessment and the following concerns were identified by the residential staff and her family: insertion of foreign objects into her vagina, self-injurious behaviour (biting and scratching self resulting in bleeding and severe scarring), smearing of faeces, rectal digging, incontinence, somatic complaints (joint aches, headaches, stomach aches), exposing herself to male staff, 'faking' of seizures, and repetitive behaviour (e.g. tearing paper and clothing).

A review of Mary's history revealed that she was born by emergency caesarean section brought on by complications of a difficult breech presentation and anoxia. In early childhood she was diagnosed with cerebral palsy, moderate learning disabilities and having a seizure disorder. She underwent several orthopaedic operations and has never been able to walk independently. Mary attended special schools and was described as a student who enjoyed school but had few friends. At 13 years of age Mary's parents requested that she had a breast reduction and hysterectomy, the reasons for which were unknown. Mary had an older sister who had two children, one of whom was profoundly learning and physically disabled. At the time of assessment, the sister and her children lived with her parents.

Since the birth of Mary, her mother had suffered from severe depression and multiple physical illnesses and was never able to care for her independently. Given the mother's poor health, Mary's father took the responsibility for all her care, including her personal self-care. Up until 5 years previously, Mary lived with her parents and attended a day programme. At this time, there was a family crisis which led to her present placement in a residential group home for four women. Although this was seen as an emergency placement, Mary was living in this home at the time of the referral. In the home, the three other women were non-verbal and severely to profoundly learning disabled. One of the women suffered from a psychiatric disorder and was often very distressed at night, screaming and awakening the household. It was reported by the staff that Mary never interacted with the other residents and chose only to interact with the staff. When Mary first arrived at the home, she was unable to carry out any personal self-care skills. Within a short time of arriving, the staff had taught Mary to carry out all her personal self-care independently. At that time, there were no concerns with her behaviour.

Approximately 3 years prior to referral, Mary was allegedly sexually abused by an uncle who then killed himself after the accusation was made. Shortly after the uncle's death Mary began to exhibit the above behaviours. Mary was having regular weekend visits with her family and the staff reported that before and after the family visits there was an increase in the above behaviours. Mary has often stated that she does not want to stay with her family but prefers to visit for the day; however, her family has requested otherwise. In terms of medical care, Mary was seen regularly by a neurologist and was on anticonvulsant medication.

Given the complexity of the case, the first phase of the assessment included the following: psychiatric interview, complete full medical work-up, interviews with parents and staff members, observations of Mary at day programme, review of Mary's day and residential programme and environment. Together with a complete history, this information was reviewed at the first internal meeting. The psychiatric interview revealed that Mary did not present with any obvious symptoms to suggest any major psychiatric disorder. There was some suggestion of anxiety symptoms but nothing to suggest a specific anxiety disorder. During the interview Mary spoke about the alleged abuse by her uncle, negative feelings aroused by her father inappropriately touching her during bathing and generally the difficult family situation at home. A complete medical examination revealed that her seizure disorder was well controlled on medication, there was some evidence of scarred tissue in her vagina probably due to insertion of foreign objects; scarring was also reported around the wrist and hands from biting and lastly she presented with early signs of arthritis in many of her joints.

Interviews with the parents revealed that they were severely stressed by the mother's ill health and growing concerns about their grand-daughter who was severely physically and learning disabled. The family also had difficulty viewing Mary as an independent woman who needed to develop a life of her own. Interviews with the staff revealed a high degree of stress, conflict among the staff about how to manage the self-injurious and sexualized behaviour and there was a growing view that Mary presented with many psychosomatic symptoms. Observations of Mary at her day programme and residential setting indicated that she was higher functioning than most of the other clients and tended to relate exclusively with the staff. The day programme involved repetitive activities that did not seem to interest Mary and often she was off task interacting with the staff. At her home, she confined herself to her bedroom or was in the kitchen with the staff. She rarely engaged in social interaction with her fellow residents and tended to leave the room when one of them came in.

After the brief presentation of Mary's case in the first internal meeting it appeared that Mary did not suffer from any major psychiatric disorder. It was hypothesized that she probably was suffering from emotional difficulties from particular life events. There were also concerns raised about the environments in which Mary worked and lived. A vocational assessment and possibilities for alternative living situations were also requested. At this time psychotherapy was suggested and an assessment for suitability was requested. In addition, more information was needed on the self-injurious behaviours that Mary was exhibiting and data collection was requested. More information was also needed with regards to the philosophies of the staff team on sexual behaviour and also what strategies they had already in place to respond to Mary. There were concerns about Mary's communication skills and a speech/language assessment was requested to evaluate her communication skills.

Once this additional information was collected the mental health team met again to discuss Mary. In this meeting all the information that had been collected on Mary was thoroughly reviewed and assessments and additional data that had been collected were reported during the meeting. The psychiatrist and psychologist reported that there seemed to be no evidence to suggest the presentation of a major psychiatric disorder. A psychotherapy assessment revealed that Mary presented with many emotional concerns related to her physical and learning disabilities, the alleged abuse trauma associated with her uncle, the conflict and dynamics in her family and her unhappiness with her current residential placement. In the assessment she seemed to respond to interpretations and there was evidence to suggest that she had some insight into difficulties. The evidence from the environmental analysis and functional analysis of behaviour suggested that both her vocational and residential environments were inappropriate. In particular, she was not interested in working full-time doing piecemeal work but instead preferred a part leisure and work programme. She showed interest and abilities to do office work such as photocopying, filing and paper shredding. In terms of her residence, she was higher functioning than the other residents and had demonstrated that she could live in a semi-supported environment with similar functioning adults. The functional analysis of her behaviours suggested

CASE STUDY 13.1 *(Cont'd)*

that they were multifunctional. For example, the self-injurious behaviour was more likely to occur after Mary had a major upset which included conflict with another resident, returning from a difficult family visit, when she was frustrated with the limits of her physical disability and her needs having to be placed on hold while the staff attended to frequent upsets from another resident. The somatic complaints were also multifunctional and often appeared to be genuine and at times also seemed to be related to situations when the staff had to attend to the needs of the other clients. Lastly, the speech/language assessment revealed that Mary did have some difficulties with clarity of speech and word-finding problems and they tended to deteriorate when she was upset.

Note how the above assessment drew on information from the family, residential and vocational staff, psychiatrist, psychologist, behaviour therapist and speech/language therapist to provide a complete profile of Mary's problems and needs.

Diagnosis in the presence of challenging behaviour

From earlier sections in this chapter, it is clear that there are potentially multiple causes for challenging behaviour. Furthermore, within the same person, similar behaviours may represent different functions at different times (Gardner & Graeber 1993). Frequently, it can be very difficult, both for clinicians and support staff, to distinguish symptoms related to psychiatric illness from behaviours arising from other causes. For example, problems arise when staff are not able to recognize the onset of a psychiatric illness, interpret the situation solely as one where the individual's challenging behaviours are getting worse and lose confidence in former strategies being effective. Similarly, complications can arise when staff fail to recognize the onset of a psychiatric illness and persist with strategies to manage the apparent deterioration in challenging behaviour (e.g. an individual with bipolar disorder who typically has problems with non-compliance, when suffering from depressed mood, is forced to go to work and complete a full day of activities).

In response to this recognition of multiple causality, there is a growing awareness that an assessment must be correspondingly sophisticated. This implies the necessity to encompass all the variables that influence an individual's behaviour (e.g. biomedical, psychological, interactional, environmental) (Gardner & Sovner 1994, Griffiths 1995).

CASE STUDY 13.2   **Complex interplay between schizophrenia, challenging behaviour and problems of adolescence**

This case study concerns a 16-year-old girl who has mild learning disabilities with a diagnosis of schizophrenia. The initial presentation was a compliant teenager with symptoms of hallucinations (hearing command hallucinations) and delusions (thinking people were out to get her) that were well controlled on medication. For the past 2 years there had been an increase in the symptoms associated with schizophrenia; she responded poorly to medication changes and reported the presence of command hallucinations to kill her mother and thoughts of wanting to hurt people in authority. She also believed that people were poisoning her food. In addition, there had been an onset of non-compliance and verbal and physical aggression. It was difficult to tease out which behaviours were associated with schizophrenia and which were challenging behaviour and also those associated with the onset of adolescence.

A comprehensive assessment revealed many causes for her aggression: auditory hallucinations telling her to hit her mother; delusional thinking that someone was trying to poison her food or wanting to hurt people in authority; frustration at her need to depend on others for tasks; anger at having schizophrenia and learning disabilities and being different; a dislike of being told what to do; and a desire to make her own decisions but being unable to make many choices.

Education was provided to the mother about the presentation of schizophrenia in adolescence and the complex interplay between schizophrenia, challenging behaviour and adolescence. The teenager also received supportive counselling to discuss issues of adolescence and schizophrenia. Medication trials were set up which were carefully controlled and monitored for changes in all areas of behaviour. Behaviour strategies were recommended to deal with non-compliance and aggression. In relation to the aggression, for example, interventions focused on reducing levels of anger with the intent to reduce the likelihood of aggressive behaviour. These included the teaching of anger management skills and helping the mother and staff to recognize potentially anger-provoking situations. Similarly, providing more opportunities for choice making and strategies for requesting assistance to make personal choices were established. In other situations, when the girl became angry because of delusional thinking or command hallucinations, interventions focused on the use of medication and psychological therapy (e.g. thought stopping). Consistent consequence strategies were established to provide appropriate feedback for aggressive episodes. Staff were also taught to use reactive strategies in critical situations.

CASE RECOGNITION

However good our assessment and treatment regimes become, it must not be forgotten that the first step to mental healthcare is to have one's problem *recognized*. In this respect, people who have learning disabilities are at a major disadvantage compared to the general population. Typically, the decision to consult a GP or other professional regarding mental illness is not taken personally by the individual who has learning disabilities (Fletcher 1993, Nezu & Nezu 1994). Seeking help and treatment for a psychiatric problem is thus dependent upon a third party first recognizing the signs and symptoms of psychiatric illness and, second understanding their significance and taking action. If the disorder is associated with the development of conspicuous symptoms such as challenging behaviour, case recognition is relatively easy. In the absence of specialized knowledge, however, it is likely that many mental health problems will not be identified. Recent studies confirm that this is indeed the case, many cases of depression and anxiety disorders remaining unrecognized and untreated (Patel et al 1993, Reiss 1990). The reasons for unrecognized psychiatric illness are often attributed to carers' lack of understanding of the cause of the behaviour and the need for referral and psychiatric assessment (Borthwick-Duffy & Eyman 1990).

The problems of case recognition are compounded by the fact that the primary healthcare system relies so heavily on a person's ability to recognize and report symptoms of ill health. People who have communication problems may not have the skills to do this, while healthcare professionals may not have the skills needed to overcome this barrier. Rodgers (1994) argues that professionals in primary healthcare in the UK may lack the communication skills needed to give appropriate care to people who have learning disabilities. Langan et al's (1993) survey of 70 GPs in the West of England reports that GPs generally lacked special expertise for dealing with people who have learning disabilities and almost half felt further training was appropriate Similar problems have been found in the US. Harper & Wadsworth (1992) argue that healthcare professionals in the US often lack the opportunity to interact with people whose ability to express and understand healthcare information is limited.

Support workers and direct care staff working with people who have learning disabilities, as well as GPs, also have a crucial role in recognizing potential symptoms. These people are in the best position to identify significant behaviour change and, potentially, to make appropriate referrals. Immediate carers are usually first to notice significant signs and symptoms but often lack the knowledge or confidence to act on this. Professionals such as community nurses and social workers often have access to more wide ranging information in relation to the person's overall functioning, yet these professionals may also lack the skills to make a truly informed decision about whom to refer for in-depth clinical assessment. A number of recent initiatives have been directed specifically towards capitalizing on this knowledge base. The PAS-ADD Checklist (Moss et al 1998) and the Mini PAS-ADD (Prosser et al 1998) are two schedules designed to help health and social service staff identify mental health problems in the people for whom they care. Training materials developed by Guy's and St Thomas's hospitals (Bouras et al 1997) have been designed to raise the awareness and understanding of staff about a wide range of issues relating to the detection, management and treatment of mental illness in people who have learning disabilities.

MENTAL HEALTH PROBLEMS ACROSS THE LIFESPAN

Children and adolescents

While there has been increasing focus and research into the understanding of mental health issues in adults who have learning disabilities, there remains a paucity of interest in the mental health needs of children and adolescents who have learning disabilities. Prevalence studies have estimated that 20–35% of children and adolescents who have learning disabilities suffer from mental health problems (Eaton & Menolascino 1982, Parsons et al 1984). In the Isle of Wight study (Rutter et al 1970) 30.4% of children with IQs less than 70 were found to have a psychiatric disorder on the parent questionnaire and 41.8% on the teacher questionnaire. Comparable rates for the non-learning disabled population were 7.7% and 9.5% respectively.

In spite of this proven need, few studies have been conducted on the identification and diagnosis of mental health problems and provision of therapeutic interventions in children and adolescents who have learning disabilities. There are currently few child psychiatrists and clinical child psychologists with any formal training within the area of learning disabilities. For many families of children who have learning disabilities, medical health services have typically involved a number of professionals investigating questions of aetiology and providing treatment for difficult behaviours. Psychiatric services are often not considered and when they are, they tend to be inadequate. Moreover, there is often no integrated multidisciplinary approach which attempts to understand fully the complexities of the individual. Assessments and treatment plans are often completed without collaboration between professionals and community service agencies and much of the care and management of the individual is left in the hands of families and the school system. Typically, intensive intervention from professionals occurs when the mental health status of the child or adolescent has deteriorated to a point where they have been placed in a residential facility and/or denied appropriate educational services.

The problems that exist in identifying and diagnosing a psychiatric disorder in children and adolescents with normal IQ exist also in children and adolescents who have learning disabilities. While in adults there is usually an established pattern of behaviours and symptoms to examine, in children and adolescents one has to be familiar with ongoing developmental issues and skilled at communicating with someone who has not reached cognitive maturation. Gathering information from family members, school teachers and workers is invaluable in formulating a diagnostic impression of the individual. Given the pattern of developmental change in children and adolescents, it is also important to provide regular follow-up and reassessment to collect information on cross-sectional symptomatology and longitudinal course to assist with accuracy of the diagnosis (see Case study 13.3). For example, it has been reported that in adolescents with normal IQ who present with psychotic symptoms, there tends to be a high rate of misdiagnosing at onset (McClellan et al 1993) where it is difficult to differentiate early-onset schizophrenia from bipolar disorder during the first two episodes (Werry et al 1994). The same is likely to be true with the learning-disabled population.

Most research that has investigated psychiatric disorders in children and adolescents who have learning disabilities has focused on individuals who have mild to moderate learning disabilities. In general, the conclusions have been that the presentation of psychiatric symptoms is similar to that in the general population. However, in most studies, individuals who have severe to profound learning disabilities were excluded, so there remains a question as to how psychiatric symptoms are characterized in that particular population.

CASE STUDY 13.3   **The potential for misdiagnosing schizophrenia in adolescence**

This case concerns a 15-year-old girl who has mild learning disabilities who presented with the following symptoms of at least 6 months' duration: significant withdrawal from family and friends, decreased verbal output, lack of interest in school work or other recreational activities, deterioration in socialization and personal hygiene, increased periods of sleep, flat affect, depressed mood and periods of crying spells. Any requests made of her were responded to by physical aggression. There were also incidents of seemingly unprovoked aggression towards classmates at school. Both the family and teachers at school reported that there were often periods where the girl appeared to be talking to and laughing with someone, but there was never anyone with her. She also used to pace up and down the hallway at school and frequently get up from her desk and go to look outside the door as if she had seen someone. There were difficulties with eating, she refused to eat any food in front of anyone and accused her mother of trying to poison her.

CASE STUDY 13.3 *(Cont'd)*

A diagnosis of early-onset schizophrenia was made and the girl was put on a combination of respiridone and Prozac. There was some initial improvement in symptoms but after 3 months the negative symptoms became worse. The Prozac was increased but the girl became manic, her symptoms including: excessive pacing, insomnia, obsessive ripping of clothing, increased aggression and increased appetite. Subsequently, the medication was reduced and there was a decrease in symptoms.

After a thorough review of her symptom profile and mood charting for several months, her diagnosis was changed to mood disorder with psychotic features. The mood charting over a period of several months helped to clarify that her psychotic features were only present during mood episodes and that her depressive symptoms were significantly predominant in her course. However, given that an increase in antidepressant medication had caused a manic episode, a caution was placed on her file to be aware of the possibility of future manic episodes that are unrelated to somatic treatments for depression.

Ageing and age-related changes

Studies of the general population of elderly people living in the community indicate that this group suffers from definite psychiatric symptoms in a high proportion, perhaps 20%, of people over the age of 65. Their psychiatric symptoms are often accompanied by physical illnesses and they are often disabled by their symptoms. Depression is by far the most common mental health problem in the general elderly population. Data vary from study to study, depending on population and criteria, although it is generally though that 15–20% of elderly people suffer from depressive symptoms (Shamoian 1985). However, only 15–20% of this depressed group will receive treatment. Severely depressed elderly people show an increased use of medical services; they take more psychotropic medications and are given multiple drugs more often. They see their doctor repeatedly, receive more special investigations and are admitted to hospital more frequently.

People who have learning disabilities also suffer from mental health problems in later life (see Day & Jancar 1994 for a review). Affective psychoses (mostly bipolar) tend to start in the over-40s and are more common in women. Paranoid psychoses are more likely to start over the age of 50, sometimes being associated with temporal lobe epilepsy, severe visual and hearing defects and interpersonal difficulties. A study carried out in Oldham showed 12 individuals out of a total sample of 105 to have a diagnosable psychiatric condition (apart from dementia), giving an overall prevalence rate of 11.4% (Patel et al 1993). Most of the disorders detected in this older population were of depression and anxiety, a picture similar to that of the general elderly population.

Social risk factors for mental illness in later life

In order to achieve successful adaptation to change, all of us need an effective support network, but in this respect many people who have learning disabilities are at a major disadvantage. By definition, they have lower intellectual abilities, so their ability to acquire effective coping mechanisms is likely to be limited. In addition, the majority (apart from those whose disability is very mild) have no spouse, no children and may have little or no contact with their relatives. Their financial circumstances are probably poor and they are certainly unlikely to have status or position in society from which they can derive a sense of self-esteem. As they age, they may suffer from poor physical health and may also lose members of their family. Since many people who have learning disabilities already have impoverished social networks, this latter aspect may have an even greater impact than on members of the general population. Overall, it is clear that the social risk factors for mental illness place many members of this population in a vulnerable position.

Dementia

The most obvious age-related mental health problem is dementia. In the general population, epidemiological studies show that the prevalence of dementia rises markedly with age, from about 2% in persons aged 65–70 to approximately 20% in those over 80 (Royal College of Physicians 1981). Alzheimer's disease is associated with a number of characteristic cellular changes which are widely distributed throughout the brain. Apart from Alzheimer's, the other most commonly occurring type is multiinfarct dementia, in which the brain is damaged in a number of localized sites by burst blood vessels.*

Most people working in the learning disabilities field will have encountered dementia principally in the context of Down's syndrome individuals. Such people are considerably more at risk of contracting Alzheimer's dementia than their peers with or without Down's syndrome. There is now considerable evidence that the brains of all people with Down's syndrome aged 35 and over show the characteristic changes associated with Alzheimer's dementia. Not all such individuals, however, show the behavioural and clinical symptoms described above. Research will no doubt eventually clarify why this should be so. In the meantime, it is important to emphasize that, despite the changes in the brain, *not* all people with Down's syndrome will develop dementia.

Despite the high risk for Alzheimer's disease in Down's syndrome, the absolute number of dementia sufferers without Down's syndrome is probably greater. This is because a disproportionately large number of people with Down's syndrome die before they reach age 50. In the Oldham study already referred to, only nine people over the age of 50 years with Down's syndrome were found in a population of 105 individuals. Although the risk for the surviving people with Down's syndrome is high, the non-Down's population over 50 years of age is about 10 times as large. These individuals have a dementia risk which is about the same as the general population. Unlike those with Down's syndrome, these people are not likely to get dementia until they are in their 70s.

Diagnosing dementia in people who have learning disabilities

The dementia syndrome involves deterioration in many aspects of mental functioning. However, the changes can be summarized under three headings: memory, other cognitive functioning and emotional changes. A full diagnosis of dementia under the criteria laid down by the World Health Organization needs clinical evidence in all three of these areas.

---

* For an account of the range of dementias, see Raskind & Peskind 1992.

- *Memory loss*. This involves both short- and long-term memory, although long-term memories are retained longer than the capacity to learn and remember new information. It must be stressed that many older people have poorer memories but this is usually a benign consequence of ageing rather than being indicative of dementing disease.
- *Other cognitive deterioration*, which can be in a variety of skill areas including the cerebral control of reading, speaking, object recognition and abstract thinking.
- *Emotional changes*, which may include wandering/pacing, aggressive behaviour, apathy/loss of drive, depressive symptoms, delusions and hallucinations.

It must be stressed that the diagnosis of Alzheimer's disease, or any other dementia for that matter, involves the ruling out of any other possible cause for the symptoms, as well as an understanding of the significance of the pattern of those symptoms. This requires a high level of clinical expertise. Due to the seriousness and poor prognosis of many types of dementia, it is essential that the diagnosis be made only when all the clinical evidence has been properly evaluated.

The issue of careful diagnosis is crucial because a number of conditions, many of them treatable, can mimic the early symptoms of dementia. These include depression, thyroid problems and sensory loss. A full clinical examination and monitoring over at least 6 months are necessary before a firm conclusion can be reached. A key publication in this respect is *Diagnosis of dementia in individuals with intellectual disability* (Aylward et al 1995), which proposes a set of standardized criteria for the diagnosis of dementia in people who have learning disabilities for use by clinicians and researchers.

TREATMENT

At present there is a lack of controlled studies that have investigated the effects of various treatments on mental health problems in individuals who have learning disabilities. Up to now, the general approach has been to assume that what works in the general population will work for people who have learning disabilities. If a multidisciplinary approach to assessment has been taken, then it naturally follows that the recommendations for treatment will be multimodal, where several treatment options are put forward. This may include one or more of the following: psychopharmacology, behaviour therapy, various forms of psychotherapy and educational intervention. It is beyond the scope of this chapter to provide a comprehensive review of the growing literature on treatments for psychiatric disorders in individuals who have learning disabilities. Instead a brief discussion will be provided on each therapy.

Psychopharmacology

There is an increasing research interest into psychopharmacology for individuals who have learning disabilities and several excellent reviews highlight current issues in the area (Aman 1991, 1993, Aman & Singh 1988). There is generally a two-fold approach to psychopharmacological treatment of individuals who have learning disabilities: (a) the treatment of a diagnosable psychiatric disorder and (b) the treatment of symptoms (Bates 1984). The treatment of a diagnosable psychiatric disorder includes schizophrenia, bipolar disorder, major depression, psychoses, attention deficit hyperactivity disorder and various forms of anxiety. However, in most cases, psychopharmacology alone does not successfully treat the disorder and other forms of intervention are necessary to augment the treatment (e.g. behaviour therapy, psychotherapy).

The second approach to psychopharmacological interventions in individuals who have learning disabilities is the treatment of specific symptoms. This approach is more problematic and obviously less clearcut. However, many symptoms and behaviours that may or may not be related to a diagnosable psychiatric illness are known to be responsive to psychotropic medications (e.g. agitation, hallucinations, self-injurious behaviour, hyperkinesis, etc.). In this instance it is important that the use of psychotropic medication be individualized to the individual and only used when such symptoms are unresponsive to other available treatments (e.g. behavioural, psychotherapy).

In general, individuals who have learning disabilities respond in a similar way to the general population to stimulant, psychotropic and antidepressant medications (Russell & Tanguay 1996). It is common practice to provide a comprehensive assessment of the problem, start medication on lower doses and slowly increase to achieve maximum benefit with minimal side effects, as individuals who have learning disabilities tend to be more susceptible to side effects. The practitioner should also be aware that individuals who have learning disabilities are also susceptible to exhibiting unusual side effects that are not always outlined in the clinical profile of the medication. It is also good practice to avoid polypharmacy and changing more than one medication at a time, to coordinate other therapies with medication changes, not to make major medication changes prior to a vacation or prolonged home visit and to monitor the effectiveness of the medication and side effects regularly (Sovner & Hurley 1985).

Several authors have outlined standards for the use of psychotropic medications in individuals who have learning disabilities (Aman 1991, Aman & Singh 1991, Sovner & Hurley 1985). Kalachnik (1988) defined a series of standards for administering medications in individuals who have learning disabilities and they include: interdisciplinary assessment of need for medications, identification of specific target behaviours (formal psychiatric diagnosis not required), written, informed consent, use of minimal effective dose, periodic attempts to reduce dosage, monitoring of side effects, integration of behavioural, medical and educational interventions, and periodic data-based evaluations of the medication.

Behaviour therapy

Contemporary behaviour therapies reflect the contributions of classical conditioning (Pavlov 1927), early reinforcement theory and operant conditioning (Skinner 1938, Thorndike 1911), observational and cognitive learning (Bandura 1977, Beck 1967, Ellis 1962, Meichenbaum 1975) and biofeedback and anxiety reduction models (Wolpe 1958). Although many studies have demonstrated the effectiveness of using behaviour therapy to treat severe behaviour disorders and to teach adaptive skills in individuals who have learning disabilities, few have examined the effectiveness of such a therapy in the treatment of psychiatric disorders in this population. However, in community settings and tertiary care facilities behaviour therapy is often used in the treatment of psychiatric disorders in conjunction with the use of medication.

As outlined in an earlier section, the assessment and treatment of psychiatric symptoms in individuals who have learning disabilities can be very difficult given the presence of challenging behaviours and multiple determinants to symptoms and behaviours. Gardner & Griffiths (1997) advocate a multimodal approach to assessment and treatment, in which a given behaviour may be regarded as having both psychiatric and behavioural antecedents. Their model attempts to provide the clinician with a framework to disentangle potential psychiatric and behavioural causes.

Cognitive therapy

Cognitive therapy is based on the study of mediating processes where the premise is that an individual's affective state is influenced by the manner in which they perceive and structure their experiences (Beck 1967, Ellis 1962). Beliefs, expectancies, plans and values are seen as making a large contribution to the maintenance of abnormal behaviour. The application of cognitive therapy in individuals who have learning disabilities is relatively new and unexplored. However, some research has been conducted and preliminary findings are promising. For example, Benson (1986, 1992) adapted Novaco's (1975) anger management model for use with individuals who have learning disabilities and found it was effective with those who have mild to moderate learning disabilities (Benson et al 1986). The model defines anger as an emotional response to a situation the individual perceives as threatening to their self-esteem. The aim of the training is to teach methods of controlling anger as well as socially acceptable ways to express anger. Training includes recognition and identification of emotions, self-monitoring of mood, relaxation training, self-instructional training and problem solving.

In relation to anxiety disorders, relaxation training has been successfully used even with people who have severe or profound learning disabilities and multiple disabilities (Hegarty & Last 1997, Rickard et al 1984). A study of people whose level of disability was moderate, and who were hence able to self-report, showed that reductions in the behavioural manifestations of anxiety were also associated with similar reductions in self-assessed experience of anxiety (Morrison & Lindsay 1997). Several studies have evaluated the effectiveness of various types of relaxation technique. Lindsay et al (1989) compared the effectiveness of behaviour relaxation training (BRT) and abbreviated progressive relaxation (APR). The conclusion was that the BRT group showed a more rapid improvement and that this technique was more effective in both group and individual formats (Lindsay & Baty 1989).

Anxiety management techniques have been successfully used in the treatment of specific phobias, usually in conjunction with desensitization, modelling and generalization components (Erfanian & Miltenberger 1990, Lindsay et al 1988). Intervention strategies for phobias in children and adolescents who have learning disabilities are reviewed by King et al (1990).

Psychotherapy

The term 'psychotherapy' encompasses a variety of therapeutic approaches including psychodynamic psychotherapy and counselling. While there are many theories of psychodynamic psychotherapy, most can be characterized by focusing on the unconscious and issues of resistance (defences) and the therapist–patient relationship (transference and countertransference).

Although there is evidence to suggest that psychodynamic therapy was used with individuals who have learning disabilities as early as the 1930s (Chidester & Menninger 1936), for many decades the common view was that cognitive deficit prevented the use of psychotherapy. Such a view tended to deny the opportunity for individuals who have learning disabilities to talk and deal with their emotional conflicts. There is now a growing awareness that individuals who have learning disabilities can benefit from psychodynamic psychotherapy.* In general, it is acknowledged that thought processes in individuals who have learning disabilities are at a concrete stage, in many ways analogous to those found in children. With the growing interest in the use of psychodynamic psychotherapy in individuals who have learning disabilities, efforts have been made to modify traditional adult psychotherapy models and borrow principles from child psychotherapy models.

Similarities with child psychotherapy models are seen not only in the concreteness of the individual's thought processes, but also in the way of life. As with children, for example, many individuals who have learning disabilities live in a 'family' made up of caregivers (e.g. staff, families, case managers, social workers, employers) who have a significant impact on their lives and their ability to make change (Levitas & Gilson 1994). In child psychotherapy, a central part of the process is to hold routine meetings with the patient's family. When working psychotherapeutically with a learning-disabled individual, it is equally important that the same consideration be given to the caregivers.

Reiss (1994) has summarized a number of recommendations for psychotherapy that have been suggested in the literature. These include the need to adapt interview techniques to the client's cognitive level and to make the therapy relatively directive and the importance of ensuring that the therapist is supportive and flexible and prepared to intervene in the client's environment. Appropriate goals should be set; issues of transference and countertransference need to be managed just as in child therapy; and the issue of learning disability as a disability should be addressed explicitly.

Counselling seeks to help people understand and work out their day-to-day problems. Counsellors are often seen as therapists who listen, encourage and offer support and advice. They can also teach the individual to distinguish between behaviours that are socially inappropriate and those that are appropriate. It has been reported that counselling is often utilized more than psychodynamic psychotherapy in individuals who have learning disabilities (Pfadt 1991).

A few studies have been published which have looked at the effectiveness of psychodynamic psychotherapy or counselling in individuals who have learning disabilities, most of which are single case studies (Matson 1984, Symington

---

* The reader is referred to Hurley (1989) for a review of the literature on psychodynamic psychotherapy.

1981). As with the use of psychodynamic psychotherapy in the general population and the current climate of threatened cuts to budgets and the growing interest in evidence-based treatment, there is a strong need for outcome-based research in the area of psychotherapy with individuals who have learning disabilities.

Educational interventions

There is significant value in providing education on mental health issues, both for the individual and for their support network. For the individuals it can help them gain some insight into their difficulties, enhance their understanding of why they behave in a certain manner and why particular treatments are indicated. This can help facilitate compliance with treatment. Education also helps to dispel myths and outdated beliefs that may be held by the individual and/or the support network. The education can cover a wide range of topics but it is important to tailor it to individuals and their particular circumstances. Topics can include: psychiatric disorders, specific symptoms, the rationale for use of different therapies, medication profiles and side effects, and monitoring of changes in symptoms.

Multimodal treatment

If more than one intervention is being adopted in the treatment plan, it is highly recommended that there is coordination of the commencement of the therapies as well as regular monitoring of their effectiveness. Although this approach may seem logical, it is often not practised and there is also often poor communication among the clinicians carrying out the treatment. It is valuable to provide a systematic structure for treatment processes, such as regular monitoring of therapies, interdiscplinary team review and follow-up steps to avoid reliance and long-term use of therapies, particularly medications.

CONCLUSION

This chapter has attempted to be very wide ranging in its coverage of the complex issues of mental health in people who have learning disabilities and so inevitably has not been able to cover every aspect in detail. It is to be hoped, however, that we have been able to provide the reader with a useful guide to this field. Where the text lacks detail, we have attempted to provide authoritative sources for further reading.

There is no doubt that advances have been made during the past 15 years, there now being a much greater awareness of the importance of addressing the mental health needs of people who have learning disabilities. Considerable progress has been made, particularly in relation to case identification and diagnosis. Much less progress has been made in relation to the systematic evaluation of treatment options. Many people who have learning disabilities receive medication for mental illness and/or challenging behaviour. However, the efficacy of such treatments has not been adequately explored (Crabbe 1994). Behavioural interventions are often specified for challenging behaviour and have proved to be very effective in some cases (Emerson 1993). Other psychological treatments, such as cognitive behaviour therapy, have not received so much attention with this population. In the future it is to be hoped that the full range of psychological treatments will be more fully evaluated for use with people who have learning disabilities and additional mental health needs.

Finally, it must be abundantly clear to the reader that the mental health needs of this population are highly complex. As a result, we must work to develop assessment and treatment models with the sophistication necessary to deal with this complexity. These models should emphasize accurate diagnosis and assessment of needs as a crucial step which provides a clear direction for biomedical and psychological interventions. Following this, however, it is important to think about *long-term* prevention of mental illness, rather than simply reducing symptoms in the short term. The development of such care models is very important for people who have learning disabilities, because the majority of them will need help to develop strategies for the long-term maintenance of their mental health.

FURTHER READING

Emerson E, Moss S C, Kiernan C K 1999 The relationship between challenging behaviour and psychiatric disorders in people with severe intellectual disabilities. In: Bouras N (ed) Psychiatric and behavioural disorders in mental retardation. Cambridge University Press, Cambridge
Provides an extensive discussion of the relationships between challenging behaviour and psychiatric disorders.

Moss S C 1999 Issues of diagnosis. In: Bouras N (ed) Psychiatric and behavioural disorders in mental retardation. Cambridge University Press, Cambridge
This chapter provides a detailed description of the theoretical issues relating to assessment.

Raskind M A, Peskind E R 1992 Alzheimer's disease and other dementing disorders. In: Birren J E, Sloane R B, Chen G D (eds) Handbook of mental health and ageing. Academic Press, London
This chapter provides a comprehensive account of the range of dementias involved for people who have a learning disability.

REFERENCES

Aman M G 1991 Pharmacotherapy in the developmental disabilities: new developments. Aust N Z J Dev Disabil 17:183–199

Aman M G 1993 Efficacy of psychotropic drugs for reducing self injurious behavior in the developmental disabilities. Ann Clin Psychiatr 5:171–188

Aman M G, Singh N N 1988 Psychopharmacology of the developmental disabilities. Springer-Verlag, New York

Aman M G, Singh N N 1991 Pharmacological intervention. In: Matson J L, Mulick J A (eds) Handbook of mental retardation, 2nd edn. Pergamon Press, New York

Aman M G, Tasse M J, Rojahn J, Hammer D 1996 The Nisonger CBRF: a child behavior rating form for children with developmental disabilities. Res Dev Disabil 17:41–57

American Psychiatric Association 1994 Diagnostic and statistical manual of mental disorders. APA, Washington DC, p xxi

Aylward E H, Burt D B, Thorpe L U, Lai F, Dalton A J 1995 Diagnosis of dementia in individuals with intellectual disability. American Association on Mental Retardation, Washington DC

Bandura A 1977 Social learning theory. Prentice-Hall, Englewood Cliffs, NJ

Bates W J 1984 Multimodal treatment of mental illness in institutionalized mentally retarded persons. In: Menolascino F J, Stark J A (eds) Handbook of mental illness in the mentally retarded. Plenum Press, New York

Beck A T 1967 Depression: clinical, experimental, and theoretical aspects. Harper and Row, New York

Beck A T, Ward C H, Mendelson M, Mock J E, Erbaugh J 1961 An inventory for measuring depression. Arch Gen Psychiatr 4:561–571

Benavidez D A, Matson J L 1993 Assessment of depression in mentally retarded adolescents. Res Dev Disabil 14:179–188

Benson B A 1986 Anger management training. Psychiatr Aspects Mental Retard Rev 5:51–55

Benson B A 1992 Teaching anger management to persons with mental retardation. IDS Publishing Corporation, Worthington, OH

Benson B A, Rice C J, Miranti S V 1986 Effects of anger management training with mentally retarded adults: II. Poor social skills. Am J Mental Defic 89:657–659

Bland R C, Newman S C, Orn H 1988 Epidemiology of psychiatric disorders in Edmonton. Acta Psychiatr Scand 338 (suppl):77

Bodfish J W, Crawford T W, Powell S B, Parker D E, Golden R N, Lewis M M H 1995 Compulsions in adults with mental retardation: prevalence, phenomenology and comorbidity with stereotypy and self-injury. Am J Mental Retard 100:183–192

Borthwick-Duffy S A, Eyman R K 1990 Who are the dually diagnosed? Am J Mental Retard 94:586–595

Bouras N, Murray B, Joyce T, Kon Y, Holt G 1997 Mental health in learning disabilities: a training pack for staff working with people who have a dual diagnosis of mental health needs and learning disabilities, 2nd edn. Pavillion, Brighton

Campbell M, Malone R P 1991 Mental retardation and psychiatric disorders. Hosp Commun Psychiatr 42:374–379

Chidester L, Menninger K A 1936 The application of psychoanalytic methods to the study of mental retardation. Am J Orthopsychiatr 6:616–625

Corbett J A 1979 Psychiatric morbidity and mental retardation. In: James F E, Snaith R P (eds) Psychiatric illness and mental handicap. Gaskell Press, London

Crabbe H F 1994 Pharmacotherapy in mental retardation. In: Bouras N (ed) Mental health in mental retardation: recent advances and practices. Cambridge University Press, Cambridge, pp 187–204

Dalton A J 1995 Alzheimer disease: a health risk of growing older with Down syndrome. In: Nadel L, Rosenthal D (eds) Down syndrome: living and learning in the community. Wiley-Liss, New York, pp 58–64

Dalton A J, Wisniewski H M 1990 Down's syndrome and the dementia of Alzheimer disease. Int Rev Psychiatr 2:43–52

Day K 1985 Psychiatric disorder in the middle-aged and elderly mentally handicapped. Br J Psychiatr 147:660–667

Day K, Jancar J 1994 Mental and physical health and ageing in mental handicap: a review. J Intellect Disabil Res 38:241–256

Demb H B, Brier N, Huron R, Tomor E 1994 The adolescent behavior checklist: normative data and sensitivity and specificity of a screening tool for diagnosable psychiatric disorders in adolescents with mental retardation and other developmental disabilities. Res Dev Disabil 15:151–165

Eaton L F, Menolascino F J 1982 Psychiatric disorders in the mentally retarded: types, problems, and challenges. Am J Psychiatr 139:1297–1303

Edelbrock C, Costello A J 1988 Convergence between statistically derived behavior problem syndromes and child psychiatric diagnoses. J Abnormal Child Psychol 16:219–231

Ellis A 1962 Reason and emotion in psychotherapy. Lyle Stuart, New York

Emerson E 1993 Severe learning disabilities and challenging behaviours: developments in behavioural analysis and intervention. Behav Cognit Psychother 21:171–198

Emerson E, Moss S C, Kiernan C K 1999 The relationship between challenging behaviour and psychiatric disorders in people with severe intellectual disabilities. In: Bouras N (ed) Psychiatric and behavioural disorders in mental retardation. Cambridge University Press, Cambridge

Erfanian N, Miltenberger R G 1990 Contact desensitization in the treatment of dog phobias in persons who have mental retardation. Behav Res Treatment 5:55–60

Fletcher R J 1993 Mental illness–mental retardation in the United States: policy and treatment challenges. J Intellect Disabil Res 37 (suppl 1):25–33

Gardner W I 1996 Nonspecific behavioural symptoms in persons with a dual diagnosis: a psychological model for integrating biomedical and psychosocial diagnoses and interventions. Psychol Mental Retard Dev Disabil 21:6–11

Gardner W I, Graeber J L 1993 Severe behaviour disorders in persons with mental retardation. A multimodal behavioral diagnostic model. In: Fletcher R J, Dosen A (eds) Mental health aspects of mental retardation. Lexington Books, New York

Gardner W I, Griffiths D 1997 Influence of psychiatric disorders on nonspecific behavioral symptoms: diagnostic and treatment issues. In: Fletcher R J, Griffiths D (eds) Proceedings of the Third International Congress on the Dually Diagnosed. National Association for the Dually Diagnosed, New York

Gardner W I, Sovner R 1994 Self injurious behaviour, diagnosis and treatment: a multimodal functional approach. Vida Publishing, Willow St, PA

Goldberg D, Huxley P 1980 Mental illness in the community. Tavistock Publications, London.

Griffiths D 1995 A holistic perspective on the diagnosis and treatment. A behavioural point of view. In: Fletcher R J, McNelis D, Fusaro L (eds) Proceedings of the Second International Congress on the Dually Diagnosed. National Association for the Dually Diagnosed, New York

Hamilton M 1960 A rating scale for depression. J Neurol Neurosurg Psychiatr 23:56–61

Harper D, Wadsworth J 1992 Improving health communication for persons with mental retardation. Public Health Rep 107:297–302

Hegarty J R, Last A 1997 Relaxation training for people who have severe/profound and multiple learning disabilities. Br J Dev Disabil 43:122–139

Holland A J 1991 Learning disability and psychiatric/behavioural disorders: a genetic perspective. In: McGuffin P, Murray R (eds) The new genetics of mental illness. Butterworth-Heinemann, Oxford

Hurley A D 1989 Individual psychotherapy with mentally retarded individuals: a review and call for research. Res Dev Disabil 10:261–275

Jacobson J W 1998 Psychological services utilization: relationship to severity of behaviour problems in intellectual disability services. J Intellect Disabil Res 42:307–315

Jawed S H, Krishnan V H, Prasher V P, Corbett J A 1993 Worsening of pica as a symptom of depressive illness in a person with severe mental handicap. Br J Psychiatr 162:835–837

Kalachnik J E 1988 Medication monitoring procedures: Thou shall, here's how. In: Gadow K D, Poling A G (eds) Pharmacotherapy and mental retardation. Little, Brown, Boston

Kazdin A E, Matson J L, Senatore V 1983 Assessment of depression in mentally retarded adults. Am J Psychiatr 140:1040–1043

King B 1993 Self-injury by people with mental retardation: a compulsive behavior hypothesis. Am J Mental Retard 98:93–112

King N J, Ollendick T H, Gullone E et al 1990 Fears and phobias in children and adolescents with intellectual disabilities: assessment and intervention strategies. Aust N Z J Dev Disabil 16:97–108

Langan J, Russell O, Whitfield M 1993 Community care and the general practitioner: primary health care for people with learning disabilities. Norah Fry Research Centre, University of Bristol

Levitas A S, Gilson S F 1994 Psychosocial development of children and adolescents with mild and moderate mental retardation. In: Bouras N (ed) Mental health in mental retardation: recent advances and practices. Cambridge University Press, Cambridge

Lindsay W R, Baty F J 1989 Group relaxation training with adults who are mentally handicapped. Behav Psychother 17:43–51

Lindsay W R, Michie A M, Baty F J, McKenzie K 1988 Dog phobia in people with mental handicaps: anxiety management training and exposure treatments. Mental Handicap Res 1:39–48

Lindsay W R, Baty F J, Michie A M, Richardson I 1989 A comparison of anxiety treatments with adults who have moderate and severe mental retardation. Res Dev Disabil 10:129–140

Lund J 1985 The prevalence of psychiatric morbidity in mentally retarded adults. Acta Psychiatr Scand 72:563–570

Matson J L 1984 Psychotherapy with persons who are mentally retarded. Mental Retardation 22:170–175

Matson J L, Kadzin A E, Senatore V 1984 Psychometric properties of the Psychopathology Instrument for mentally retarded adults. Appl Res Mental Retard 5:881–889

Matson J L, Gardner W I, Coe D A, Sovner R 1991 A scale for evaluating emotional disorders in severely and profoundly mentally retarded persons. Br J Psychiatr 159:404–409

McClellan J M, Werry J S, Ham M 1993 A follow-up study of early onset psychosis: comparison between outcome diagnoses of schizophrenia, mood disorders and personality disorders. J Autism Dev Disord 23:243–262

McLoughlin I J, Bhate M S 1987 A case of affective psychosis following bereavement in a mentally handicapped woman. Br J Psychiatr 151:552–554

Meichenbaum D 1975 A self-instructional approach to stress management: a proposal for stress inoculation training. In: Sarason I, Spielberger C D (eds) Stress and anxiety, vol. 2. Wiley, New York

Meins W 1993 Assessment of depression in mentally retarded adults: reliability and validity of the Children's Depression Inventory (CDI). Res Dev Disabil 14:299–312

Meins W 1995 Symptoms of major depression in mentally retarded adults. J Intellect Disabil Res 39:41–45

Morrison F J, Lindsay W R 1997 Reductions in self assessed anxiety and concurrent improvement in cognitive performance in adults who have moderate intellectual disabilities. J Appl Res Intellect Disabil 10:33–40

Moss S C 1995 Methodological issues in the diagnosis of psychiatric disorders in adults with learning disability. Thornfield J (University of Dublin) 18:9–18

Moss S C 1999a Issues of human rights for the mental health for older people with intellectual disabilities. In: Herr S, Weber G (eds) Aging, rights and quality of life for older persons with developmental disabilities. Paul Brookes, Baltimore

Moss S C 1999b Issues of diagnosis. In: Bouras N (ed) Psychiatric and behavioural disorders in mental retardation. Cambridge University Press, Cambridge

Moss S C, Patel P, Prosser H et al 1993 Psychiatric morbidity in older people with moderate and severe learning disability (mental retardation). Part I: Development and reliability of the patient interview (the PAS-ADD). Br J Psychiatr 163:471–480

Moss S C, Prosser H, Ibbotson B, Goldberg D 1996 Respondent and informant accounts of psychiatric symptoms in a sample of patients with learning disability. J Intellect Disabil Res 40:457–465

Moss S C, Ibbotson B, Prosser H, Goldberg D P, Patel P, Simpson N 1997 Validity of the PAS-ADD for detecting psychiatric symptoms in adults with learning disability. Social Psychiatr Psychiatr Epidemiol 32:344–354

Moss S C, Prosser H, Costello H et al 1998 Reliability and validity of the PAS-ADD Checklist for detecting psychiatric disorders in adults with intellectual disability. J Intellect Disabil Res 42:173–183

Murphy G 1994 Understanding challenging behaviour. In: Emerson E, McGill P, Mansell J (eds) Severe learning disabilities and challenging behaviours: designing high quality services. Chapman and Hall, London, pp 37–68

Nezu C M, Nezu A M 1994 Outpatient psychotherapy for adults with mental retardation and concomitant psychopathology: research and clinical imperatives. J Consult Clin Psychol 62:34–42

Novaco R W 1975 Anger control: the development and evaluation of an experimental treatment. Lexington Books, Lexington, MA

Oliver C, Head D 1990 Self-injurious behaviour in people with learning disabilities: determinants and interventions. Int Rev Psychiatr 2:101–116

Parsons J A, May J G, Menolascino F J 1984 The nature and incidence of mental illness in mentally retarded individuals. In: Menolascino F J, Stark J A (eds) Handbook of mental illness in the mentally retarded. Plenum Press, New York

Patel P, Goldberg D P, Moss S C 1993 Psychiatric morbidity in older people with moderate and severe learning disability (mental retardation). Part II: The prevalence study. Br J Psychiatr 163:481–491

Pavlov I P 1927 Conditioned reflexes: an investigation of the physiological activity of the cerebral cortex (trans. W H Grant). Oxford University Press, London

Pfadt A 1991 Group psychotherapy with mentally retarded adults: issues related to design, implementation, and evaluation. Res Dev Disabil 12:261–285

Prosser H, Moss S C, Costello H, Simpson N, Patel P, Rowe S 1998 Reliability and validity of the Mini PAS-ADD for assessing psychiatric disorders in adults with intellectual disability. J Intellect Disabil Res 42:264–272

Raskind M A, Peskind E R 1992 Alzheimer's disease and other dementing disorders. In: Birren J E, Sloane R B, Chen G D (eds) Handbook of mental health and ageing. Academic Press, London

Reid A H 1982 The psychiatry of mental handicap. Blackwell, Oxford

Reiss S 1982 Psychopathology and mental retardation: survey of a developmental disabilities mental health program. Mental Retardation 20:128–132

Reiss S 1987 Reiss screen for maladaptive behavior. International Diagnostic Systems, Chicago

Reiss S 1990 Prevalence of dual diagnosis in community-based day programs in the Chicago metropolitan area. Am J Mental Retard 94:578–585

Reiss S 1994 Handbook of challenging behaviour: mental health aspects of mental retardation. IDS Publishing Corporation, USA

Reiss S, Benson B A 1985 Psychosocial correlates of depression in mentally retarded adults: I. Minimal social support and stigmatization. Am J Mental Defic 89:331–337

Reiss S, Rojahn J 1993 Joint occurrence of depression and aggression in children and adults with mental retardation. J Intellect Disabil Res 37:287–294

Rickard H C, Thrasher K A, Elkins P D 1984 Responses of persons who are mentally retarded to four components of relaxation instruction. Mental Retardation 22: 248–252

Ritvo E R, Jorde L B, Mason B A et al 1989 The UCLA University of Utah epidemiologic survey of autism: recurrence risk estimates and genetic counseling. Am J Psychiatr 146:1032

Rodgers J 1994 Primary healthcare provision for people with learning difficulties. Health Social Care 2:11–17

Royal College of Physicians 1981 Organic mental impairment in the elderly: implications for research, education and the provision of services. J Roy Coll Phys London 102:141–167

Russell A T, Tanguay P E 1996 Mental retardation. In: Lewis M (ed) Child and adolescent psychiatry. A comprehensive textbook. Williams and Wilkins, Baltimore

Rutter M, Graham P, Yule W 1970 A neuropsychiatric study in childhood. Spastics International Medical Publications and Heinemann, London

Shamoian C A 1985 Assessing depression in elderly patients. Hosp Commun Psychiat 36:338–339

Skinner B F 1938 The behaviour of organisms: an experimental analysis. Appleton-Century, New York

Sovner R, Hurley A D 1985 Assessing the quality of psychotropic drug regimes prescribed for mentally retarded persons. Psychiatr Aspects Mental Retard Rev 8/9:31–38

Sovner R, Fox C J, Lowry M J, Lowry M A 1993 Fluoxetine treatment of depression and associated self-injury in two adults with mental retardation. J Intellect Disabil Res 37:301–311

Spitzer R L, Endicott J, Robins E 1978 Research diagnostic criteria: rationale and reliability. Arch Gen Psychiatr 35:773–782

Symington N 1981 The psychotherapy of the subnormal patient. Br J Med Psychol 54:187–199

Szymanski L S 1988 Integrative approach to diagnosis of mental disorders in retarded persons. In: Stark L A, Menolascino F J, Albarelli N H, Gray V C (eds) Mental retardation and mental health. Classification, diagnosis and treatment services. Springer-Verlag, New York

Tasse M J, Aman M G, Hammer D, Rojahn J 1996 The Nisonger Child Behavior Rating Form: age and gender effects and norms. Res Dev Disabil 17:59–75

Thorndike E L 1911 Animal intelligence: experimental studies. Macmillan, New York

Varley C K 1984 Schizophreniform psychoses in mentally retarded adolescent girls following sexual assault. Am J Psychiatr 141:593–595

Werry J S, McClellan J M, Andrews L K, Ham M 1994 Clinical features and outcome of child and adolescent schizophrenia. Schizophrenia Bull 20:619–630

Wolpe J 1958 Psychotherapy by reciprocal inhibition. Stanford University Press, Stanford, CA

Zung W W K 1965 A self-rating scale for depression. Arch Gen Psychiatr 12:63–70

14 Life transitions and personal change

Jeanette Thompson and Sharon Pickering

KEY ISSUES

- Transition and change
- Personal change
- Life events
- Changes in role, status and place
- Models for managing change
- Personal tasks and skills in managing change

Change is a process that all of us experience at some time or another in our lives. We experience formal adaptation processes as part of the developments in our working lives, we experience change by virtue of growing up and growing older and we therefore frequently make adjustments in both role and function in our personal day-to-day lives. Whilst we clearly acknowledge the inevitability of some of these changes we do not always recognize that people who have a learning disability will be involved in the same changes and on some occasions additional changes to those that the rest of us experience.

Transitions can be stressful as a result of the feelings of confusion that can exist. Williams & Walmsley (1990) talk about a sense of dislocation in association with life adjustments. For most of us change can be something we wish for, for example leaving school, getting married, moving to a new job, as well as something that may be unexpected, unplanned for or unpleasant. On those occasions when we expect change there are many things we can do to plan and prepare for it. In order to more successfully manage all transitions it is important to identify the key elements of any change and our subsequent responses in order to incorporate these into future actions. On this basis it is also important to consider how people who have a learning disability can manage the experience of change that they may have.

Williams & Walmsley (1990) identify two reasons for studying transitions. The first of these is the belief that by exploring our own transitions and those experienced by others, we will be better placed to understand the needs of people who have a learning disability. Second, by examining and understanding the process of adaptation to change, we may be better able to identify ways of managing personal change more successfully, both for ourselves and for people who have a learning disability. In achieving both these goals a significant contribution can be made to the empowerment of each individual.

In order to achieve the above, this chapter will explore what is meant by the terms 'transitions' and 'personal change', the types of changes people experience, the internal and external factors that influence our approach to managing change and both personal and process models for managing change. Throughout this chapter the meaning of these changes will be considered in the context of people who have a learning disability, particularly in relation to the impact of transitions upon a person's health status.

TRANSITION AND CHANGE

This chapter is concerned with personal change – ordinary, everyday change such as birth, death, illness, marriage, divorce, unemployment, moves and promotion. Transitions can be defined in the context of those brief and unsettled periods of time that mark the movement from one developmental stage to another. Consequently this chapter will focus upon the short sharp events that are called life transitions as well as some of the more fundamental changes that can be experienced. These events require individuals to take risks and cope with uncertainty and fear, part of which relates to the uncertainty as to where the change will lead (Hopson & Adams 1977).

There are a number of different types of change that can affect our lives: social, economic, institutional, political, ideological, demographic and technological (see Box 14.1).

During the last 30 years the amount of change that Western society has been exposed to has gained in momentum. The pace of change shows no indication of slowing down as we enter a new century. The speed of change and the impact it has on the lives of individuals is no less profound for people who have a

BOX 14.1	*Types of change*	
	Social	Includes issues such as the introduction of community care
	Economic	Includes the changes to benefit systems
	Institutional	Includes changes to the structure and delivery of statutory services such as health and education
	Political	Includes those areas that are typically the focus of pressure groups and development agencies and may include agendas such as valued employment for people who have a learning disability
	Ideological	Includes the involvement of people who have a learning disability in developing, delivering and evaluating the services they use
	Demographic	Includes changes in the size, nature and age structure of the population. From a learning disability perspective, this not only includes the increasing older population but also the increasing numbers of younger people who have extremely complex health needs
	Technological	Includes the communication revolution and the increased use of the Internet to create informed consumers of health and social care services

learning disability. In some instances the perception that we are on the interface between the postindustrial and the information technology era can bring particular difficulties for people who have a learning disability. Nowhere is this more evident than in the growth of a credit card and consumer society. Whilst many of us would now be lost if we were not in possession of a credit card and did not have a credit rating, many people who have a learning disability are denied access to parts of society because they do not have either of these things. This development is parallel to earlier difficulties that were experienced when people who have a learning disability were unable to access a personal bank account.

In addition, change can involve a psychological and/or a biological aspect. This particularly relates to the changes that each individual experiences as they progress through the developmental stages of life as well as the ways in which our body physically changes as we progress from childhood through to old age and death.

All the above factors create a transition. It has been suggested so far that transitions involve periods of personal or psychological adaptation to change. This process of adaptation or adjustment is influenced by the context in which the change is taking place. In this way some of the transitions we experience will present as monumental while they are happening, whilst later reflection may indicate a somewhat reduced level of significance. Conversely, some changes that appear almost insignificant at the time can at a later date be identified as having great relevance to our life.

PERSONAL CHANGE

Individual change can be influenced by a number of different factors. Williams & Walmsley (1990) identified the following:

- The person's own psychology, including their self-esteem, self-value, identity and confidence
- Belief systems and how they inform what is and is not acceptable for oneself and for people who have a learning disability
- The socioeconomic conditions
- Unpredictable events.

In addition, personal change can have a number of different foci; the most useful structure for considering these is in relation to role, status and place. Role transitions can include changes to a person's roles that may be in terms of themselves, their family and significant others and also their role in society. This includes roles such as sister, brother, son, daughter, parent, husband, wife, boss and employee. The latter may be expressed as a professional role, such as teacher, manager, sales person, nurse, etc. Role transition can include moving out of a role as well as into one; for example, the move from employment to either unemployment or retirement.

Unemployment or retirement can also be seen as a change of status, as can the move from adolescence to adulthood. Changes to a person's perceived status can have a significant impact upon their self-esteem and self-worth with the implicit ramifications for their health status, particularly their mental health and well-being.

Change of place can either be seen as a positive or negative experience or possibly a combination of both. In part this relates to the level of control and involvement that a person has over the actual transition. Most of us feel that relatively few changes are imposed upon us, though the reality of this may be somewhat different. However, what makes us feel in control is our ability to capitalize on what may be an enforced change and to identify the opportunities within that situation, particularly ones that will be to our advantage. For a person who has a learning disability many more changes of place will be imposed upon them. This may be the result of a hospital closure, a relocation programme, a rationalization of existing services, the sale of a business or going concern such as a private residential service, abuse from another person or, more positively, a desire to move on, get married and have a family.

LIFE EVENTS

This section utilizes the structure of changes outlined above to explore some of the more specific issues relating to people who have a learning disability.

Change in role

A change in role can be considered within the immediate family unit and within the wider context of the society in which we live. Changes within the family unit may include the birth of a sibling, the death of a parent or significant other. It may also include leaving the parental home to live on your own, getting married and becoming a husband or wife, having children and becoming a family unit. It may also include the breakdown of personal relationships, including those with a partner or spouse. From the perspective of the extended family, it may also mean becoming an aunt, uncle or cousin as well as taking on other family roles. These roles and the responsibilities that go with them may vary depending upon the cultural background of the person and their family.

For people who have a learning disability the roles and responsibilities within each of these areas may bring both similar and different challenges and opportunities to the remainder of the population.

Birth

The birth of a sibling is one such event that can change the position of the person who has a learning disability within the family or household unit. It means that they are taking on the role of older sister or brother. This role has many unspoken responsibilities attached to it at home, in the school playground and playing in the street. People who have a learning disability may require some support in understanding these dynamics. The greatest risk from the person's point of view comes when those around them do not expect them to fulfil any of these roles because they have a learning disability. In addition, there may be particular difficulties associated with this role especially if they are the cause of taunting and bullying experienced by their sibling.

Death

The death of an important person in one's life is clearly acknowledged as one of life's major stresses (Holmes & Rahe 1967). For some people who have a learning disability, particularly those who still live in the parental home, this can be a particularly difficult transition. If the individual has received little or no support from statutory services and their social contacts have predominantly been mediated by their parents, this time of life can be extremely traumatic. In such circumstances the death of the last surviving parent can result in the convergence of a number of major life transitions and potential stressors.

CASE STUDY 14.1

William is 67 years old and has lived at home with his mother since the death of his father 32 years ago. William has had an emergency referral made for him to the local community team for people who have a learning disability, as his mother, Gladys, has just died. The immediate response of the team is to consider William's safety. As a result William is admitted to a local respite service prior to the assessment of his self-help skills and other needs.

In the above case study, it can be seen that William is potentially facing three major life stressors: the loss of his mother, the loss of his home and familiar surroundings and potentially the loss of his support networks. All of these stressors can have a major impact upon William's health status.

ACTIVITY 14.1

How else might William's situation have been planned for? What are the difficulties with implementing these plans and how can they be overcome?

In order to minimize the likelihood of three life events of this enormity converging at one point in a person's life, much more proactive interventions are required. These include working with people at an earlier stage in their life to facilitate the development of personal social networks that are not dependent upon family members (Thompson & Pickering 1998). In addition, it means allowing, supporting and facilitating people who have a learning disability to grow up and leave home in the same way as other young people. In the situations where this does not occur, primary healthcare and learning disability services need to work together to put the appropriate person-centred plans into place.

The difficulties that may be experienced with all the above can be summarized in two areas: resources and partnership. All services are regularly working within limited resources and to full capacity. The impact of this can be seen in the development of priority matrices that allow professionals to identify which people have the most urgent level of need. It may be as a result of situations like this that William has not received appropriate input until a crisis is imminent.

Whilst working in partnership is a central part of all government agendas, the reality can be difficult to achieve. This may be because of overstretched resources but may also be as a consequence of limited understanding and awareness of both the role and function of respective partners as well as the complexity and urgency of the situation in which William and others find themselves. It is therefore incumbent upon professionals in all areas to focus more upon meeting the needs of service users than upon the barriers and difficulties of interprofessional working.

Relationships

Within society there is a widespread expectation that people will develop long-term relationships that lead to setting up home together. Often this relates to marital status but this does not exclude long-term relationships, either heterosexual or homosexual, that do not result in marriage. Marital status has been consistently shown to have a direct relationship with health and well-being, with married couples demonstrating lower levels of psychological distress (Hope et al 1999), whilst gender has been identified as a significant influence on the levels of distress, with depression and anxiety disorders being more prevalent in married women (Meltzer et al 1995, Weissman et al 1991).

Implicit within the above is the understanding that stable personal partnerships are on the whole a positive experience that people actively seek out. It is therefore surprising that people who have a learning disability can experience so much opposition and prejudice when they express the wish to engage in a long-term intimate relationship or marriage. Whilst this is not the experience of all people who have a learning disability who wish to get married, it continues to be a significant challenge for some professionals, service providers and families.

CASE STUDY 14.2   Karl and Karen are both in their late 20s and have been in a serious relationship for 4 years. Currently, Karl lives with his parents and Karen lives in a small group home. Karl has recently asked Karen to marry him and after making him wait for more than a week, Karen has finally said yes.

ACTIVITY 14.2   What actions do you think Karl and Karen will need to take? How do these compare with any wedding plans you may have been involved in?

Having agreed to marry, Karl and Karen decided that they would discuss this with Karl's parents and Karen's key worker. Karl's parents were initially a little concerned though not particularly surprised. However, Karen's key worker was very concerned about whether Karen really understood what a big commitment marriage was, where she and Karl would live and how they would manage.

ACTIVITY 14.3   If Karen lived in the service you work in, what sort of response do you think she would have received when she announced that she and Karl wanted to get married?

The response Karen received does not appear to be uncommon. Often people who have a learning disability announcing a marriage are greeted with all the problems and difficulties they may face rather than the celebrations that others would experience. This is all the more ironic because many of these difficulties are equally real for the rest of society and many marriages within the general population do end in divorce.

Psychological distress has been shown to relate to role changes that arise as a result of divorce or separation. These are believed to relate to contact with children, financial support and social contacts or support (Bordow 1992, Kelly 1994).

Parenting

As a natural consequence of the increased involvement of people who have a learning disability in their communities and the subsequent development of social contacts and relationships, there is an increase in the number of children being born to parents who have a learning disability. This situation in itself causes a significant number of issues both for the people involved and for the services providing support to them.

All too often the involvement of learning disability services is requested at the stage where people are about to go to court and risk losing their children to statutory services, with all the inherent complexities of that course of action. Often the request to services is to provide assessment data to demonstrate whether a person is able to look after their children properly or has the cognitive ability to learn to do so. The difficulty with these situations is not only the willingness of the parents or parent to cooperate at such a stressful time, but also the task of defining what constitutes good parenting, particularly as good parenting can be affected by any number of variables. These include major life stressors, the quality and level of support from partner and family members, environment, financial circumstances and many others.

A key issue when resolving such complex situations is the imperative to balance the needs of both the parent(s) and the child. Within this are the complexities of the different professionals and organizations working together when each of them operates from a potentially different value and philosophy base (Nocon 1989). The challenge is to resolve the issue in a way that ensures optimum health status for all those involved.

Valued employment

A great deal of research exists concerned with the transition from youth to adulthood (Coffield et al 1986, Jenkins 1982, 1983). Within this literature there is a recognition that the process of becoming an adult is structured by many things: gender, marriage, parenthood and also the place of the person within the work environment. This is particularly prevalent in Western societies where the Victorian work ethic predominates.

For people who have a learning disability the value of employment is no less important than for the rest of society. However, for many people valued employment continues to be extremely difficult to achieve. Emerson et al (1999) identified that less than 5% of people who have a learning disability are in such employment. The difficulties they experience may arise from the economic health of the country. In times of recession and instability people who have a learning disability find more difficulty in sustaining or gaining employment. In addition, the perceptions of society as to the value of people who have a learning disability will impact on their ability to gain entry to the workforce. Finally, the complexities of the benefit system can mean people are trapped in a position of being unable to afford to go out to work.

Such discrimination is difficult enough to counteract but there may also be indirect discrimination by professionals and service providers if they believe that people who have a learning disability cannot work or should not take the jobs of other people. In addition, there may be a belief that day centres and similar projects are equivalent to work. Within this situation additional complexities have arisen with the introduction of the minimum wage. This has resulted in some people having their jobs redefined as voluntary, in order to escape the parameters of the legislation. Other people have found themselves in situations where 'work' is now being combined with therapeutic interventions, such as 'healthy lifestyles' programmes, in order to redefine the function of the organization as therapy rather than work. This is another way in which financial remuneration is able to remain below the agreed minimum wage. The absence of valued work opportunities for people who have a learning disability can impact upon the person's health status in much the same way as the physical and mental health of any person who is unemployed for a long period of time.

A crucial role for professionals and service providers working with people who have a learning disability therefore is to work towards valued employment in order to improve their health status. Where this is not achieved then consideration should be given to supporting people with the individual difficulties they experience within their physical and psychological well-being as a result of effectively being unemployed.

Change in status

This section is concerned with the position of people within both society and their immediate family. Hareven (1982) argues that the status and position people experience are moulded by their cumulative histories and by the specific conditions which affect their lives. This is also illustrated by Warner et al (1998) who describe the central position of genetics, age and gender upon life experience along with lifestyle factors and other sociopolitical influences which mould the person. The adaptation of individuals and families to these factors is dependent upon the interrelationship of all the factors at each given point in time. Key factors known to have a bearing upon successful adaptation include experiences of family relationships, the expectations of family support and the ability to interact successfully with the wider society, particularly public agencies and large bureaucracies.

This aspect of transitions typically includes the changes we experience as we move through the developmental stages of life. This includes the transition from childhood to adolescence and then into adulthood, the movement through mid-life and into old age, with associated changes such as retirement.

Childhood to adolescence

The transition from childhood to adolescence is traditionally a very tempestuous time in a person's life. This stage in life is characterized by dramatic physical changes as well as enormous psychological and emotional challenges (Rutter & Hay 1994). From the perspective of a person who has a learning disability each of these changes can have increased complexities, particularly in relation to understanding and articulating the changes to other people around them. Also this is the beginning of that crucial developmental stage of finding your own identity and persona. Professional involvement at this time may focus upon sexual health, lifestyle choices and choices about education, jobs and other opportunities.

Adolescence into adulthood

As already noted, it is crucial during adolescent years that each of us asserts our own personality and rejects the characteristics of our parents. For the person who has a learning disability this may not be so easy to achieve. This can be because of difficulties with verbal communication but more often relates to limited role models and a lack of control over their own lifestyle. This can mean not being able to go out with friends for the evening either because they do not live locally or because this is not presented as an option for the person due to problems with safety or overprotection.

The progression from adolescence to adulthood is also often marked by an increase in the stability of a person's lifestyle, with choices being made to leave home, establish relationships, set up home and maybe start a family. Additional elements of this transition include the right to vote, gaining control over your finances and the changing relationship with your parents. Once again, for people who have a learning disability something that appears 'simple' enough for the rest of us to achieve can become significantly more difficult; for example, as has already been discussed in relation to credit cards and credit rating.

Middle years

Mid-life transitions are increasingly recognized as normal features of adult life rather than deficiencies of character or acute situations that need to be tidied up (Levinson et al 1978, Wolf & Kolb 1980). The mid-life transition is a time which bridges two major areas of life: early adulthood and middle age. It is a very important time for a person's career, family and sense of self.

At the same time as the above psychological and emotional transition, a number of physical changes may also begin to take place. These are particularly relevant for women as they begin to enter the menopause. The menopause can be an extremely significant time for many women, particularly as they adjust to their inability to continue bearing children. Situations such as this will implicitly have a knock-on impact for women's psychological and mental health.

For men the physical changes may not be so obvious but there is a growing body of evidence to support the existence of a male menopause or mid-life change (Bowskill & Lineacre 1976). This period of transition can be characterized by some men changing their behaviour to reflect activities that are more consistent with younger men; for example, buying a large motor bike or going clubbing.

For people who have a learning disability these changes may often have been ignored. More consideration is given to supporting women entering the menopause but the picture is by no means consistent. Some of the more subtle life changes do, however, still appear to be largely ignored, with little support made available. This may be because of the hidden nature of some of the changes which can only be identified by talking to people and determining their experiences.

Old age and retirement

There are many transitions that an individual who is growing older will experience. It could be suggested that older people are much better at adjusting to these changes as they have had a great deal of experience of them. However, this is not necessarily the case and there is evidence that some people are better equipped to adjust than others (Bromley 1988). The factors that appear to have an impact upon successful transitions are:

- a positive approach to life
- a full and active life, with hobbies
- good social networks
- healthy lifestyle.

Fitzgerald (1998), when considering the needs of people who have a learning disability during the transition to old age, identified the importance of where people lived, how they spend their time, friends, family and the existence of real choices. Ward (1998) also noted that people who have a learning disability value being able to talk about the old days and having staff work with them who will listen and to whom they are able to talk.

Harris et al (1997) suggest the factors associated with a successful transition to old age for people who have a learning disability include a healthy lifestyle, a healthy living environment, a positive mental attitude towards becoming older, positive support networks and a feeling of safety, security and stability.

Fennell et al (1988) suggest that retirement is an essential part of old age, particularly as it is seen as a sign that old age has begun. The process of the transition to retirement is complex. Atchley (1976) divides it into a series of stages including preretirement, where expectations are formed, honeymoon, which immediately follows the retirement, disenchantment, which is often seen when people fail to develop satisfying new roles and routines. The next stage is reorientation where stock is taken and choices are made. This is followed by stability, in which an individual begins to deal with the changes brought about by the retirement. The final stage is termination when the process of retirement is no longer important. The catalyst for this stage is often disability and poor health.

ACTIVITY 14.4   How may the experience of retirement be different for people who have a learning disability? How does this differ from the experience of other members of society?

These differences predominantly focus upon the often very different employment experience of people who have a learning disability. Many people will not have worked from leaving school to the age of retirement. Those people who have been employed for any or all of this period will not always have had a meaningful salary that equates with that of their non-disabled peers. This can lead to differences in retirement in relation to finances available to support hobbies and activities during this period of life.

Change in place

Essentially this section involves the concept of moving home, one of the biggest stressors in life (Holmes & Rahe 1967). For most of us moving home is a conscious decision that we make, with an understanding of the implications of our choice and a level of control over the decision and the stages within the process.

For people who have a learning disability these stressors can be magnified as a consequence of a number of factors. These can range from the earliest point in the process when the person first became aware that they were to move home. This awareness may have been raised in a generalized way, based around the hospital or institution closing rather than the person being specifically told they were moving. It may be related to the limited amount of control and involvement people have had over the decision that they were to move.

It may relate to factors which influence the different places the person would like to live as well as when they would like this to happen by. It may also relate to discussions around the type of house and how they would like it decorated or issues about how they would still see their friends and where they may go to work.

ACTIVITY 14.5   What might be the impact on a person if they are not involved in discussions or supported in making decisions about life changes?

The impact this can have upon the health and well-being of a person is significant, particularly in terms of self-esteem, confidence and self-worth. There are also important messages about power and control that may have ramifications for relationships between the person and professionals. The remainder of this chapter will explore these reactions in more depth by considering the individual's reactions to change, the meaning of life changes and the strategies people who have a learning disability and professionals can use to work through these transitions.

REACTIONS TO PERSONAL CHANGE

As already stated, change is an extremely personal experience which affects each individual in a different way. Personal responses to change may include one or more of the following emotions: fear, anxiety, indifference, anticipation, excitement, guilt, resentment or pleasure.

ACTIVITY 14.6   Think about an event that changed your life significantly. Write down your thoughts and feelings at the time. Now consider your current thoughts and feelings about the situation. Do they differ?

Your thoughts and feelings about significant life events were very likely centred on how this change was going to affect the rest of your life. This is even more likely if that event involved a perceived loss such as the loss of your job or leaving school. These feelings may have resulted in a sense of confusion and an element of uncertainty regarding future choices. At the time these feelings may have been overpowering and caused significant confusion. However, as time progresses these will often subside, leaving you with a generalized feeling that the situation was manageable and on occasions even positive.

PERSONAL MEANING OF TRANSITIONS

For many of us our perception of transitions is often focused upon the big events in life that are obvious to outside observers. It is in this way that professionals and others often view the life transitions experienced by people who have a learning disability. Whilst this can be extremely important and its value in supporting people to manage those major transitions cannot be overestimated, it is equally important to consider those smaller, less obvious transitions that often take place within the person. These changes can include important aspects of a person's life such as the beginnings of empowerment or disempowerment. These situations may initially be completely imperceptible to other people, including professionals working with that individual. It is only by asking a person and listening to their response that you will be able to identify a change in how they think and feel about themselves and their current experiences and the way in which this will affect them in the future.

Crucial to understanding this is an ability to interpret, with the person, their verbal and non-verbal communication, combined with an understanding of our own communication skills and style.

CASE STUDY 14.3   Sally, 23 years old, is a happy person who enjoys going out with her friends and enjoys her college course; she is studying catering and life skills. One day at college she is confronted by a new teacher who does not know Sally very well and does not realize how much reassurance Sally needs with the things she is doing, particularly when asked to speak up in front of her fellow students. During the day Sally is asked to discuss what she has done over the weekend; when she struggles to make herself clear the teacher moves on to the next person, without making sure Sally is all right. When talking to Sally afterwards it is clear that this situation has significantly undermined her confidence. This is particularly difficult as Sally is only just beginning to believe she can assert herself in a public forum. Observations of Sally afterwards indicate that this situation has had an impact in other parts of her life, including home where she also stops speaking up for herself for a while.

It would have been preferable had the above situation never happened. This would only have been possible through very skilful understanding and observation of both the person and their communication skills. It was skilful communication skills that helped resolve the situation and place Sally back on the road to becoming more assertive. It is, however, impossible to estimate how much such a situation impacted upon her overall development and self-esteem.

Of note within this context is the similarity with situations that we are all exposed to. However, most of us have developed strategies to deal with these situations in a way which allows us to preserve our self-esteem and feelings of self-worth.

COPING WITH CHANGE

One way of effectively managing life transitions and the inherent changes within them is to develop appropriate levels of personal response to those changes. Some of the responses that we can develop are adjustment, coping, renewal, transformation and transcendence (Brammer 1991).

Adjustment

Brammer (1991) describes adjustment as an automatic adaptational response to environmental pressure. On experiencing environmental pressure to change, the initial decision that has to be made by the individual is whether to resist the change or to adapt to it. Resisting change, or doing nothing, could be seen as the easy option in that it may save the person the time and energy required to make a positive choice. Conversely, it may result in significant danger for an individual; for example, a decision not to make a change in lifestyle by a person who is overweight, smokes, has high blood pressure and leads a sedentary life can have ramifications regarding their long-term health status and quality of life.

Making a positive choice and adjusting to the situation may be the best thing to do when something is unimportant, dangerous or futile to resist. Once we have decided that adjustment is the best response it is necessary to consider the appropriate strategy to achieve the optimum outcome.

Coping

The use of coping strategies is a more active problem-solving approach than the process of adaptation and may include questioning, the appraisal of danger, the setting of goals and option appraisal (Lazarus & Folkman 1984). Coping strategies include some fundamental attitudes and skills, such as:

- developing a positive attitude to change
- identifying opportunities within the situation
- taking control and responsibility for what is happening
- building support through family, friends and professional networks
- managing stress constructively by solving problems and appraising potential danger

- identifying the manageable elements of the change process and working with these
- making what appears unmanageable manageable by reconstructing the problems and issues involved.

The assumptions that underpin the development of a coping strategy include the belief that we have a huge reservoir of untapped potential which can be utilized to proactively cope with life changes. In addition, it is predicated upon the belief that we are able to learn and develop more appropriate approaches to coping and that we are able to grow from such challenges. Implicit within this is the understanding that we will become more able to cope with the future as a result of each experience.

Renewal

Renewal can be defined as a proactive attempt to direct change in a creative direction to the advantage of the individual (Brammer 1991). The renewal process is not effective as a response to enforced transitional change; it is more usefully employed in situations where a person seeks to change as a response to life becoming dull, repetitive and potentially boring. Such an approach to change is extremely risky and requires the individual to be able to manage that risk. Renewal involves having new goals and planning a new life direction; these can be either personal or professional.

It is possible to consider the relevance of this approach to initiating life changes in the context of people who have a learning disability and behaviour that challenges services and society. It is acknowledged that challenging behaviour is a form of communication for many people and that it may be a response to physical or psychological pain. For this group of people it may also be a coping mechanism and a way of changing a life that is inherently boring to one that they feel is more stimulating and over which they have more control.

Transformation

Transformational change can be seen as a fundamental shift in the way a problem, issue or situation is viewed either by an individual or by society. An example of this may be the way in which many of us reconstruct the recent death of someone significant in our lives. This often takes on the guise of focusing upon the benefits to the individual who has died, such as no longer being in pain or suffering indignity.

From the personal perspective, for many individuals the transition from employment to retirement might be viewed as a negative life event, particularly as a person no longer goes out to work and may see themselves as having no economic usefulness. However, a person may transform this view and see retirement as a great opportunity to learn new things and have new and different experiences. In this way, therefore, the transition changes from an unhappy event to a new time of challenge.

Brammer (1991) suggests that such shifts in thinking are a coping mechanism that can be learnt. However, it is necessary to interface concepts such as this with the overall philosophies and belief systems operating within learning disability services. It would not currently be seen as appropriate to use this approach to restructure a person's concept of adult training centres as a positive experience when the service user's preference was valued employment. Essentially, therefore, the transformational approach to managing transitions is appropriate with enforced or unavoidable changes, rather than where the person's personal preference is known but very difficult to achieve.

Transcendence

With this type of change and transition an individual may begin to develop their understanding of the meaning of their lives. In this way it has similarities to self-actualization (Maslow 1954) and some of the inherent complexities of this concept. Understanding at this level is believed to be related to the process of reflection and the development of self-awareness. Despite this it is not seen as a highly intellectual function but more as a feeling and a level of understanding which relates to a fundamental insight and perception of your own life and raison d'etre.

ANALYSING LIFE TRANSITIONS

Reflection upon transitions that have been key in your own life will identify the fact that transitions have a 'life of their own'. Essentially this means they have a beginning, a middle and an end with a clear turning point at some stage within this cycle. Brammer (1991) notes that transitions have the following stages.

- Beginning
- Between
- Present
- Future
- Finish

By placing the present in the middle of the overall process, Brammer (1991) is acknowledging that during any transition there comes a point when each individual recognizes that they are experiencing life change. In recognizing this, they also actively engage in considering future options. However, the use of the term 'present' in this context is confusing, as each stage will essentially be 'present' at the time it is taking place.

An alternative approach to analysing transitions can be seen in the model shown in Figure 14.1. This can be utilized to inform the interventions of professionals when supporting people who have a learning disability during any life transition.

If we are to be able to support people who have a learning disability through any life transitions then it is essential to understand the different stages of the transition. In addition, we need to develop the skill of analysing each transition in a way that will inform useful action planning and the understanding of the service user.

FIGURE 14.1   *Model for analysing transitions*

Beginning

This stage represents the initial point at which the transition begins. As the individual involved, you may or may not be aware of this starting point of the life change. The awareness of this initial point may come as a consequence of stage two of this model where a feeling of discomfort prompts the individual to reflect upon past events.

↓

Confusion

Confusion will not necessarily be represented within all life changes, but for some people this stage will form a significant part of the process. This stage can be characterized by feeling out of control and disempowered. As such, the first point of understanding by the person that they are experiencing a life transition can occur at this stage.

↓

Reflection

This stage is essentially about asking question of ourselves with regard to what is happening and why, what feelings we are having, and what the event/transition means for ourselves and for others. In essence, reflection is about how we can use this information for personal growth.

↓

Engagement

This stage in any transition could be seen as a turning point for the individual. Within this there is an acknowledgement that a transition is happening and a change is taking place. At this point a person can decide to take control of the process or not. A person who feels empowered may be more likely to make this an active decision, where someone is disempowered they are less likely to do so.

↓

Action planning

Once a person has decided to take control of the experience, then they will decide on their coping strategies and any future actions they are going to take. Action planning should include the following: assessment, identification of the problem, clarifying the problem as a real issue, appraisal of the options available, selection of preferred option, goal setting, planning to achieve the goal, identifying strategies to ensure the goal is achieved, implementation, monitoring and evaluation.

↓

Resolution

Within this part of the process, there is a feeling of completion. This can be either external or internal, external resolution being easier to achieve than internal. The internalization of a change may depend upon the outcome and what this means to the person.

MODELS FOR MANAGING TRANSITIONS AND CHANGE

Pearlin (1982) identifies a range of variables that need to be considered when supporting individuals through the change process. These include the individual's coping mechanisms, the availability and quality of support systems and the social context in which the change is taking place. From the perspective of people who have a learning disability, consideration of these issues can identify a number of factors important both at the time of a transition and in preparation for coping with transitions.

In the context of a transition that is taking place, it is important to assess the coping mechanisms that the individual feels able to use. These need to be assessed in the context of the forces affecting the change and the individual's ability to use these mechanisms to live through the change, imposed or otherwise. It is equally important to assess the person's social network with a particular emphasis upon the quality, availability and flexibility of that support, particularly in relation to its role in restoring and ensuring mental well-being. Assessment of the social context in which the change is taking place necessitates consideration of issues such as poverty, unemployment and social deprivation along with the impact that these may have upon the individual's ability to cope.

An additional strategy for assisting people to cope with transitions is to consider each of these areas as part of the long-term emotional development that is important for people who have a learning disability. This would include consideration of an individual's coping strategies, their social support network and the context in which they live as part of an ongoing involvement and not just as a response to an emergency.

Hopson & Adams (1976) focus on the impact of transitions upon the individual's self-esteem. They identify seven different stages, the first of these being immobilization. This includes an inability to act and to understand what is happening and can be typified by a sense of being overwhelmed. Classically, transitions of which we have little experience tend to provoke intense feelings at this time. Minimization is the second phase and can include significant feelings of denial. The purpose of this is to provide some time during which we can retreat from reality, thus allowing us to regain strength and develop our understanding of the change. The third stage is that of accepting reality. At this point the individual begins to make the most of their new situation and to let go of what existed before.

The energy released by acceptance leads the individual in to stage five. This is characterized by the testing out of new behaviours that are designed to cope with the new order. Stage six seeks meaning; this is essentially a reflective stage during which people aspire to work out how and why things have changed. The final stage is that of internalization, during which the changes become part of the person and their behaviour.

Throughout this model, the person's self-esteem will fluctuate, with stage three typically seeing a significant reduction in the value a person places upon themselves. Acceptance of reality and letting go of what has been can be a turning point with a subsequent gradual increase in feelings of self-worth.

IMPLICATIONS FOR SERVICE DELIVERY

As has been demonstrated above, transitions can be extremely complex periods in an individual's life. In order to minimize the disruption and the damage that can be done to a person's health status and/or quality of life, it is essential that professionals consider their role in supporting service users. Interventions that can be useful when supporting people through life changes or transitions include assisting them to deal with the initial crisis and to initiate coping strategies. Also, giving and receiving support, assisting them to release their emotions through the use of counselling approaches, listening to and expressing feelings through the use of effective counselling skills such as those outlined by Heron (1990). In addition, there is a need to provide reassurance when relevant and to support people through the different stages of the grieving process. Other strategies include supporting people to maintain their self-esteem and their health and well-being as well as working towards stabilizing the person's lifestyle. Finally, other interventions can include reinforcing efforts that are being made, clarifying perceptions, reaffirming positivity, goal setting, linking people into support groups and supporting the individual in defining and analysing life goals.

CONCLUSION

This chapter has provided a framework which can be used to consider the various aspects of change as experienced by individuals both with and without a learning disability. It has provided a structure for identifying and analysing life transitions that should prove useful to professionals when working with individuals. In addition, the chapter has adopted the framework of change in role, status and place. Once an area of change has been identified it is necessary to assess the individual in order to explore the meaning of the change for that person and also their personal reactions to the change. This information forms the backdrop to the way in which the professional both interprets any subsequent data and develops any intervention plans. These individual plans will also be informed by a more detailed analysis of the transition by using one of the models outlined in the latter part of the chapter. This process will lead the professional and the service user into a more systematic exploration of what is happening in the person's life and begin the process of effectively planning action to meet the service user's needs. Successful interventions in this area can support the service user in achieving optimum health and an enhanced quality of life.

FURTHER READING

Brammer L M 1991 How to cope with successful life changes: the challenges of personal change. Hemisphere Publishing, New York
This book explores the issues around transitions from a generic perspective. It provides a good basis from which readers can further develop their understanding of this area. In addition to providing a good theoretical base

from which to understand transitions, the book also provides some good practical examples as to how to deal with them.

Thompson J, Pickering S 1998 Social networks in old age. In: Pickering S, Thompson J (eds) Promoting positive practice in nursing older people. Baillière Tindall, London
This chapter, whilst being in a book about nursing older people, has much to offer. The book itself focuses upon all people who are older including people who have a learning disability. The chapter considers issues around social networks and not only suggests ways in which practitioners can assess people's networks and social contacts but also demonstrates ways in which people's social contacts can be developed.

Ward C 1998 Preparing for a positive future: meeting the age related changes of older people with learning disabilities. ARC Publications, Chesterfield
This document is the result of a national project designed to identify what constitutes a positive future for older people who have a learning disability. A key message within it is the need to listen to what people want and what people are telling service providers. It provides the reader with a range of practical strategies in order to achieve more positive futures for people including service standards, reflective exercises and useful addresses.

REFERENCES

Atchley R 1976 Selected social and psychological differences between men and women in later life. J Gerontol 31:204–211

Bordow S 1992 An analysis of defended custody judgements. Family Court of Australia, Office of the Chief Executive, Sydney, NSW

Bowskill D, Lineacre A 1976 The 'male' menopause. Muller, London

Brammer L M 1991 How to cope with successful life changes: the challenges of personal change. Hemisphere Publishing, New York

Bromley D B 1988 Human ageing: an introduction to gerontology. Penguin, London

Coffield F, Borrill C, Marshall S 1986 Growing up at the margins. Open University Press, Milton Keynes

Emerson E, Robertson J, Gregory N et al 1999 Quality and costs of residential supports for people with learning disabilities. Hester Adrian Research Centre, Manchester

Fennell G, Phillopson C, Evers H 1988 The sociology of old age. Open University Press, Milton Keynes

Fitzgerald J 1998 Time for freedom? Services for older people with learning difficulties. Centre for Policy on Ageing and Values into Action, London

Hareven T K 1982 The last stage: historical adulthood and old age. In: Erikson E H (ed) Adulthood. Norton, New York

Harris J, Bennett L, Hogg J 1997 Ageing matters. BILD Publications, Kidderminster

Heron J 1990 Helping the client: a creative practical guide. Sage Publications, London

Holmes T H, Rahe R H 1967 The social readjustment rating scale. J Psychosom Res 11:213–218

Hope S, Rogers B, Powers C 1999 Marital status transitions and psychological distress: longitudinal evidence from a national population sample. Psychol Med 29:381–389

Hopson B, Adams J 1976 Towards an understanding of transition: defining some boundaries of transition dynamics. In: Adams J, Hayes H, Hopson B (eds) Transition: understanding and managing personal change. Martin Robertson, London

Hopson B, Adams J 1977 Transitions: defining some boundaries. In: Adams J, Hayes H, Hopson B (eds) Transition. Allenheld and Osman, Montclair, New Jersey

Jenkins R 1982 Hightown rules: growing up in a Belfast housing estate. National Youth Bureau, Leicester

Jenkins R 1983 Lads, citizens and ordinary kids: working-class youth life-styles in Belfast. Routledge and Kegan Paul, London

Kelly J B 1994 The determination of child custody. Children Divorce 4:121–142

Lazarus R, Folkman S 1984 Stress, appraisal and coping. Springer, New York

Levinson D, Darrow D N, Klein E B, Levinson M H, McKee B 1978 The seasons of a man's life. Knopf, New York

Maslow A H 1954 Motivation and personality. Harper and Row, New York

Meltzer H, Gill B, Petticrew M, Hinds K 1995 The prevalence of psychiatric morbidity among adults living in private households. HMSO, London

Nocon A 1989 Forms of ignorance and their role in the joint planning process. Social Policy Admin 23(1):31–47

Pearlin L I 1982 Discontinuities in the study of ageing. In: Hareven T, Adams K (eds) Ageing and life course transitions: an interdisciplinary perspective. Tavistock, London

Rutter M, Hay D 1994 Development through life: a handbook for clinicians. Blackwell Science, Oxford

Thompson J, Pickering S 1998 Social networks in old age. In: Pickering S, Thompson J (eds) Promoting positive practice in nursing older people. Baillière Tindall, London

Ward C 1998 Preparing for a positive future: meeting the age-related changes of older people with learning disabilities. ARC Publications, Chesterfield

Warner M, Longley M, Gould E, Picek A 1998 Healthcare futures 2010. Welsh Insitute for Health and Social Care, Pontypridd, Glamorgan

Weissman M M, Bruce M L, Leaf P J, Holzer C 1991 Affective disorders. In: Robins L N, Regier D A (eds) Psychiatric disorders: the epidemiologic catchment area study. Free Press, New York

Williams F, Walmsley J 1990 Transitions and change: work book 3. In: Mental handicap: changing perspectives. Open University Press, Milton Keynes

Wolf D M, Kolb D A 1980 Beyond specialization: the quest for integration in mid career. In: Derr C (ed) Work, family and career. Praeger, New York

4 DEVELOPING PARTNERSHIPS

Not only is 'partnership' a buzz word at the moment, it is essential in order to deliver effective services for people who have a learning disability. This is going to be no less crucial in the future as we have now moved very clearly into an era where generic services are having to consider the needs of people who have a learning disability more and more. Carers are being acknowledged as central in the whole picture and the need to work with communities is not only increasingly important in learning disability service delivery but also from a public health perspective. It is for these reasons that this section addresses working with carers, communities and other professions and agencies.

SECTION CONTENTS

15 **Supporting the supporters – some reflections on family caregiving**
   Gordon Grant

16 **Working with communities**
   Angela Butcher with Jeanette Thompson and Sharon Pickering

17 **Interprofessional and multiagency working**
   Peter Mathias and Tony Thompson

15 Supporting the supporters – some reflections on family caregiving

Gordon Grant

KEY ISSUES

- Stress and coping
- Family resilience
- Family systems perspectives
- Lifespan
- Health

INTRODUCTION

This chapter reviews evidence about the varied ways in which families support and care about children and relatives who have learning disabilities. It suggests that over time there has been a shift from an emphasis on understanding the everyday stresses and problems families face to the ways in which they manage these. As a consequence there has been growing interest in what makes some families apparently more resilient than others. This shift in focus is quite important for nurses and other healthcare professionals in that it begins to offer some insights into the nature of resilience in families and into ways of reinforcing it with the aim of supporting the positive health status of all family members.

It is important to address key theoretical perspectives about family care as these provide different 'cognitive maps' for nurses and other healthcare professionals about possible ways of intervening with and supporting families. Accordingly the first part of this chapter provides a brief review of stress-coping theory, family resilience and family systems theory. It also suggests that constructions of caring and the lifespan need careful consideration by professionals if family support is to be holistic and extend seamlessly from 'cradle to grave'.

The second part of the chapter draws from empirical research evidence to reinforce these points. It summarizes key findings and offers some principles to guide nurses and other healthcare professionals in supporting families.

This chapter has a close affinity with Chapter 5 about the new public health agenda, Chapter 16 on working with communities and Chapter 17 which concerns interagency and multiprofessional working.

THEORETICAL PERSPECTIVES AND FAMILY CARE

Stress-coping theory

For a long time family caregiving has been informed by an understanding of stress as a central part of the caregiver experience, reflecting the continuing influence of a deficit model which implies a pathology within family functioning. Studies, for example, report that family carers quite often suffer psychological and physical stresses including psychiatric disturbance (Burden 1980, Grant et al 1990, Quine & Pahl 1991). The fascination with stress in families extends to studies of the care of people with specific syndromes (Hodapp et al 1998) and to families at different stages of the life cycle (Baxter et al 1995).

Yet it is not always made clear what theoretical perspectives underpin studies of family stress so it is often difficult to offer reasoned explanations as to why caregiving is stressful for some people and not others. Some studies appear to assume a direct connection between the personal characteristics of the person who has learning disabilities (their medical diagnosis, social skills, behaviour, for example) and the existence of stress within family carers. Such a 'stimulus–response' model (Robinson 1983) is rather too simplistic to be useful as it assumes that circumstances and events are either:

- stress provoking all the time
- equally stress provoking
- not mediated by other factors like coping skills and support networks.

Life events theorists, by contrast, see stress as stemming from interactions with the environment. Here stress is seen as the result of the cumulative effects of major life events like divorce, moving house, the birth of a disabled child, the onset of serious illness or bereavement (Dohrenwend & Dohrenwend 1974). The assumption is that life events like these, if occurring close together, are more likely to result in physical or psychological stress than single events. A 'life events' approach to understanding stress may be particularly useful at key transition points in people's lives, whether these be related to the onset, course and outcome of a person's disability, changes in their support networks or service transitions, particularly those between health, education and social services agencies. More is said about this later in relation to lifespan perspectives.

In a third model, generally credited to Lazarus & Folkman (1984), stress is construed in terms of a relationship between the person and the environment that is appraised by the person as relevant to their well-being and in which the person's resources are taxed or exceeded. In this model people are seen as constantly appraising transactions within their environment; those seen as stressful (i.e. as a threat or challenge) require coping to regulate distress (emotion-focused coping) or to manage the problem causing distress (problem-focused coping). Termed the 'transactional model', this approach emphasizes the cognitive appraisals people bring to situations and to the secondary and consequent appraisals made of the coping resources they can call on to deal with these. The validity of this model has been confirmed in studies of families supporting people who have very varied types of disability or chronic illness (Nolan et al 1996, Quine & Pahl 1991).

BOX 15.1	*Practice implications of stress theory*

- Importance of understanding significant life events (i) within the family history or (ii) that can be anticipated, for their effects on stress and coping.
- Recognizing that family members will perceive 'stressors' in different ways, i.e. apparently adverse circumstances will not necessarily be seen as stress provoking.
- Important factors shaping the experience of stress in family carers (Grant et al 1990, Orr et al 1991, Quine & Pahl 1991):
  - interpersonal relationship with care recipient
  - perceived social support
  - household finances
  - challenging behaviour
  - access to coping strategies and coping resources.
- Requirement to look beyond traits in carers or 'cared-for' persons for reasons as to why stresses are experienced.

Two important factors stand out in this model: first, the emphasis on the need for an improved understanding of how subjective appraisals mediate the experience of stress since these seem to be better predictors of stress than people's objective circumstances; and second, the explicit link made between stress and coping in ways that can be empirically tested. There are still some inconsistencies in the literature about whether dependency factors in care recipients, for example challenging behaviour, physical capacity, carer traits, family characteristics or environmental factors are most important in explaining stress. However, a number of general points can be made (Box 15.1).

Family resilience

More recently, literature has been emphasizing a strengths-based model which acknowledges that families can cope extremely well under conditions of apparent adversity (Hawley & DeHaan 1996, Schumacher et al 1998). These studies suggest that families frequently 'bounce back' from challenging situations and that they may have many kinds of resources for coping which mediate the experience of day-to-day stresses associated with caregiving (Quine & Pahl 1991). There is earlier evidence from studies such as that by Carr (1988), amongst others, that families commonly display a resilience and assert that things have worked out well and without major trauma for many years despite the 'daily grind'. This has led to interest in the nature of resilience and expertise within families, including families whose parents have learning disabilities (Booth & Booth 1998), and how these qualities are best recognized and reinforced.

Not only do uplifts and gratifications occur within families supporting offspring who have learning and other disabilities but they also seem to be more widespread than had previously been supposed (Grant et al 1998, Wilson et al 1998). Even in the unlikely context of caregiving partners of men with AIDS,

Folkman (1997) found that positive and negative psychological states coexisted in the midst of enduring and profoundly stressful circumstances. She concluded that we need to know more about the coping processes that trigger the search for positive psychological states and the intensity and duration of such states necessary to help sustain individuals in coping with everyday challenges. The indications are that even momentary experiences of gratification or uplift in caregiving can have long-lasting, stress-alleviating and life-enhancing effects.

Beresford (1994) identified two main sources of reward in families with disabled children: the child's successes or achievements and aspects of the caring role. Amongst the former, Beresford identified the 'precious' value to parents of the smallest achievements made by their children, these being all the more remarkable when they contradicted the prognoses of doctors. Pleasures were also associated with being able to enjoy a 'normal' everyday life. Among rewards associated with the caring role were those intrinsic to the role itself, some parents expressing the view that it was preferable to a career or a return to employment. Beresford also found that rewards may also be dependent upon the course of a child's disability, families of children with better prognoses 'drawing strength' from the expectation of decreased demands upon their energy and resources.

Culture undoubtedly has an important place in family resilience with race and ethnicity in particular being influential in shaping caregiving norms. Hence, placing a child in a prone sleeping position or sleeping in the same room as the child appears to be more accepted in the Asian community in Britain and is associated with a lower incidence of sudden infant death syndrome (Farooqi 1994). This points to the dangers of pathologizing behaviours that are culturally normative for different ethnic groups. It also emphasizes the importance of seeking to understand, from the perspectives of family members, what works for them in their own terms. In this sense it may help front-line professionals to make new discoveries which can be used to improve how families are supported. There is, however, a long way to go in addressing the linguistic, economic and cultural barriers that can still prevent families from black and ethnic communities taking up health and social services they may need (Fatimilehin & Nadirshaw 1994).

Hawley & DeHaan (1996, p 293), after reviewing diverse literature on family resilience, have suggested that resilience describes 'the path a family follows as it adapts and prospers in the face of stress, both in the present and over time'. They argue that family resilience should be viewed therefore through short- and long-term lenses, recognizing that time and development are contributing factors. It is further suggested that resilience is affected by the unique context of each family, including developmental factors, risk and protective factors, cultural and world-view considerations (see Box 15.2).

Clearly, such factors are never going to be static, hence the importance of acknowledging the developmental focus of the resilience model. This would suggest that nurses and other front-line workers should never assume that not hearing from a family previously judged to have been coping well necessarily implies that this is still the case. Most families, including those managing self-sufficiently, value proactive visiting and a listening ear from professionals even though they may not need further practical support (Grant et al 1994).

BOX 15.2	*Exploring resilience in coping among family carers would suggest that nurses and healthcare professionals will need to address a number of dispositions and capacities in family carers*

- Accessible external coping resources (e.g. income, social support, services).

- Accessible internal coping resources (e.g. analytic capacity, time, expertise).

- The capacity to use instrumental (problem-solving) and cognitive (reframing) coping strategies.

- The ability to select an appropriate coping strategy from a pool to fit the nature of the demand or challenge.

- The capacity to continuously reappraise which coping strategies work – an initial response involving escape or withdrawal might, for example, be a necessary first step towards solving a problem (Brown 1993).

- The ability to locate uplifts and rewards within apparently adverse circumstances.

- The ability to 'make sense' out of what often appear to be 'non-normative' conditions.

Family systems theory

One of the undoubted limitations of much family care research, especially that involving people who have learning disabilities, is that evidence has been drawn principally from mothers. There are probably two associated reasons for this: first, mothers are often correctly assumed to occupy the primary caregiving role within families so their views and experiences are usually judged to be authoritative; and second, much of the empirical research has been based on models emphasizing individual psychopathology with mothers being seen as most at risk. Family systems theories, on the other hand, suggest the need for a greater focus on family interaction and adaptation. Broadly speaking, three theoretical orientations have been exploited in this connection.

Social support and social network theory emphasizes the importance of relationships among social units and how different relationships promote or impede the flow and exchange of resources and social support (Dunst et al 1986). Social support networks are typically defined in terms of their structural properties such as their size, density, membership, proximity and frequency and direction of contact whilst social support has usually been defined in relation to physical and emotional content, attitude transmission and information sharing. The general view is that social support networks nurture and sustain linkages among people that are supportive on an everyday basis and at times of need or crisis. Studies of people who have learning disabilities and their families in this mould have demonstrated that support networks can undergo quite major transitions in relatively short periods of time (Grant 1993) and that more supportive social networks are usually associated with better personal (carer) well-being, family cohesion and improved child behaviour and development (Dunst & Trivette 1988, Dunst et al 1986).

Closely related to social support and social network theory is *human ecology theory*. Bronfenbrenner (1979) contends that it is necessary to view social units topographically, rather like a set of concentric circles, each embedded within another. Hence, at the inner level would be a circle comprising the individual and their family members. The family unit is further embedded within wider ecological systems including relatives, friends, neighbours (the informal system), and then within wider formal systems including neighbourhood organizations, statutory and independent sector organizations. The basic idea is that events within any ecological unit do not occur in isolation. Rather they interact, directly or indirectly, within and between levels. Hence, membership change within a person's support network (death of a father, for example) may have immediate direct effects on the spouse (bereavement, reduced income, loss of a valued source of support) and short-term indirect effects on maternal caregiving (increased responsibility, sense of isolation) which may have long-term consequences (reappraisal of caregiving role, abrogation of caring responsibilities). This is a rather basic example but it draws attention to the dangers of viewing an individual in isolation from their social and ecological context.

The third systems perspective is based on *help-seeking/help-giving theory* which suggests the need to pay closer attention to the conditions under which help-seeking and help-giving exchanges occur (Gourash 1978). Here the idea is that there are definable characteristics of these exchanges that are necessary for help-giving to have positive consequences. Help seekers are likely to respond favourably if:

- positive attributions are ascribed to help givers by help seekers
- help seekers have the opportunity to reciprocate, though delayed reciprocity may be necessary
- any exchanges minimize social differences between help seekers and help givers
- help seeking neither implies lost freedoms nor threatens self-esteem or autonomy.

As people who have learning disabilities grow older, patterns of interdependence with parents and other family members can undergo significant shifts, with role reversals taking place as caregivers become more physically and emotionally dependent (Magrill 1997, Walker & Walker 1998). However, there is still very little empirical evidence about how people who have learning

---

BOX 15.3	*Practice implications of family systems theories*

- A requirement to view families as a part of wider social systems.
- The scope for enlisting additional or complementary help from within a family's social network.
- The need to address how reciprocities and interdependencies can be maintained between family members.
- The importance of addressing shifts in interdependencies over the life course.
- The need to hear the 'voice' of all family members, especially the person with learning disability, in determining best ways of supporting families.
- The potential for recognizing that family carers and their disabled relatives may not always have compatible needs and wants.

disabilities experience family care or about what practical, psychological and economic contributions they make to sustain families. Examples of these experiences are described in Chapter 9.

Constructions of caring

At a common-sense level everyone knows what caring is. At a conceptual and operational level it is much more difficult to pin down. For a long time there has been a tendency to view caring along two dimensions, according to Parker (1981): first, as in 'caring about' someone through expressions of generalized concern or in expressed emotion, financial assistance or gift giving; and second, in 'tending', as seen in more practical and personal helping. Although quite a lot of research seems nevertheless to have emphasized the instrumental dimensions of caring, that is in terms of physical and practical tasks, there has been growing recognition from feminist and other writers of caring as emotional and organizational labour as well as physical work (Arber & Ginn 1995), as something capable of providing a sense of identity for individuals (Lewis & Meredith 1989), as something which is set within a hierarchy of obligations, responsibilities and position in the family life cycle (Finch & Mason 1990) or as something which is perhaps better understood in terms of its purposes rather than its content (Nolan et al 1996).

There is, evidently, no unitary or predominant view about the nature of caregiving at the present time. All the foregoing formulations provide helpful insights and broadly speaking suggest the need to pay attention to content issues (tasks), functional issues (purposes and outcomes) and shaping/constraining phenomena (obligations, sanctions, life cycle position) if a more embracing view of caregiving is to be adopted. This in itself carries important implications about how nurses and other health and social care professionals set about assessing family care. The next section will explore this area within the context of lifespan approaches and perspectives.

Lifespan perspectives

Lifespan perspectives attempt to take into account the changing roles, functions, obligations, development, resources and coping strategies of families over the lifespan. Such perspectives have received little attention from researchers possibly because of the costs, time commitments and difficulties of securing the necessary funding for primary research. There are, however, different theories or, perhaps more accurately, assumptions about what happens as people age.

Years ago Birenbaum (1971) suggested that family coping becomes more difficult as the child ages and as families face support network shrinkage over time, supporting the notion of the 'wear and tear' hypothesis. However, the 'adaptation' hypothesis, by contrast, suggests that people adjust to caregiving over time and acquire skills and competences which help them to cope better, even when their own support networks may indeed be more depleted (Grant 1993, Seltzer & Krauss 1989). Supporting this last hypothesis is growing evidence about strengthened reciprocities as the 'cared-for' person becomes a support to the family in their own right.

BOX 15.4	*Four lifespan dimensions or 'trajectories' seen to be relevant to the way healthcare professionals assess and seek to work with families*

- *The family life cycle* – the effects of shifts in intergenerational ties, in support network membership.
- *The caregiving trajectory* – the effects of the 'stage' family carers have reached in moving from 'novice' to 'expert' carers.
- *The service trajectory* – the effects of transitions on development and adaptation as individuals move between health, education, social services and independent sector services.
- *The development/disability trajectory* – the effects of construing disability as an ongoing process with landmarks, transition points and changing demands.

The whole point of thinking longitudinally in these ways is to increase the prospects of predictability for families. If developmental stages can be anticipated and planned for then families are likely to feel more secure and it is probable that more tailored and effective interventions will follow. Not to do so runs the risk of leaving families in limbo and facing uncertain futures (Walker & Walker 1998).

FORMAL AND INFORMAL CARE RELATIONS AND HEALTHCARE: PRACTICE ISSUES

In this section, case study and survey data about family caregiving are reported in an attempt to bring to life the theory and practice implications reviewed so far. It is hoped that they will help to illustrate the considerable resilience that can be found in families, something of the insights and expertise they can possess, the centrality of maintaining reciprocities within their caregiving and patterns of differentiation in coping. The illustrations underline the relevance of a family resilience model, of family systems thinking, of the gendered basis of caregiving and of life course dimensions in family coping. As such, they help to suggest important parameters for professional assessment frameworks.

Resilience in coping strategies

The Brown family provide a good example of resilience in family coping (Grant et al 1998). Despite having had an upsetting experience with a health visitor over the manner in which disclosure of Sue's cerebral palsy and learning disability had been staged many years ago, Jan and Frank Brown had become determined advocates for Sue. Now, some 20 years after Sue had been given a diagnosis, Jan and Frank were helping Sue to locate daytime training and employment opportunities. Life at home was still quite difficult even when everyone pulled together, helped also by Sue's younger sister Mel. Particularly difficult for the family to manage were Sue's temper tantrums but Jan's account about how she tried to contain these were very revealing about the complex strategies involved.

> Then we have the challenges of ... these temper tantrums. Sometimes they can last a couple of minutes, sometimes they'll last an hour, so you've got to be prepared for that. So, whilst that's going on I'm thinking about something else. I'm keeping cool. I'm pretending it's not happening. I'm singing to myself or I'm thinking about something totally different so that I don't let her know she's winning. You can't let her win. You've got to be in control all the time, so that's very difficult. I mean, some days she's a joy. You can sit with her and you can't get enough of looking at her, she's so lovely, and then, another day, you're looking for the 666 on her forehead because she's like a beast from hell! Sometimes it can be very, very hard, but as I say, most of the time I'm able to cope with that, but if I lose my cool, then I've lost, she's won and I may just as well give up.

This description from Jan provides some clues supporting a family resilience model: the capacity to utilize both problem-solving and cognitive coping, the ability to select from a pool of coping options, the capacity to identify rewards in the midst of constant challenges, the characteristic 'bouncing back' from the ups and downs of the daily grind and the underlying commitment to maintaining a sense of control whatever the circumstances. In addition, Jan had a supportive husband and daughter. Together they had also developed a 'private' language to help them communicate with Sue who had no discernible speech so they were able to support one another and Sue directly in responding appropriately to her gestures, expressed emotion and other signals. In these respects they had talents and capacities only one other person (Sue's schoolteacher whom they had tutored so that she in turn could help Sue) possessed.

Despite Sue's apparently profound communication difficulties, neither Jan, Frank nor Mel had any difficulties viewing Sue's occasional signals of pleasure and appreciation as a form of reciprocity. Although Sue could manifestly do little in practical terms to help her family, such material reciprocity was not expected. The family's efforts to ensure Sue's personal integrity and dignity under all circumstances seemed to act both as a driving force in their caregiving efforts, giving meaning to their lives, and as a kind of proxy for reciprocity. The family were also able to recognize seemingly small gains in Sue's development and behaviour which might in other contexts pass unnoticed. This is encapsulated in another comment from Jan.

> Well, for one thing, she's lovely to look at. She's got a lovely soul. I know that sounds a bit blasé, but she has. She loves everybody. She's not spiteful or selfish or nasty. She's got a genuine love for people. She's got a great joy of life, and considering the amount of handicap she has, I mean I've got nothing but admiration for her. I'm very proud of her. I know just how much it takes for the kid to try and turn over or to try and pick something up with her hand or even to adjust herself ... I mean, she makes me laugh, she's got a wonderful sense of humour, she's very funny and she's just a joyful person.

This short case illustration also suggests some support for the relevance of help-seeking/help-giving theory in the way that positive attributions about caregiving come to be assumed and reciprocities are found to exist. The capacity of the family to view Sue as a unique and giving personality – indeed, as a person first – seemed to typify a commitment to caregiving which neither implied lost freedoms on Sue's part nor threatened her self-esteem or personal integrity.

Despite their knowledge, skills and expertise the Browns still required lots of support from their key worker in sorting out day opportunities and short-term breaks for Sue and even in being helped to 'let go' a little more so that Sue could lead a more independent life. This throws into relief one of the possible corollaries of expertise in family care; realizing that they are able to provide highly personalized care and support, such families are likely to be very critical of services which do not come up to their own exacting standards. For this reason they may also be very reluctant to relinquish responsibilities for continued caregiving.

Mediating factors and family coping

Not all families exhibit the expertise shown by Jan and her family in the way that caring and coping are orchestrated. However, few attempts have been made thus far to examine dimensions along which coping strategies might be differentiated. One very recent exception was the author's own small-scale study of 41 family carers drawn from 27 families in Wales (Grant & Whittell 2000) who were supporting children or adults who have severe learning disabilities. Below some brief details are reported about the relationship between coping strategies and gender, family composition and stage in the life cycle.

Gender

Women identified a higher proportion of useful coping strategies than men. Contrary to received wisdom, they used more problem-solving strategies than men, as evidenced by their focus on fully exploiting their coping repertoires until they find something that works (88% women, 53% men), their ability to establish priorities and concentrate upon them (88% women, 53% men) and their reliance on personal expertise (100% women, 67% men). However, they also to some extent used cognitive coping strategies more effectively than men, as shown in reliance on strong personal and religious beliefs (46% women, 13% men), their acceptance of the situation (88% women, 60% men) and self-belief (96% women, 73% men). Examining interview narratives, it became evident that there were a number of possible reasons for these differences.

- Though not in every case, men (husbands/male partners) tended to defer to the 'expertise' of their female partners. This was even more pronounced amongst stepfathers who had acquired new families.

- Men were less involved than women in the direct care of their relative but appeared to derive more benefit from maintaining interests outside of caring. The division of labour therefore placed women in the role of primary carers with many men playing 'secondary' caring roles.

- Emotional displays in front of the 'cared-for' person seemed to be seen as a sign of weakness or a 'lost battle' so there was likely to be a heightened dependency on cognitive coping under such circumstances, which would bear upon more women than men.

Family composition

There were 10 lone carers in the study sample, including people at all stages in the lifespan; unmarried or separated persons as well as those who had been widowed. Interestingly, every single one of these carers placed a strong emphasis on cognitive coping. All of them found the following coping strategies useful.

- Seeing the funny side of the situation.
- Realizing that their family member was not to blame for things.
- Taking one day at a time.
- Accepting the situation as it was.
- Believing in themselves and in their ability to handle the situation.
- Looking for the positive things in each situation.

Such high dependency on cognitive coping marked them out from other family carers. Although some had siblings or other relatives on whom they could depend there were disparities in perceived helpfulness (20% lone carers, 55% other carers). As the main or sole providers of support, lone carers found meeting all their commitments very demanding. This was more pronounced among younger lone carers for reasons that will become apparent shortly. This was exacerbated when respite and home care support services were lacking or seen to be inflexible in responding to expressed needs. Circumstances such as these combined to reinforce a dependency on carers' abilities to make sense of the way things were.

One lone parent, Vicki, supporting six children, including Richard who was severely disabled, summed up her feelings about the use of relaxation techniques as a coping device by commenting succinctly 'I haven't got the time!'. Richard, 14 years of age, had heightened tactile sensitivity which appeared to be linked to his uncontrollable head banging which Vicki had found very difficult to deal with. She was constantly reappraising what to do but found herself going for weeks unable to sleep at night. 'It's like my brain won't switch off. I'm mulling over everything and I'm putting the world to rights, you know.' Frustratingly for Vicki, she had received no professional help designed to assist her to manage these coping difficulties, apart from respite care services.

> Over the years, no, I've had nobody coming up to me and saying, well, you know, how do I feel? I've had none of that; nobody coming up to me and saying, well you know this situation, you could deal with it in such and such a way so that you don't get affected, you don't get stressed – no, I've had none of that. The only help I do get is the respite and that basically is to give me a break, to give me a rest from Richard, and also to introduce Richard into a different family.

Dual carer and other families presented a vast range of caring arrangements and were far from free of the difficulties that lone parents like Vicki described. Things were easier where there was an agreed division of labour for household and caregiving between partners. However, there could be occasions when respective parents took up very different value positions about the best way to cope. When this occurred, frustration and conflict could ensue with at times rather dire consequences for family harmony and the well-being of children and relatives.

Lifespan considerations

Findings from the same study pointed towards a number of lifespan differences in family coping. Parents with preschool children were far less sure about their experience and expertise as carers (69%) than other carers. They had less self-belief and a lower opinion of their ability to handle situations (69%). They were less assertive with their child (46%) though it is not clear whether this was due to their relative inexperience as carers or to cultural norms surrounding child rearing in the early years. Parents of younger children tended to rely much more on stress alleviation techniques than other carers. All these indicators would suggest that such carers represent a priority group for services.

At the other end of the spectrum, family carers supporting disabled relatives aged 40 years or over were quite different in coping terms. They were much more resigned to their roles, placing less emphasis on information seeking (41%) than other carers, having a well-developed capacity to reframe the meaning of situations (100%), and generally more accepting of the way things were, all of which would suggest some support for the adaptation hypothesis. Nevertheless, a number of these carers felt they ought to have been more assertive than they had been in the past to get what they wanted from services. They emphasized personal and religious beliefs (67%) more than other carers, suggesting a more philosophical stance in later life.

Carers of school-aged children and younger adults can be viewed together as they seemed to share coping traits. Generally speaking, these carers placed greater importance on problem-solving methods, including things like the usefulness of having a routine and sticking to it (93%), a 100% dependency on their own experience and expertise, trying several coping strategies until one is found that works (93%) and working to a clear set of priorities (93%). These carers typically had multiple demands placed on their time and resources – other children, the needs of other relatives, employment and their own further education or retraining in some cases – so structures, routines and worked-out strategies for dealing with situations were at a premium.

As already stated, family carers of preschool children appear to be less confident about their skills and expertise, which is hardly surprising. It seems very important indeed that greater effort is made to provide such families with information, networking them to other families who can share their expertise and designing interventions to build confidence and expertise in their coping work. Project SHaRE in the US (Dunst et al 1989) is a model example of how this can be accomplished, based as it was on the principles of enabling and empowering families to identify their own needs and unique strengths in order to help them mobilize resources by themselves, thereby assisting them to become more self-sufficient and independent.

However, by the time children are well into their schooling, family carers seem to have acquired genuine 'particularistic' expertise about their offspring and how best to support them. It is at this point that professionals perhaps need to acknowledge who the true experts are and what implications this has for best professional practice in supporting families.

Recognizing knowledge and expertise in families

Given the sheer diversity of coping strategies that are used and seem to work for families, it would be none too surprising if these were not all recognized by front-line professionals. To test this out in the Grant & Whittell (2000) study, the main carers from the 27 families and their care managers (where we were able to match them) were asked respectively to complete a coping inventory, CAMI (Nolan et al 1996), about the carer's coping strategies.

The findings suggested that care managers, both nurses and social workers, underestimated the range of coping strategies which family carers found useful. Cognitive coping strategies used by carers were most likely to be unrecognized by care managers; that is, strategies in which carers depend very much on reframing the significance of challenges to them. This is perhaps predictable since cognitive coping is representative of 'internal' coping resources which are by definition concealed from the outside world, reflecting dispositions, analytic capacities and frames of reference which individuals bring to their everyday caregiving.

However, there were also signs that nurses and social workers underestimated the decision-making, problem-solving capacity of families. Three coping strategies were particularly discriminating here: thinking about a problem and overcoming it, establishing and concentrating on priorities, and relying on one's own experience and expertise. With these being more manifest strategies for coping than cognitive coping, the explanations for difference here probably lie elsewhere. Our interviews with nurses and social workers suggested that these were to do with 'structural' issues connected with the organization of care management. The front-line workers we interviewed were struggling with large caseloads; they were facing additional responsibilities for planning in the wake of local government reorganization; there were some local difficulties with workloads, staff burnout and staff turnover; frameworks for assessment were not all that they could be; and there were acknowledged service shortfalls. In other words, there were plenty of organizational factors preventing closer attention to family care needs. Most of the time workers were having to operate in crisis-response mode. A full elaboration of these factors and their effects is beyond the scope of this chapter.

Interestingly, the one coping strategy that care managers significantly overestimated was the capacity of carers to maintain interests outside caring. It cannot be assumed merely because carers engage in paid employment or voluntary organized activity that they necessarily benefit from this in coping terms.

BOX 15.5	*Practice implications*
	■ Avoid prejudging which coping strategies work for families without speaking to them first.
	■ Pay closer attention to the range of cognitive coping strategies upon which families are reliant. Not only are these more concealed, they are often used when problem solving fails.
	■ Invite carers to use self-administered coping interventories like CAMI as a part of assessment and review work, especially with their availability in the form of a practitioner guide (Nolan et al 1998).

Many are forced to go to work through economic necessity but it may be poorly paid, offer little intrinsic satisfaction or add to difficulties with time scheduling.

Families' views about practice gaps

In bringing this section to a close, an attempt is made here to summarize what family-based studies suggest about other gaps in current practice.

Recent evidence from a study by Robinson & Williams (1999) about the impact of the Carers Act 1995 on people who have learning disabilities and their family carers does not paint an encouraging picture about present assessment practice. Far fewer families had received a full carer's assessment than would be indicated by their expressed needs; some key areas of carers' lives were not discussed including their health, housing, work and ability to continue caring and information dissemination to carers about their rights and entitlements left much to be desired. Even in Wales where the much-vaunted 1983 All Wales Strategy promised so much, only a small minority of people who have learning disabilities and their families had been party to an individual plan (IP) (Felce et al 1998) despite the fact that the entire strategic planning system originally depended on these becoming fully operational. The operational effectiveness and coverage of IPs continue to present serious challenges.

However, the mere existence of an IP is not a sufficient guarantee that families will perceive things in a positive light (Grant et al 1994). On a more positive note, the same study suggested that families did not necessarily want the highly structured arrangement of an IP but rather a close and empathic relationship with a professional worker from any health or social care discipline who understood their needs and wants.

One of the major areas of unmet need lies in relation to fears and anxieties about future caregiving arrangements, supporting the findings of Robinson & Williams (1999). This is not restricted to older carers (Hogg & Lambe 1998) and to issues about what will happen after family carers die. It applies to many stages of the family life cycle where transitions could be anticipated but uncertainties about the processes and outcomes remain; for example, in relation to moves from child to adult services, from segregated to community-inclusive services where risk taking may be involved or from a dependency on informal to formal care. Alternatively there were occasions when families needed external help to renegotiate caring arrangements within the family in the light of changes in support networks. This once again reinforces the need for an emphasis by professionals on lifespan factors in family care.

Despite the rapid development of many family support services in Wales, the 'multiple careers' of families are still not fully recognized, meaning all the familial, social and economic roles with which family members were often juggling (Todd & Shearn 1996). It is still quite rare for support to be 'identity affirming'; that is, culturally sensitive and addressed to families' valued aspirations.

There continue to be difficulties in persuading some families to strike a more liberal balance between protection and community inclusion in how they orchestrate and manage caregiving. As caregivers age they seem to be less enthusiastic about providing their relative with opportunities outside the home (Shearn & Todd 1997). It is important to understand the reasons rather than readily assuming that they are embedded in family psychopathology. Families can be forgiven for being a trifle protective if the entire education system still cannot decide on a policy of segregated, integrated or inclusive schooling for at its very root this is really a question about society's preparedness to tackle the very forces that create separations in people's lives. One of the basic challenges for health and social care practitioners, then, is the difficulty of helping families to find meaningful pathways through health, education and social services which do not necessarily have consistent inclusive policies. This once again draws attention to the impacts of service trajectories within the family life course.

DISCUSSION

It is considered that transactional stress-coping theory, family resilience models and family systems theories all provide complementary and relevant insights into the private world of family care. Front-line practice needs to be informed by such theoretical perspectives so that genuine knowledge-building, evidence-based practice can develop. Despite the Carers Act 1995 and the *Caring about carers report* (DoH 1999), there are still no unifying principles in the UK to guide nurses and other healthcare workers in their work with families.

However, many of the findings from family studies affirm the need for interventions with families based on competence-enhancing principles (Dunst et al 1993). This basically means an orientation which directly addresses the strengths families can bring to their everyday caregiving so that these can be enhanced in efforts to achieve better child, personal (carer) and family outcomes.

At the practice level this would involve an emphasis on:

- use of *active and reflective listening skills* as a basis for understanding a family's needs and concerns
- forms of help which are based on *the family's own appraisal of resources and problems*
- support which recognizes and strengthens each family's *unique and effective styles of coping*
- support which addresses *incompatible coping strategies used by different family members*
- support which acknowledges and seeks to overcome *factors that mediate or constrain effective coping in families*
- support which concentrates on helping families to *realize caregiving rewards and uplifts*
- help which is *proactive* rather than a response to crisis
- help *compatible with family culture*; that is, each family's rules and norms, beliefs and cultural practices, routines and structures for coping
- support which builds on and strengthens a *family's skills, expertise and decision-making capacity*
- help which acknowledges how effective coping is embedded within *social network and social support arrangements*
- support which takes account of *lifespan factors which can disrupt the predictability of family coping efforts.*

Such principles act as a guide to practice and are likely to have a number of implications for already hard-pressed front-line professional workers. If they are taken at face value they reflect and emphasize partnership and competence enhancement but such approaches do bring challenges for practitioners. Recognition and respect for expertise in families may challenge professional wisdom and practice. Identifying the more concealed but effective coping strategies in families is likely to require patience as well as skill. Recognizing and reinforcing the subtle shifts that take place in family coping over the lifespan means making a commitment to long-term relationships with families but instabilities and turnover in community support teams may make this difficult. Bringing decision making out into the open will place a higher premium on professional negotiating and brokerage skills. And there remains the question of the best ways of representing the carer's and cared-for person's needs and concerns when these differ.

In the meantime, replication of American-style family-oriented case management (Dunst et al 1993), which has had such startlingly good outcomes, would seem to represent a promising way of learning what works for families in multicultural Britain. An emphasis on supporting family strengths through reviewing coping strategies and how they work for individuals is likely to lead to an *expansion of coping repertoires*, affording families more choice and control over possible options. Some coping strategies, however, appear not to be used for reasons to do with lack of skill or competence rather than preparedness, suggesting in these circumstances the need to assist families in *strengthening coping mastery*. If coping mastery can be strengthened it is very likely that this will provide carers with an important source of reward, thereby leading to *caregiving enrichment* and possibly to the prospects of a more committed caregiving future. However, just as it is important for professionals to avoid an undue emphasis on stress in families, it is vital to avoid a blinkered focus on coping. Families typically face stresses and rewards, as discussed at the beginning of this chapter. An assessment of stresses and rewards in families will help to address 'push–pull' factors which are very much a part of the lived reality for many carers; for example, the strong expressed wish to continue caring versus the experience of isolation, fatigue, chronic strain and the desire to escape such circumstances. Hence, placing family strengths and resilience in the framework of assessment will help families to *acknowledge contradictions* in their everyday caregiving.

Though vital, getting frameworks for family needs assessment right is only one necessary step in securing improved family support. As the brief review of practice gaps has demonstrated, there is a chasm between rhetoric and reality. The patchiness of many family support services, the very labour-intensive nature of individualized work practices and the challenges of inter-agency collaboration can leave community nurses and their professional colleagues as victims of a deficient service system. Good professional practice in supporting families therefore can only flourish if related questions about economics, evidence-based practice and organization development are tackled in parallel.

FURTHER READING

Booth T, Booth W 1998 Growing up with parents who have learning disabilities. Routledge, London

Provides perspectives on resilience, competence and adaptation in families whose parents have learning disabilities.

Department of Health 1996 Carers (Recognition and Services) Act 1995: policy guidance. DoH, Wetherby, Yorkshire
Describes national policy guidance about supporting family carers following the 1995 legislation.

Department of Health 1999 Caring about carers: a national strategy for carers. DoH, London
Describes the national strategy for carers as an example of 'joined up' policy thinking; comes complete with a report of a consultative conference on the national strategy and a guidebook about the provision of short-term breaks.

Dunst C J, Trivette C M, Deal A G (eds) 1994 Supporting and strengthening families: volume I – methods, strategies and practices. Brookline Books, Cambridge, MA
Demonstrates the application of 'family support principles' to the design of tailored interventions to support families with disabled children.

Mittler P, Mittler H (eds) 1994 Innovations in family support for people with learning disabilities. Lisieux Hall, Chorley
Reviews a range of initiatives for supporting families.

Nolan M, Grant G, Keady J 1998 Assessing the needs of family carers: a guide for practitioners. Pavillion Publishing, Brighton
Describes three instruments for assessing stresses (CADI), rewards (CASI) and coping strategies (CAMI) among family carers; provides background about the development of the instruments, illustrative case studies and practice applications.

REFERENCES

Arber S, Ginn J 1995 Gender differences in informal caring. Health Social Care Commun 3:19–31

Baxter C, Cummins R A, Polak S 1995 A longitudinal study of parental stress and support: from diagnosis of disability to leaving school. Int J Disabi Dev Education 42(2):125–136

Beresford B 1994 Positively parents: caring for a severely disabled child. HMSO, London

Birenbaum A 1971 The mentally retarded child in the home and the family life-cycle. J Health Social Behav 12:55–65

Booth T, Booth W 1998 Think of the children: growing up with parents who have learning difficulties. J Learning Disabil Nursing Health Social Care 2(3):138–143

Bronfenbrenner U 1979 The ecology of human development: experiments by nature and design. Harvard University Press, Cambridge, MA

Brown J 1993 Coping with stress: the beneficial role of positive illusions. In: Turnbull A P, Patterson J M, Behr S K et al (eds) Cognitive coping; families and disability. Paul H Brookes, Baltimore

Burden R L 1980 Measuring the effects of stress on mothers of handicapped infants: must depression always follow? Child Care Health Dev 6:111–125

Carr J 1988 Six weeks to twenty one years old: a study of children with Down's syndrome and their families. J Child Psychol Psychiatr 29:407–431

Department of Health 1999 Caring about carers: a national strategy for carers. DoH, London

Dohrenwend B S, Dohrenwend B P 1974 Stressful life events: their nature and effects. Wiley, New York

Dunst C J, Trivette C M 1988 Toward experimental evaluation of the family, infant and pre-school program. In: Weiss H B,

Jacobs F H (eds) Evaluating family programs. Aldine de Gruyter, New York, pp 315–346

Dunst C J, Trivette C M, Cross A H 1986 Mediating influences of social support: personal, family and child outcomes. Am J Mental Defic 90(4): 403–417

Dunst C J, Trivette C M, Gordon N J, Pletcher L L 1989 Building and mobilising informal family support networks. In: Singer G H S, Irvin L K (eds) Support for caregiving families: enabling positive adaptation to disability. Paul H Brookes, Baltimore

Dunst C J, Trivette C M, Starnes A L, Hamby D W, Gordon N J 1993 Building and evaluating family support initiatives. Paul H Brookes, Baltimore

Farooqi S 1994 Ethnic differences in infant care practices and in the incidence of sudden infant death syndrome in Birmingham. Early Human Dev 38(3):209–213

Fatimilehin I, Nadirshaw Z 1994 A cross cultural study of parental attitudes and beliefs about learning disability. Mental Handicap Res 7(3):202–207

Felce D, Grant G, Todd S J et al 1998 Towards a full life: researching policy innovation for people with learning disabilities. Butterworth Heinemann, Oxford

Finch J, Mason J 1990 Filial obligation and kin support for elderly people. Ageing Society 10:151–175

Folkman S 1997 Positive psychological states and coping with severe stress. Social Sci Med 45:1207–1221

Gourash N 1978 Help seeking: a review of the literature. Am J Commun Psychol 6(5):413–423

Grant G 1993 Support networks and transitions over two years among adults with a mental handicap. Mental Handicap Res 6(1):36–55

Grant G, Whittell B 2000 Differentiated coping strategies in families with children or adults with intellectual disabilities: the relevance of gender, family composition and the life span J. Appl Res Intellect Disabil 13: 256–275

Grant G, Nolan M, Ellis N 1990 A reappraisal of the Malaise Inventory. Social Psychiatr Psychiatr Epidemiol 25:170–178

Grant G, McGrath M, Ramcharan P 1994 How family and informal supporters appraise service quality. Int J Disabil Dev Education 41(2):127–141

Grant G, Ramcharan P, McGrath M, Nolan M, Keady J 1998 Rewards and gratifications among family caregivers:

towards a refined model of caring and coping. J Intellect Disabil Res 42(1): 58–71

Hawley D, DeHaan L 1996 Towards a definition of family resilience: integrating lifespan and family perspectives. Family Process 35:283–298

Hodapp R M, Fidler D J, Smith A C M 1998 Stress and coping in families of children with Smith-Magenis syndrome. J Intellect Disabil Res 42(5):331–340

Hogg J, Lambe L 1998 Older people with learning disabilities: a review of the literature on residential services and family caregiving. Foundation for People with Learning Disabilities, London

Lazarus R S, Folkman S 1984 Stress, appraisal and coping. Springer, New York

Lewis J, Meredith B 1989 Contested territory in informal care. In: Jeffreys M (ed) Growing older in the twentieth century. Routledge, London

Magrill D 1997 Crisis approaching: the situation facing Sheffield's elderly carers of people with learning disabilities. Sharing Caring Project, Mencap, Sheffield

Nolan G, Grant G, Keady J 1996 Understanding family care: a multidimensional model of caring and coping. Open University Press, Buckingham

Nolan G, Grant G, Keady J 1998 Assessing the needs of family carers: a guide for practitioners. Pavillion Publishing, Brighton

Orr R R, Cameron S J, Day D M 1991 Coping with stress in children who have mental retardation: an evaluation of the double ABCX model. Am J Mental Retard 95:444–450

Parker R 1981 Tending and social policy. In: Goldberg E M, Hatch S (eds) A new look at the personal social services. Policy Studies Institute, London

Quine L, Pahl J 1991 Stress and coping in mothers caring for a child with severe learning difficulties: a test of Lazarus' transactional model of coping. J Commun Appl Social Psychol 1:57–70

Robinson B C 1983 Validation of a caregiver strain index. J Gerontol 38(3):344–348

Robinson C, Williams V 1999 In their own right: project about the Carers Act 1995. Norah Fry Research Centre, University of Bristol

Schumacher K L, Stewart B J, Archbold P G 1998 Conceptualisation and measurement of doing caregiving well. Image: J Nursing Scholarship 30(1):63–69

Seltzer M M, Krauss M W 1989 Ageing parents with mentally retarded children: family risk factors and sources of support. Am J Mental Retard 94:303–312

Shearn J, Todd S 1997 Parental work: an account of the day to day activities of parents of adults with learning disabilities. J Intellect Disabil Res 41:285–301

Todd S, Shearn J 1996 Time and the person: the impact of support services on the lives of parents of adults with learning disabilities. J Appl Res Intellect Disabil 9:40–60

Walker C, Walker A 1998 Uncertain futures: people with learning disabilities and their ageing family carers. Pavillion Publishing and Joseph Rowntree Foundation, Brighton

Wilson S, Morse J, Penrod J 1998 Absolute involvement: the experience of mothers of ventilator-dependent children. Health Social Care Commun 6(4):224–233

16 Working with communities

Angela Butcher with Jeanette Thompson and Sharon Pickering

KEY ISSUES

- The concept of community
- Citizenship
- Social networks
- Building alliances
- Developing inclusive communities
- The culture of service delivery

INTRODUCTION

Learning disability services are now almost completely based within local communities. This has been as a direct consequence of both policy directives and philosophical changes about the way and the context in which services should be provided to people who have a learning disability. Having achieved the physical move into the community, services have by no means been as successful in engaging with the community in order to support people to have meaningful and valued lives. Kinsella (1993), amongst others, notes the re-creation of small-scale institutions within the community setting.

This chapter sets out to explore the ways in which meaningful interaction within local communities can be stimulated and how people can be supported to maintain these contacts. In doing this, it is also important to note the link that meaningful contacts within one's own community can have in relation to an individual's mental health and well-being.

As a consequence of moving services into the community, the challenge now facing service providers is to find creative and innovative ways of empowering and enabling people who have a learning disability to participate in a meaningful way in the activities taking place within their communities. In order to facilitate the achievement of this, this chapter will discuss what a community is, what citizenship means to individuals and how an understanding of these issues can be used to support people who have a learning disability in building relationships in their community. It will also discuss the relationship that professionals have with people who have a learning disability and ways in which our practice can become more centred around people's needs, wishes and ambitions, in order to improve their health and quality of life.

THE CONCEPT OF COMMUNITY: A SENSE OF BELONGING

The first part of this chapter examines some of the wider issues that professionals working with people who have a learning disability need to consider when they are supporting someone to become integrated into their community. One of the first questions we have to ask is: what is community? Community has been defined as 'the free space where people think for themselves, dream their dreams and come together to create and celebrate their common humanity' (Ludlum 1993, p 32). As such, community is not just about bricks and mortar; it is also about feeling as if you belong and are valued by the people around you.

Wertheimer (1996) said, 'Community is people not places'. By focusing upon Wertheimer's approach to defining community, it is possible to see how strong community networks are able to provide emotional, physical and mental support for people and therefore improve their health status. Schwartz (1997) also discussed the idea that people are tribal and the contribution that this makes to our sense of happiness and well-being. By being part of a tribal system, Schwartz suggests, we gain a sense of mutual support from our fellow tribe members which in turn has a positive impact upon our health.

ACTIVITY 16.1   Think about who belongs to your tribe.

When thinking about this you may have included parents, partners, siblings, children, friends, other family members, neighbours, acquaintances and work colleagues, to name a few. Your tribe may include a small number of people or it may be more extensive as represented in the concept of the extended family. For people who have a learning disability, their sense of tribe may be skewed by the environment in which they live, particularly those who live in institutions or similar establishments. The sense of belonging they feel will be significantly influenced by the number of relationships they can sustain with people who are not paid to support them.

Belonging in a modern community

Modern life can be isolating for many people. As towns get bigger, people seem to become more cut off from each other. As Sarason (1977) suggested, physical proximity and psychological closeness can be amazingly unrelated. He discussed the idea of the loss of a psychological sense of community, where more and more people are feeling alone, unwanted and unneeded. Out-of-town shopping centres, use of cars and large housing estates have all added to the degeneration of the local community.

This has created a situation in which the shops, community centres and other places that used to be the hub of any community have dwindled in number. As a direct consequence, relationship building and the opportunity to develop a psychological closeness with people within the community has been seriously undermined. The absence of places and opportunities to develop these community links will in turn impact upon the health and well-being of individuals, for example, in relation to the person's sense of self and feelings of self-worth. Of particular relevance are situations when people are feeling low and do not have any friends to act as reference points in order to make them feel valued and important again.

Oldenburg (1989) wrote about the importance of these places and referred to them as 'third places'. He referred to their role in both creating and sustaining relationships and referred to home as the 'first place' and work as the 'second place'. Further examples of third places are buildings that are open for anyone in the community to use, such as pubs, cafes and community centres. Within these places people can become 'regulars' and build important social relationships. Modern lifestyles can, as already suggested, mean that people often do not have these third places in their lives.

ACTIVITY 16.2   What are the third places in your life? How do these compare with those in the life of someone you know who has a learning disability?

The third places in your life may include pubs, clubs, sport centres, etc. The importance of these environments is the way in which they enable us to meet and connect with new people who we can build relationships with and which have the potential to outlast the duration of the initial social contact.

Conversely, some environments used for recreational purposes do not provide the same opportunities to develop friendships. These include places like cinemas, theatres and restaurants. The difficulty with these environments is that they do not have a focus around meeting and communicating with people whom you do not already know.

When discussing with a person who has a learning disability how they wish to spend their leisure time, it is important to consider what they wish to gain from the experience. If the goal is to meet new people and develop friendships then places such as the cinema are not necessarily appropriate. This does not mean that people should not go to these places but that the outcomes of the experience should be clearly identified. This is particularly important from a professional or supporter's perspective if the goal they have contracted to work upon with a service user is that of developing friendships, as in order to achieve this it is necessary to go to places where people can meet and connect with others.

The impact of the institutions upon the experience of community

Historically many people who have a learning disability have been denied opportunities to engage in their own community as they have been hidden away in institutions and have been without a voice. Some people who have a learning disability may have experienced their sense of community only in the context of large total institutions in which they had clear roles and routines identifi, for them (Goffman 1961). People living in these institutions had to adapt the way they lived to fit in with institutional systems. This meant that people who have a learning disability were seen as patients who needed to live in a hospital because they were ill and in need of medical care. However, as Hogg (1998) stated, whilst specialist support may be needed for people who have specialist needs, this does not mean people have to go into specialist environments for these needs to be met. *Signposts for success* (Lindsey 1998) reinforced this when it stated that people who have learning disabilities do not have to live in hospital in order to have their health needs met.

Many people have now moved out of the institutions and are living in smaller houses in the community. The ethos behind this is that people have more chance to integrate into their community if they are living in an ordinary house in an ordinary street. However, as Kinsella (1993) pointed out, many of these smaller environments are very similar to the bigger institutions in the way that they operate. Barr & Fay (1993) state that just because a place is smaller and located in the community does not stop it from being a total institution as institutional practices and cultures can just as easily be transferred to a smaller building. Sinson (1990) called this phenomenon 'micro-institutionalization' and identified that once again management structures and routines were assuming control over people's lives.

Dowson (1991) further develops this concept by identifying that people who have a learning disability living in ordinary houses are as unlikely to make connections with the community as they did when living within the institution. Whilst they may not be physically contained in a total institution, it is notable that their day is often dominated by movement between different parts of a service system or different service provision, in a way which envelops them almost completely.

ACTIVITY 16.3

Think about the lifestyle of the people who have a learning disability you work with. What do they do during their daily lives? Who do they connect with? Who do they get the chance to develop friendships with?

You may have been very lucky and been able to focus upon a person who spends much of their time actively engaged in valued employment opportunities and has a varied social life to complement this. In other words, you may have thought about a person who lives an everyday lifestyle with everyday opportunities and responsibilities, a lifestyle that supports the person as a citizen. Conversely, you may have thought about a person whose life is still very much controlled by organizations and service systems and despite the fact they are now living in the community in a small group home or supported living environment, they are still experiencing a predominantly institutional lifestyle.

Citizenship: the right to be listened to

Jefferson & Hall (1998) suggest the term 'citizenship' was used to define the establishment of statutory conditions whereby all members of society would be able to take a full and productive role in their society. Marshall (1951) describes the concept of citizenship as an achievement of a number of different 'rights'. These include civil, political and social rights. Civil rights can be seen as including legal, contractual and property rights as well as freedom of thought and speech and choice of religious practice. Political rights are set in the context of universal suffrage and the right to organize oneself and society within a political framework. Social rights encompass the right to an acceptable standard of living in line with current social expectation as well as access to welfare services and benefits.

These social rights need to be considered in the context of meaningful roles in life and inclusion within one's own community, having clearly identified that a 'community' is about relationships and citizenship is about having equal rights. All people should be able to be citizens and as such should have the following rights.

- To follow their dreams and ambitions.
- To be able to contribute to and receive support from the community.
- To have their opinions, needs and talents respected alongside those of any other citizen.
- The same opportunities for education and employment and the security that results from sufficient income.

Consideration of all these issues is essential for each of us in the context of our overall health and well-being. Issues such as this are so integral to our individual expectations of life that we often fail to understand their fundamental importance and therefore they may not be given sufficient attention by those who provide services to people who have a learning disability.

The following section explores some of the ways in which people can be supported to become citizens and be more involved in their community.

STRATEGIES FOR DEVELOPING INCLUSIVE COMMUNITIES AND INCREASING COMMUNITY PARTICIPATION

Community connections

Valued participation comes when people have started to build up relationships in the community, through joint interests and sharing routines and leisure pursuits. It is only then that people who have a learning disability can start to contribute to and change the community in which they live.

The first step towards community integration is having a presence within that community, which means physically living within it. In addition to living in that environment, it is also necessary for people to positively engage in the activities of that community. One way of doing this is for people to go out and use the local amenities; this does not just mean people going to the shops or supermarket but also giving people the opportunity to interact with the shopkeeper or with other customers. These need to be the amenities that all the community use and at a time when they are open to everyone.

All too often people pass through the community but are not actually part of it (Dowson 1991). Examples of this can include homes where service users use the local milkman for their milk deliveries but because the night staff are on duty, the milkman gets paid at 4am when he delivers the milk, rather than returning when service users are awake and can be actively involved in the process. A further example is having food delivered from local shops because it saves time and energy and because it allows for bulk buying and thus saves money. The cost of such savings must be set against against the loss of opportunity for people who have a learning disability to meet people and become involved in their community and through this, the opportunity to enhance their mental health and well-being.

Due to their treatment in the past, some people who have a learning disability may have had little or no involvement in speaking up for themselves and being listened to or may have had some very negative experiences. Consequently people need support in how to communicate with other people and how to behave in group situations, particularly when this involves meeting new people and establishing connections and relationships within their community. People have been without a voice for so long that they cannot suddenly be expected to speak up for themselves without some form of support.

ACTIVITY 16.4   Think of a time when you were not listened to. How did it feel?

The feelings that such an experience provokes can be very powerful. You may have felt angry, worthless, undervalued, isolated, to name but a few. It is very disempowering not to be listened to and can have a detrimental effect upon a person's self-esteem and psychological well-being. For many people who have a learning disability, not being heard is an everyday occurrence. Anya Souza in Chapter 9 describes her experience and what it feels like not to be listened to.

Self-advocacy

To be part of the community and to be able to take up full citizenship, people need to have a voice. To know that they are not alone and that they have a peer group supporting and listening to them. Self-advocacy is a good way to support people who have a learning disability to find their voice. A member of a self-advocacy group described the experience as 'Standing up and talking about our feelings, speaking up for yourself, trying to get things done, letting people do it for themselves and speaking up for ones that can't talk' (March et al 1997, p 78).

To be able to take part in a self-advocacy group, people have to know that it is OK to dream, to begin to see that they are people who have options and a future and equal rights with the rest of the citizens in the community. To be able to advocate for themselves, people have to have an idea of self, so self-awareness is important, alongside an understanding that they are allowed to have a view of their own and a say in their lives. These are concepts that health professionals should promote and help people to develop by supporting them to gain a sense of self. This can be achieved in a number of ways, such as encouraging people to make decisions in their lives and ensuring that those decisions are acted upon.

At a recent meeting of a Sussex self-advocacy group, one person spoke about the courage needed to speak out. They said that the role of health professionals is to encourage the people to be brave enough to speak out. It is important that professionals are aware that their presence can influence how people behave. Professionals do have power over people's lives and it is understandable that people who have a learning disability may be concerned that they may be punished if they criticize the services. Self-advocacy groups allow people to experience turn taking, to demonstrate feelings of respect for other people and to be shown respect by others. As one group member said, 'The group gives me somewhere I can talk over my problems ... I don't have to shout any more' (Preston 1998, p 29). Self-advocacy groups are about sharing problems with people who really know how you feel because they have had the same or similar experiences. They are not necessarily about providing solutions but providing support and being there for each other.

Self-advocacy groups can also empower people to have input into the services. As a member of the Bognor and Chichester self-advocacy group 'Voice' said, 'We need to make people in authority aware that we can't be shoved from pillar to post and we have the right to decide for ourselves'. Self-advocacy is a way to enable people to participate in society and so by participating we are able to change the society in which we live (Whittell 1998).

Citizen advocacy

A citizen advocate is defined as a valued citizen who is unpaid and independent. It is a person who creates a relationship with an individual who is at risk of social exclusion and finds a way to understand, respond to and represent that person's interest without interpretation and influence. This brings their partner's gifts and concerns into circles of ordinary community life (O'Brien 1987). As Schwartz (1992) said, citizen advocates help 'the client' to be seen as a citizen. A citizen advocate can be:

- a friend
- a link to the wider community
- a reliable person outside the services
- a person who is committed to the client
- a defender of the client's rights.

The citizen advocate's role and function in each of these areas provides the person who has a learning disability with the support that they need in order to engage within their community in a meaningful way. This in turn provides opportunities to build valued relationships and contacts which allow the person concerned to develop a personality and character that is not overly influenced by organizations and the constraints that institutions can impose upon people. Essentially, this allows the person to develop a sense of self based upon a wider variety of influences, much the same as occurs for other members of the general population. For the majority of people, the opportunity to develop as a person occurs during adolescence where individuals challenge society and test out the boundaries of different relationships. This period in our lives may be crucial not only in developing our sense of value and self-worth but also in establishing the baseline for our mental health and well-being.

Developing inclusive communities

Health professionals can further contribute to the process of building inclusive communities and supporting the work of advocacy groups by helping people build networks of friends and connections within their community. Shafik Asante (1997) identifies a number of different strategies that may be useful in building inclusive communities. He uses the terms 'villaging', 'building alliances' and 'quilting' to illustrate ways of developing a variety of relationships. Whilst identified as separate approaches within his work, these approaches have significant overlaps and as such they should be used together.

Fundamental to the concept of 'villaging' is the belief that people need people and that all people should be supportive of each other at all times. Villaging is a strategy that can be used to create a solution to a commonly shared problem and operates from the premise that by acting together we are stronger and better than when we act in isolation. The first step in the process is wanting a village. This may be the wish of one person or a group of people. In order to develop a cohesiveness around the group of 'villagers' there are a number of actions that need to be taken. These include the importance of creating a feeling of being wanted and being important. This can be achieved by considering factors such as hospitality, communication, reciprocity and positive valuing of the contributions individuals are able to make.

Within this it is also important to consider strategies for building alliances; the focus for building these relationships may vary depending upon the central purpose. For example, if the aim of the alliance is to support the achievement of a collective goal, then it will need to be built with people who have similar concerns. If the alliance is about building someone's involvement within their community then the target people may well be individuals who have similar interests and who have strong networks throughout their community. Identifying key partners and building support are therefore important parts of this process. Key partners can provide resources both physically by their expertise and psychologically by supporting the person who is trying to build different alliances.

Quilting is again part of the process of building relationships or alliances and developing inclusive communities. A quilter's purpose in life is to end fragmentation, have a recognition that together we are better, to build a better society for everyone and to ensure that diversity is valued. A key focus of the work of quilters is to increase the educational work in relation to inclusion and diversity. The focus upon education emanates from the belief that in order to truly change what people do, you need to change what people think. The most effective way to achieve this is the educational system, particularly during a person's formative years. An additional aspect of this is the ability to utilize the many and varied skills and abilities that each person brings with them in order to create a more inclusive community.

In essence, therefore, Asante (1997) is highlighting a number of strategies that can be enlisted to help build a more inclusive community. These include considering the public health role of the professional by exploring ways in which they can educate the community about the needs and aspirations of people who have a learning disability, in order to challenge the segregated and exclusive nature of our society. On a more local scale, it involves considering who are the key community builders within the area and utilizing them and their skills to assist a person who has a learning disability to become involved in their community. Quite often, this person is not part of the circle of professionals paid to provide a service to people who have a learning disability. Building contacts with this person is about mobilizing the forces that exist within communities to the advantage of people who have a learning disability. Asante also discusses the power and effectiveness of people who come together to address the common challenges that we as individuals experience. The outcome of all these approaches is to enhance the social networks of the person who has a learning disability.

Social networks: the importance of friendship

Having said that community integration is dependent on developing relationships and friendships with people in the community, we need to examine what friendships are and how they are formed. There are many types of friendship, from lifelong best friends to acquaintances. Friendships offer us psychological, emotional and physical support when we need it. They should be interdependent relationships, where both people have something to bring to the friendship. They should help us to have a positive view of ourselves and the effect we have on others. Balkizas & O'Hare (1994) suggested that 'we discover our personhood in relationships and this is experienced as a gift from others' (p 46). This is a view in which we are recognized and treated as whole and not as a collection of defects or an easily analysed personality.

How do people make and maintain friendships?

Most people make friends with people they have met at school, college, university, work, social clubs, evening classes and sports activities. We often meet new friends through being introduced to someone by another friend. People who have a learning disability may have been moved away from their home to go to a special school. When they leave school they may then be moved into residential care where they may not be able to choose where they live or who they live with. This lack of control means that it is very difficult to maintain friendships and build social networks. Maintaining friendships involves money, transport, access to a telephone and being able to write and post letters. So the opportunities that learning-disabled people have to establish friendships can be very limited.

ACTIVITY 16.5
Think about your friends, how you met them and what they mean to you. Explore these questions with someone who has a learning disability. How do the two experiences differ?

Understanding social networks

A way of understanding the types of relationships that people have is to compile a picture of a person's social network. A social network consists of all the people that a person comes into contact with both personally and professionally

(Thompson 1995). People's social networks can vary greatly and Thompson & Pickering (1998) describe several ways of assessing the quality of someone's social network based upon the characteristics of a network as identified by Atkinson & Williams (1990).

- *Range* – the amount of people in the network
- *Density* – frequency of contacts between people in the network and contact with person at the centre of the network
- *Multiplexity* – whether contact is characterized by several different types of exchange or just one type
- *Intensity* – strength of the relationships in the network
- *Durability* – whether the relationships will last over time
- *Reciprocity* – whether the relationship is one of mutual support
- *Symmetry* – the balance of power in the relationships in the network

The social network of people who have a learning disability may have a large range of people within it. For some people this may be positive but for many it means an overemphasis upon the presence of paid professionals. This can mean that the symmetry, reciprocity and multiplexity of these relationships may be low which in turn may impact on the qualitative experience of these relationships from the perspective of the person who has a learning disability. Looking at someone's social network like this allows you to see where the gaps are and which areas need to be discussed with the service user in order to identify how they wish to see their network develop and to agree any future goals.

ACTIVITY 16.6

Try thinking about your own social networks and what qualities they have. Consider this information in the context of someone who has a learning disability; what qualities do their social networks have? What might this mean in terms of their health and their quality of life?

You may have considered how your social networks and the qualities that they have impact upon your own quality of life; this is particularly relevant when thinking about how others support you and how you support others in their everyday lives. For many people who have a learning disability, there is often an imbalance between the amount and depth of the support that they receive and what they give to others within their network. If someone has severe physical impairment they are more likely to be dependent on professionals and as such there may be little reciprocity. This can and does impact upon a person's self-esteem and has a direct result upon that person's health status.

Circles of support

Circles of support are another approach to developing the inclusion of people who have a learning disability into their community as well as supporting them to take more control over their lives. As we have already suggested, many people who have learning disabilities live unfulfilled, isolated lives. They and their families sometimes live under great stress and they do not have the energy or hope to be able to plan for the future, but a circle of supporters and friends can help to share the load (Mount 1995). Often people who have a learning disability lack of friends due to the lifestyle that care systems force upon them. Circles of support are one way of helping to establish a social network.

Circles of support are built on the idea that friendship is a basic human need and if people are put in contact with each other, friendships will flourish. Circles are not owned by the services or professionals; they try to rebalance the sense of individual and community responsibility for vulnerable people in society. A person who has learning disabilities may not be able to identify many people who could form their circle, so first there has to be a committed person to try to encourage other people to join the circle. The circle does not have to be large; it just takes one person, maybe a health professional, to say they are going to set up a circle and get one other person to join and then see what happens.

Schwartz (1997) discusses the idea of 'askers'. These are people who, on behalf of a learning-disabled person, can ask other people for help. They are the go-betweens in society, who link strangers and get clubs and associations started. People who have disabilities and people in need have become invisible to us; they are surrounded by professional services and we do not have to take responsibility for them, because the service will do it. As Schwartz (1997) said, institutions relieve people of the obligation to provide charity and love to fellow human beings. The role of the asker is to offer the opportunity to people to be responsible for each other. The asker must be prepared to take the rejections that will inevitably come from asking people. By entering someone's life, the asker opens up areas that can be very painful if the person is rejected. For a long time that person may not have dared to hope that their dreams could come true (Schwartz 1997). So the asker must absorb any rejection and come to the person only when they are sure that they have made a strong connection with others who are prepared to be involved in the person's life.

An important part of the circle is that it is lead by the person at the centre of the circle and should go at their pace. It is not about people solving problems for someone, it is about working together; this is aptly described as 'walking with the focus person'. Hope for the future and empowerment of the individual are the important parts of the circle (Wertheimer 1995, p 53). A fundamental element of circles is that people are there for each other; sometimes all anyone can offer is to be there (Ludlum 1993). The person at the centre of the circle may just need someone who will listen whilst they talk about their experience of isolation and exclusion; the reality is that 'we can't always make it all right for people' (Wertheimer 1995).

If a circle is working well it should be a relationship of mutual support where everyone has gifts and abilities to contribute. It should create a community that the person can belong to and play a valued role in. Circles are based on the idea that everyone needs support and a sense of belonging. Common to all circles should be a sense of interdependence (Mount et al 1988). As Schwartz (1997) stated, there is enormous power in simple friendship. Mount (1995) identifies friendships as being able to give hope to people and so helping them to have the courage to change things.

Circles need a facilitator to hold the circle together and to keep it on the right track. The first thing the facilitator does is to clarify what change the focus person wants to see and who they would like in their circle. It is the facilitator's job to 'keep the dream going' (Ludlum 1993, p 11) and to stop other people from changing the dream. To be a facilitator you need to be someone who listens to people and is willing to share ideas and find solutions to problems. Circles are also about having fun, going to the cinema, having meals together and socializing.

Circles are for vulnerable people. As a result some people worry that a circle of support is a way in which the unscrupulous could take advantage of vulnerable people. The reality, however, is often that the more people who are involved in a person's life, the safer the person is. Schwartz (1992) has listed the fundamental things that can help to keep vulnerable people safe in their community.

- Having unpaid relationships with people outside where they live.
- Belonging to community groups.
- Knowing people in their community who might help them if something goes wrong.
- Having someone they can trust to help them with their money.

Circles of support do not work for everyone; as Ludlum (1993) states, 'The most effective way to kill a good idea is to have it catch on'. If circles become something that everyone in care should have they will lose their integrity, creativity and spontaneity. Circles can only come about and last if people are genuinely committed to the idea and not attending because it is part of their job and their supervisor has told them to be there.

Such ways of working can help to integrate people who have disabilities into the community but they are not the only solution and, as already said, they do not suit everyone. Circles are effective because they deal in the fundamental needs of all humans: to be loved and to belong. As Vanier (1979) said, for the handicapped person who had felt abandoned, there is only one reality that will bring him back to life: an authentic, tender and faithful friendship. That person must discover that he is loved and important to someone and only then will his confusion turn to peace.

CONCLUSION

Circles of support, citizen advocates and self-advocacy groups are not tools to be used without thought or effort; they do not work to set formulae. Each circle, citizen advocate partnership and self-advocacy group is unique and shaped by the people who are in them. They are not systems safeguards but they have the capacity to help people shift their centre of gravity from the service world to the real world (Sanderson et al 1997). Citizen advocates are free to move between professional boundaries and to speak and act in ways that professionals may feel unable to do. They can be valuable allies in helping to remove the obstacles that care systems can create in which people are seen as 'service users' rather than individuals.

In addition, the approaches highlighted within this chapter focus on ways to more effectively integrate people who have a learning disability within their own communities. In doing this, the links to a person's quality of life and overall mental health and well-being are inextricable. The existence of a variety of relationships within a community that vary in terms of purpose, durability, reciprocity, etc. can only increase the strength of an individual. As such, this reinforces who they are as a person and subsequently builds their resilience to ill health, both physically and mentally.

FURTHER READING

Collins J 1992 When the eagles fly. Values into Action, London
Book about people leaving long-stay institutions and moving into the community.

McIntosh B, Whittaker A 2000 Unlocking the future. King's Fund Publishing, London
Ideas about how to develop new lifestyles with people who have complex learning disabilities.

McIntosh B, Whittaker A 1998 Days of change. King's Fund Publishing, London
A practical guide to developing better day opportunities with people who have a learning disability.

Mount B 1991 Dare to dream. Communitas, Manchester
How to help people to achieve change in their lives. Contains many examples and practical advice.

Mount B, Ducharme G, Beeman P 1991 Person centred development: a journey in learning to listen to people with disability. Communitas, Manchester
Advice about how to form a circle of support.

Murray P, Penman J 1996 Let our children be. Parents with Attitude, Sheffield
Book of stories, pictures and poetry about families' experiences of having a family member with a disability.

Nunkoosing K, John M 1997 Friendships, relationships and the management of rejection and loneliness by people with learning disabilities. J Learning Disabil Nursing Health Social Care 1(1):10–18
Research examining the factors that hinder or enable people who have a learning disability to develop friendships.

Perske R, Perske M 1990 Circles of friends. Abingdon Press, Nashville
Stories about people's circles of support.

REFERENCES

Asante S 1997 When spiders webs unite: challenging articles and essays on community, diversity and inclusion. Inclusion Press, Toronto

Atkinson D, Williams P 1990 Networks. Open University Press, Milton Keynes

Balkizas D, O'Hare M 1994 The helping hand of God. Nursing Stand 9(9):46–47

Barr O, Fay M 1993 Community homes: institutions in waiting? Nursing Stand 7(41):34–37

Dowson S 1991 Moving to the dance or service culture and community care. Values Into Action, London

Goffman E 1961 Asylums. Pelican Books, London

Hogg J 1998 Competence and quality in the lives of people with profound and multiple learning disabilities: some recent research. Tizard Learning Disabil Rev 3(1): 6–14

Jefferson J, Hall M 1998 Promoting choice, autonomy and independence with older people. In: Pickering S, Thompson J (eds) Promoting positive practice in nursing older people. Baillière Tindall, London

Kinsella P 1993 Supported livings a new paradigm. National Development Team, Manchester

Lindsey M 1998 Signposts for success. Department of Health, London

Ludlum C D 1993 Tending the candle: a booklet for circle facilitators. Communitas, Manchester

March J, Steingold B, Justice S 1997 Follow the yellow brick road! People with learning difficulties as co-researchers. Br J Learning Disabil 25:77–80

Marshall T H 1951 Citizenship and social class. Cambridge University Press, Cambridge

Mount B 1995 Capacity works: finding windows for change using personal futures planning. Communitas, Manchester

Mount B, Beeman P, Ducharme G 1988 What are we learning about circles of support? Communitas, Manchester

O'Brien J 1987 Learning from citizen advocacy programs. Georgia Advocacy Office, Atlanta

Oldenburg R 1989 The great good place: cafes, coffee shops, community centres, beauty parlours, general stores, bars, hangouts and how they get you through the day. Paragon, New York

Preston A 1998 Developing self advocacy skills in adults with learning difficulties and challenging behaviour. Br J Learning Disabil 26:27–30

Sanderson H, Kennedy J, Ritchie P, Goodwin G 1997 People, plans and possibilities. SHS Ltd, Edinburgh

Sarason S 1977 The psychological sense of community prospects for a community psychology. Jossey-Bass, San Francisco

Schwartz D B 1992 Crossing the river: creating a conceptual revolution in community and disability. Brookline Books, Pennsylvania

Schwartz D B 1997 Who cares? Rediscovering community. Westview Press, Oxford

Sinson J 1990 Micro-institutionalisation? Br J Mental Subnormality 36(2):77–86

Thompson J 1995 Fostering integration. Nursing Times 91(9):55–59

Thompson J, Pickering S 1998 Promoting positive practice in nursing older people. Baillière Tindall, London

Vanier J 1979 Community and growth: our pilgrimage together. Griffen House, Toronto

Wertheimer A 1995 Circles of support: building inclusive communities. Circles Network, Bristol

Wertheimer A 1996 Changing days. King's Fund Publishing, London

Whittell B 1998 The all Wales strategy: self advocacy and participation. Br J Learning Disabil 26:23–26

USEFUL ADDRESSES

British Institute of Learning
Disabilities
Wolverhampton Road
Kidderminster
Worcestershire DY10 3PP
01562 850251

Circles Network
Pamwell House
160 Pennywell Road
Upper Easton
Bristol BS5 0TX
0117 939 3917

King's Fund Institute
11–13 Cavendish Square
London W1M 0AN
0207 307 2569

National Development Team
St Peter's Court
Manchester M1 5LW
0161 228 7055

Norah Fry Research Centre
University of Bristol

3 Priory Road
Bristol BS8 1TX
0117 923 8137

Parents with Attitude
c/o 44 Cowlishaw Road
Sheffield S11 8XF

People First (Manchester)
5 Fourways House
57 Hilton Street Manchester M1 2EJ
0161 236 6418

Tizard Centre
University of Kent
Beverley Farm
Canterbury
Kent CT2 7LZ
01227 764000

Values into Action
Oxford House
Derbyshire Street
London E2 6HG
0207 729 5436

17 Inter professional and multi-agency working

Peter Mathias and Tony Thompson

KEY ISSUES

- The need for interprofessional working in order to contribute to the provision of services focusing on the health needs of learning-disabled people
- The interface between the differing professional and non-professional support systems
- Strengthening and supporting the helping systems
- Changes in the welfare and educational structures which affect the total provision of learning disability services
- Organizational change in relation to contemporary social policy

WHY WE NEED TO WORK ACROSS PROFESSIONAL AND ORGANIZATIONAL BOUNDARIES

No one can doubt the paradox that reflects the world of working within learning disability services as it is experienced by professionals and others. Quite often, this can be seen to be the result of the interaction of a wide variety of conflicting changes in economic conditions, social values, rapid information flows, technological and sociopolitical changes. The origins of many of these changes can be found in the demand for greater choice as well as better quality and equality of service provision by service users. In addition, there is an increased demand amongst human service providers for market share, resulting in provider competition across both organizational and geographic boundaries. Associated with this are changes in the nature of jobs available to the workforce. This is particularly related to the need to develop a competent and qualified workforce in health and social care (TOPSS 2000). Finally, there are widespread expectations of improved social and environmental conditions, together with adequate rewards for work undertaken with disadvantaged groups.

In the past decade professionals have been under particular pressure to balance the risks and opportunities which arise from demands at both strategic and operational level. The nature of this balance is complex as it involves the understanding of many of the features of change which are interrelated and can often seem beyond the control of the professional undertaking their everyday work.

The reformation of health and social care systems is high on most of the political agendas of Western Europe. This reformation tends to reflect structural

and organizational changes in the delivery of services, together with the introduction of either competitive or collaborative mechanisms into the public sector
agencies. These changes are often reflected in the push for developments in the
health and social care field and have affected the drive towards care delivery
within the primary care sector and a reconfiguration of the acute care services.
This is reflected particularly in England with the advent of primary care groups
and primary care trusts and these developments are bringing in their wake a
drive for a more cost-effective training solution which should lead to better
provision of individualized care.

The context within which these changes are taking place is once again
increasing the pressure on professionals and agencies to work together with
a common aim of ensuring better services for those who are labelled as
having a learning disability. The recent policy changes in England, such as
those contained in *The new NHS: modern, dependable* (DoH 1997) propose
that a strategic duty to work in partnership should be placed on those commissioning and providing health in local authority services. These principles are
also replicated in equivalent documents within other parts of the United
Kingdom.

All of the above, and other policy initiatives supporting these changes,
such as the Health Act (1999), point firmly to a new demand that agencies
and services have to pursue partnership within a political and legal agenda. It is
also true that in the last decade the theory basis of interagency working has
gathered momentum. However, in order for learning disability services to be
delivered in a really effective way such theories have to be operationalized. In
doing this they have to be considered against a backcloth of workers coping
with the contemporary demands of society and the physical and psychological
demands which can be experienced when working with people who have a
learning disability.

It has become apparent that there is disenchantment with regard to the delivery and provision of these and other services. This was highlighted during the
latter part of 1998 when the Labour administration became quite explicit in its
message to those who manage the services that both the public and those who
use the service have lost confidence in the ability of the contributing agencies to
deliver effective care.

At the beginning of the millennium it is likely that the pressure will increase
for agencies to provide a seamless service based upon a public health model in
order that each will add value to the respective contribution. If this is to be the
case then new and maybe novel competencies will have to emerge within the
workforce, particularly if it is to be successful in meeting the expectations of
those who need a holistic service. The core of new initiatives and policy guidance is that a far greater emphasis is to be placed upon delivering services that
are both more responsive and meet the quality standards that users and carers
would expect to see.

The quality agenda

It is interesting that the need for professional self-regulation is seen as an essential component of the delivery of services of a high quality. Therefore, it is
crucial that the professional standards developed on a national basis have to be

responsive to the changing needs of that service and at the same time tally with the expectations of the general public.

Clinical governance within the health sector reflects most of the ideals contained within the recent policy debate, but it really boils down to the process of delivering quality through a model of participation and shared decision making. A somewhat novel responsibility is being placed upon chief executives and boards of health trusts in relation to accountability for clinical care and the vicarious liability for the decisions made by clinical practitioners. It is highly likely that health practitioners, and those who contribute to the process, will have to offer proof of continuing professional development and they will have to be aware of mechanisms available which form part of the national framework to support quality and effectiveness within the health services.

The initiatives in relation to governance fall into two main categories: those that have advisory roles, such as the setting of standards, and those that have regulatory roles that focus on ensuring performance and monitoring of that performance in order that these standards can be met. These frameworks will cover all areas of specialist work and treatment and will be drawn up by expert reference groups that draw upon the best evidence of clinical and cost effectiveness. In addition, the government has given clear messages that there will be user representation with regard to interpretation of such effectiveness. These reference groups will guide service commissioners and providers on how to ensure that specific services are provided. Each particular framework will include:

- information with regard to supporting programmes that are required; for example, lifelong learning, training, continuing professional development and workforce planning
- information to support the bench marking needed to ensure that interventions are correctly implemented
- identification of key interventions and practices together with associated costs
- the evidence base for selected interventions.

It is envisaged that each of these approaches will contribute to the overall quality and effectiveness agenda. In doing so it will invariably increase the need for effective interprofessional and interagency working.

Partnerships between statutory organizations

Local Authority Social Services and the NHS have, since their inception, been the primary form of protection and support for people who have a learning disability. This responsibility continues to be important in the context of the current government, with the need for integrated policy in support of multiprofessional working becoming increasingly obvious. Successive attempts have been made to address the public interpretation and perception, together with sensitivities regarding the provision of such services. In doing this it is important to realize the impact that health and social care policy across the board has upon the individual lives of people who have a learning disability.

It is sometimes difficult for those at the chalk face of delivery to accept that the central role of government is an exacting and complex one and includes balancing strategies for operationalizing service delivery within a framework of legislation and the overall constraints associated with the totality of public service.

Given the above scenario, it would be understandable if professionals became complacent about the fact that contemporary learning disability services do not always fulfil the expectations for everyone who uses those services. It would be equally easy to passively accept that there are inequalities in the health services, particularly with regard to access to proper services that are matched to client need.

Certainly in the past four decades there has been an increasing evidence base identifying the unacceptable variations in the performance of services and associated outmoded practices which continue to show up on occasion (DoH 1999). All too often such variations are brought to light through the publicity associated with adverse enquiries and reviews.

It is still the case, within the health service particularly, that any strategies which could assist families, groups and communities in providing mutual help are rooted in legislative frameworks which were designed when most care was provided in institutions and can no longer support the delivery of such care. One very important feature emerging in the 21st century is the bridging of the gap between what occurred between the hospital closure period of the 1970s and 1980s and the new emphasis on public health. This revolves around the need to have sound primary care systems in place through the concept of primary care groups and primary care trusts or their equivalent. If learning-disabled people are to benefit from raised public awareness and responsibility then there has to be a shift in the attitude of professionals in relation to the way in which they are prepared to work together within a professional framework. These frameworks will in the future involve more risk, they will be exposed to a greater degree of public scrutiny and be based upon a far more accountable relationship with their own client population.

In order to place the contemporary provision of service on a strong strategic foundation, professionals will require preparation associated with effective clinical teamwork. The objective will be to ensure that services at least meet the aim of protecting the public, particularly in relation to those individuals defined as having challenging behaviour. The aim will also be to deliver cost-efficient and effective ways of providing services based upon guidance from national bodies responsible for monitoring the activities of such services, such as the National Institute for Clinical Effectiveness (NICE).

Other features will include the:

■ involvement of service users and carers in their specific care pathways and within the planning of services overall
■ continuing of efforts to forge sound operational partnerships within education, employment, health, social care and housing
■ creation of supportive services and ancillary workers who will assist the learning-disabled person and their families or carers to build communities that are healthy in the widest possible context

- integration of services within primary care in order that primary care groups work closely with specialist clinical teams to deliver services within a sound planning framework
- accurate assessment of individual health needs which would be aimed at delivering better treatment within care, either in a domiciliary or institutional setting which will enable 24-hour access to services
- development of systems of information which support the delivery of healthcare and the accurate management of health resources.

From the above it can be seen that paradox will undoubtedly emerge and that practitioners working within new services will have to learn how to handle conflicting demands made upon them. Not least will be the need for them to play their part in effective service delivery which is based upon good clinical evidence but which is cost effective. This will have to occur at the same time ensuring that they cope with the bureaucratic and communication processes associated with public services who are generally trying to provide a seamless service. It should be apparent that the monitoring of health services particularly will be placed in the arena of collaboration and partnerships between the statutory organizations and indeed the users of the service themselves. For these efforts to be successful, user involvement has to be recognized at all parts of the continuum of care. The next section further explores the concept of user involvement, along with other issues relating to the achievement of effective interprofessional and multiagency working.

THE REALITIES OF INTERPROFESSIONAL WORKING

Collaborating with service users

Recent policy initiatives clearly acknowledge the importance of collaborating with service users in determining the nature and quality of the service they receive. This is of particular importance in order to ensure that the service provided meets the needs of those it is intended for. In order to achieve this it is essential to consider the ways in which professionals and others support service users and work towards creating an equal relationship.

ACTIVITY 17.1

Consider how you and the team you work in, collaborate with the people who use the service.

Thompson & Saunders (1999) identify the need for service users to be involved at all levels of the process of determining care delivery, including planning, managing and evaluating care and service developments. It is possible to identify five distinct types of service user involvement:

1. The user's opportunity to influence, coordinate and manage their own care.
2. The personal involvement of service users in the running and overall management of the service.
3. Engagement of service users in the development of new services.

4. Use of surveys and other forms of consultation.
5. The use of citizen advocates.

ACTIVITY 17.2   What skills do you think are essential to achieve effective collaboration with service users?

In order to achieve a high level of collaboration with service users you may have identified some of the following skill sets:

■ Active listening
■ Negotiation
■ Augmented and facilitated communication skills
■ Interpersonal skills
■ Relationship building
■ Verbal and non-verbal communication skills
■ Enablement and empowering skills
■ Facilitation skills.

Policy documents and advisory bodies are actively promoting partnership of this kind, at every level from the strategic perspective of central administration and policy to the operational level both within and between statutory and non-statutory organizations.

Developing partnerships

The current policy agenda puts the development of sound and effective partnerships across agencies at the very heart of service delivery (DoH 1997, 1998, 1999). The development of good working relationships across the different organizations that people who have a learning disability use, aims to ensure that the care they receive has continuity and is consistent with individual needs.

ACTIVITY 17.3   Identify some of the key partnerships that you feel are necessary in developing healthcare for people who have a learning disability.

Key areas of collaboration not only include nursing and healthcare providers but also employment, education, housing and personal social services, all of which are underpinned by the need to work collaboratively with planners and commissioners of services.

Some of the key areas in which relationships of this nature are beginning to develop are the health action zones, education action zones and health improvement programmes. Crucial to the success of these initiatives is effective teamwork and good professional relationships both within and across boundaries (Weinstein 1998). Many of these initiatives are community based and as such require effective primary care services that are able to commission and provide appropriate services to the local population and contribute to the development of inclusive communities.

Community inclusion

Community participation has long been a goal of learning disability services but more recently there has been a clear acknowledgement that this has not been achieved to the level people believed to be possible. This growing acknowledgement within learning disability service provision has been matched with a gradual change in policy initiatives. Policies such as health action zones, regeneration programmes and health improvement programmes are all examples of where broader public policy can work towards positive outcomes for people who have a learning disability as well as other sectors of society.

ACTIVITY 17.4   Why is interdisciplinary working important in ensuring community inclusion for people who have a learning disability? Why might ineffective working between professionals prevent community inclusion?

The effective working of all those involved in service delivery can only enhance the achievement of the positive goal of community inclusion. This is particularly important for those individuals providing the day-to-day support for people who have a learning disability. For these service providers the possession of community-building skills will be essential. Within this the ability to motivate, influence and negotiate with others will be key. However, there are some serious threats to the development of community inclusion for people who have a learning disability, including the inability of professionals to work in an interprofessional way by valuing and respecting the diversity that exists within professional groups.

Nowhere is this respect and value more important within the current political agenda than within primary care service delivery. In order to create a genuinely inclusive community for a person who has a learning disability, it is essential to ensure the services they require are delivered on a fair and equitable basis. Current research evidence indicates this is not entirely the case in primary care services.

Primary care services

Once again, the current policy agenda indicates a clear commitment to a primary care-led NHS (DoH 1997). Whilst clearly stating the role of primary care organizations in delivering healthcare across the United Kingdom, comparatively little information has been available relating to their role in commissioning and providing services for people who have a learning disability, despite the fact they will have a pivotal role in this area. In some instances this area has received very little focus due to the competing demands created by other priorities, such as coronary heart disease, mental health and accidents.

As the primary care organizations, of whatever configuration, become more established then they are more able to divert their attention to other areas. In some places this will inevitably be learning disability services. Examples already exist of health authorities considering merging community learning disability teams with primary healthcare teams. When considering initiatives such as this it is important to explore the opportunities as well as the threats that are created in such circumstances. In order to ensure the success of such developments it is essential that professional structures and ideologies are explicitly articulated as well as strategies for dealing with professional tribalism. Failure to do so can result in substantial difficulties for users of learning disability services.

Individual health needs

Within all of this, it is essential that the health needs of an individual are accurately assessed. The assessment process has traditionally been a uniprofessional activity but within the current policy climate this is unsustainable. This is further reinforced by the developments in various areas that are promoting not only joint commissioning but also joint care planning processes. The process of joint planning is further challenged by the current philosophies around person-centred planning and person-centred service delivery, which place the service user at the centre of all processes.

ACTIVITY 17.5	How do you and your team assess the health needs of service users? You may wish to think about the roles and responsibilities of each team member as well as the team as a whole.

Within a culture that places the client at the centre of service delivery, it is essential that individual practitioners are able to clearly articulate their role and contribution to both the assessment process and meeting the service user's care and support needs. Once again, it is essential that this is done in a climate of openness and honesty where service users, carers and professionals are acknowledged and valued for their expertise. The contribution of user experience to the assessment process can be said to be fundamental to the delivery of a service that meets individual needs. Crucial within this is the accessibility of information to the service user and other stakeholders.

The development of information systems

Within learning disability services it is vital to ensure that practitioners and clients have access to appropriate and user-friendly information. This is particularly important because of the wide range of professionals, organizations and agencies that are involved in delivering an effective service. Fundamental to this is the need to have communication strategies that are fast and effective and that work not just across professional boundaries but also across different organizations and agencies.

Although current technology can ensure that information is accessible to practitioners and clients at the point of need, there are significant resource and policy issues that impact upon the achievement of this. As a result there is a need to think broadly and creatively about strategies that can be used to ensure that interprofessional and interagency communication is effective. One of the ways in which effective communication can be achieved is through the use of interprofessional care notes.

The advantages of such systems are enormous, particularly in relation to the prevention of duplication of information. In addition, such measures also give increased opportunity for sharing vital information about clients and also the team goals. Ultimately it can be argued that without shared methods of communication, particularly interprofessional records, care will be fragmented, not person centred and therefore ineffective. Shared methods of communication are, as already stated, essential in the development of effective teamwork but they are also extremely important when considering the current emphasis in policy upon the development of partnerships across professions, with users and across other agencies. This next section will briefly consider the key issues in relation to effective teamwork.

EFFECTIVE TEAMWORK

The main framework through which multiprofessional care is delivered is that of multidisciplinary teams. Teams of this nature fall into a number of discrete categories including community teams, primary healthcare teams, person-centred planning teams, etc. The level at which the team operates will be influenced by its focus, e.g. whether it is client or project focused.

Irrespective of the focus of any team, certain common characteristics can be identified that facilitate the development of effective teamworking. These include the need to ensure a full understanding of systems and roles across both the different professions and organizations. This can be particularly difficult when considering the different professional backgrounds between, for example, nurses and social workers or nurses and psychiatrists. In order to ensure that collaboration is effective there should be a clear plan of what is necessary to deliver the service, which may include clear statements in terms of service contracts and staff objectives. This will help each team member understand their role in relation to that of other members of the team.

ACTIVITY 17.6   How does your team ensure that effective teamwork is developed and maintained? You may wish to think about how clear individual roles and responsibilities are within the team and to the users of the service.

Bicknell (1988) suggests there are specific measures that can be used to support and encourage effective teamwork. For example, valuing the contribution of each individual as unique and important, identification of core and shared skills within the team and the utilization of this information to create a positive team feeling as well as to manage workloads. Weinstein (1998) identifies the following as the key considerations in achieving an effective team.

- Common understanding and common goals/objectives
- Clear, jargon-free communication
- Effective leadership
- Regular interaction between members

- Equal participation by and valuing of all members
- Meaningful and challenging tasks for all members
- Joint evaluation and action planning
- Clear decision-making processes
- Small enough number of people to facilitate thorough and regular communication
- Open acknowledgement of power issues
- Open acknowledgement and resolution of conflict
- Recognition of the unique contribution of each member of the team

All the above areas should be considered in the context of any teamwork and in order to achieve the more strategic aims identified within this chapter.

THE INTERFACE BETWEEN SUPPORT SYSTEMS

The holes in the net of service provision are now quite well identified by practitioners, policy makers and users of services. With the advent of primary care groups and primary care teams, the differing priorities of localities are likely to reflect the progress which they wish to achieve in attempting to meet the challenge of service development. Of fundamental importance with regard to support systems are the priorities clearly identified by the Department of Health (1993). These include:

- Ensuring that housing agencies are properly integrated into planning, purchasing and service delivery systems

- The engagement of providers in the statutory and independent sectors in ways which will ensure more robust and creative market management

- Developing the capability of organizations, emphasizing cross-agency needs assessment and the development of joint commissioning

- Shifting the balance of care so that more resources are progressively made available for non-residential forms of care and treatment

- Enabling user and carer participation in decisions on planning, service delivery and quality control

- The development of care management with the necessary components of budget and managerial devolution of responsibility taken into account

- Consolidation of basic systems around assessment, discharge, contracting and communication. The evidence suggests that interagency working is easier to achieve where there is a history of working together and where there are shared organizational mission statements (Shaw 1998).

These points of progression that agencies and support staff have to achieve are complex. They have to be prepared to spend time together and share values, attitudes and views to help to establish a common language. In order to assist this process, collaborative working and training is now central to government initiatives that hope to enhance interprofessional collaboration and ensure that supporting services are accountable to those they seek to serve.

In order to ensure that the various support systems are in place for those people who offer support to a person who has a learning disability, dialogue has to take place which recognizes them as equal and important partners. This dialogue has to be centred around the need to maximize benefits for the disabled person who can look towards health services in meeting their health needs. The scenario also demands that the local community impacts upon the provision of services that meet the overall health need associated with individuals who have a variety of different disabilities.

Professionals who provide services will have to consider what will drive the changes necessary within their respective health systems and having identified this, they need to know how to harness effort targeted towards need reduction. In the past some of the solutions offered to the recipients of a service have not been fit for the purpose they purport to provide. We have to learn lessons from the past and professionals working together as supporters of people who have disabilities need to avoid taking measures that in the past have proved to be problematic.

Whilst professionals are working within existing government policies, as identified earlier in this chapter, some of these are still emerging and will continue to emerge throughout the next decade. These policies will provide new opportunities for improving the quality of health services and the general population's health needs should be better met. It is against this backcloth that the learning-disabled person will be drawing from the total resource. The intention is that people will be given greater scope and opportunity, both through and across the traditional boundaries. Health and local authority workers in particular will need to take on new opportunities to establish and improve working relationships, enhance role development and play their part in creating organizations that are capable of maximizing improvements in health and healthcare services for local people, wherever they are.

It is sometimes easy for individual practitioners to be unaware of the more overarching features of health provision. There is thus a vital need for health service professionals to work in partnership with all their local agencies to optimize and add value to current resources which are required to deliver improvements in healthcare. These are likely to be through health improvement programmes and regeneration schemes. This is not an easy task and it is therefore understandable when professionals feel isolated. Health and Local Authorities are not yet coterminous and have to be seen within the context of a variety of structures and organizations within local government; for example, county, district and unitary authorities. When the total regional resource is observed, the situation becomes more complex, particularly when trying to align regional health authorities with the regional development agency, national assemblies, government office and the NHS Executive. The latter scenario can involve numerous health authorities being included within a region and it is they that are responsible for assessing the health needs of the total population, including those who have a learning disability. They are also responsible for commissioning health services to meet those needs, thus necessitating effective working across a multiplicity of organizations. It is only in this way that the local community will be established as a healthy resource.

Reference has already been made to primary care groups and trusts, which will be responsible for improving and promoting the health of the local population and for delivering primary and community health services. They will eventually take on the full responsibility for commissioning the majority of community and secondary care services. Those working within the field of learning disability have to be aware of the development of health improvement programmes which are drawn up by health authorities in partnership with primary care trusts, local authorities and NHS trusts. These are an important feature for addressing local healthcare priorities. The practitioner concentrating on the needs of the learning disabled who wishes to make an impact will have to utilize the many vehicles which are part of the improvement programmes.

It is likely that the establishment of the NICE will also provide a valuable resource to individuals and organizations when promoting both clinical and cost-effective services. Learning disability nurses have had to make tremendous changes within their practice over the past 10 years and in the past 3 years alone they have had to adapt to changes in the ways in which healthcare services are planned, organized and delivered. It is only relatively recently that they have had to respond to central demands to abolish the concept of an internal marketplace and replace it with a system of integrated care based on partnership between the NHS and local organizations.

The interface between the different professional and non-professional supports, taken together with strengthening and supporting the helping systems, will be affected greatly in the 10-year programme which recent legislation has established. The major features which have a direct effect upon the person who has a learning disability are those associated with equality of access to services and the quality of these services. The anticipated outcomes for providing these needs to maximize the use of the total resource. It is apparent that the central administration is not only endeavouring to ensure that NHS policy impacts on these areas but also that the wider government agenda, such as social inclusion and regeneration schemes, can be seen to promote a healthy community.

The contemporary nurse and healthcare worker continue to see changes in clinical practice and the way in which services are delivered which demand new organizational structures associated with the quest for quality, efficiency and the modernization of the total service. A key issue for workers within health and local authority care services is that of improving the ability to focus on the community which they serve with all relevant stakeholders, whilst maintaining coherence and effective working within their own specific teams.

THE FRAMEWORK FOR STRENGTHENING AND SUPPORTING THE HELPING SYSTEMS

Access to knowledge and information continues to be a particular need for those who support people who have a learning disability. Shared learning and joint training have emerged as a useful vehicle to enhance such knowledge. Key features are emerging which can be selected from relevant policy initiatives which will inform the provision of training. Whilst not all of these on the surface appear to relate to learning disability provision, they do have significant implications for those who work within the totality of health or local authority provision. These issues include:

- Health authorities will be expected to serve populations of sufficient size to enable them to provide strategic leadership to that population within the local health system, and have the ability to commission specialized services.

- The removal of statutory constraints to improve opportunities and incentives to ensure that joint working occurs between health authorities, social services and local government. For example, the first national planning and priorities guidance issued in Health Service Circular 1998/159, Local Authority Circular (98) (22) and The Health Act (1999).

- Primary care trusts will eventually take on responsibility for providing and commissioning a range of services. This will have direct consequences for the health authorities and health service trusts who currently provide these.

- There has been an indication in legislation that some learning disability services currently attached to acute trusts may be relocated as more specialist mental health trusts emerge.

Coterminosity is likely to be a key feature of future planning, which means that local authority boundaries will form the foundations on which health authorities and community services will be built. These and related issues are bound to vex the minds planning a strategic organization of care which concentrates upon those people who have a learning disability. Amongst the issues they will have to consider will be the shape of future organizational arrangements which will affect the direct care provision within health and local authority. Additional issues are reflected in the questions below.

- In the light of all these policy changes, where will the pressure points arise for the nurse working in the learning disability system?

- Will the implementation of these policies impact on the care workers' organizational structures?

- Is it possible for the practitioner to identify a clear statement with regard to policy on who will be able to manage specialized and strategic learning disability services to a timescale?

- What will be the impact of the processes put in place to facilitate and operationalize the changes?

The original White Paper and subsequent legislation have indicated that the primary care trusts may not be able to take responsibility for specialist learning disability services. This is further reinforced where health and social care boundaries are not fixed and where joint work is particularly important and where an integrated range of services from community to hospital care is required. In this care scenario specialist trusts could prove to be the better mechanism for coordinating the delivery of these services. As the National Service Framework on Mental Health verifies, such a policy is likely to be pursued at least at the outset.

New services and new understandings

In order to consider the effects of working across boundaries and organizations, together with ensuring competent interprofessional working, the contemporary practitioner cannot avoid the culture of quality which is impacting upon learning disability services. Such quests for quality bring their own demands for the respective agencies and organizations and how they are managed to make progress. For the health service alone some key change drivers can be identified:

- Responding to information from the Commission for Health Improvement
- Responding to the demands for informed evidence from the National Institute for Clinical Excellence
- Strategies for the local implementation of the National Service Frameworks and other national strategies
- The demand for a local system of quality through the provision of clinical governance frameworks.

The enhancement of services and the associated planning of how these services are to be provided will rely heavily upon the teaching and research of those people delivering the service for people who have a learning disability. These demands will be highlighted in the need to demonstrate that their service or clinical practice is based on sound contemporary evidence of its effectiveness. The need to train and develop staff from the point of view of lifelong learning will continue and it will create its own demands to meet current and future change in practice. As this becomes a greater priority, the emphasis will have to be placed upon providing high-quality teaching, support for research, development and dissemination across health and local authorities.

There are still unacceptable variations in the quality of care provided to those who use the service and in turn those who support them. A common aim for health and social care staff in their quest to bring about high-quality services for those people who have a learning disability is developing a learning environment which supports effective working relationships, reflected in practical measures to ensure that professional preparation reinforces the role of the services.

The respective roles of health and social services as envisaged in the evolving learning disability provision are well described in two circulars on social and healthcare: LAC (92) (15) and HAG (92) (42), both of which are expected to form the basis of the forthcoming White Paper. These circulars have been reinforced by the practice guidance relating to planning, commissioning and the provision of health services for people who have learning disabilities (DoH 1998, 1999). If these documents are taken together with the Social Services Inspectorate Service Review of People with a Learning Disability who require coordinated care (DoH 1998), the key areas for attempting to add value to the respective health and social care agencies can be clearly identified.

The service of the future will continue to require an explicit value base. Such a base must reflect that the service is person focused, that it counters social exclusion by access and support. Services themselves will have to be designed so that there is clear indication of the needs of local people who have a learning disability, including those from ethnic and minority backgrounds who will require a variety of input at different phases in their lives. It will be important that such a service enables participation by local people who have learning disabilities in shaping the quality and level of service to be provided. Future practitioners will need to be outcome focused in their work so that such outcomes can be utilized to identify the progress of services for people who have disabilities. Quite simply, any future services must take account of natural communities that make clear sense to their population and this will be reflected in such areas as the provision of language, culture fair services, transport links and meaningful participation.

The flexibility of the services will be reflected in the way in which the general healthcare needs of people who have learning disabilities are met through their various milestones of development, including old age, and this will be seen in the accessibility of primary healthcare services, dental care and, whenever it arises, the need for acute physical care provision. Typically this will include health promotion, accurate screening programmes, audiology, ophthalmic provision, physiotherapy, chiropody, sexual health, pharmaceutical provision and continence maintenance services, amongst others.

It is likely that services will have to address the needs of people to develop mobility, communication and living skills, to cope with mental health conditions, offending behaviours, physical and sensory disabilities. It is possible that in the next decade we will see some re-engineering of services which will include access to inpatient assessment and treatment facilities, residential and respite care for those people who have a learning disability with a significant healthcare need.

The bottom line for supporting such services is that the practitioners working within them will have to provide health and social care which is adaptable and responsive and be able to lead and work effectively in teams where role boundaries are becoming more flexible. The outcome of these efforts should be that service users are able to access an integrated system of care which will not be constrained by organizational or geographic boundaries.

FURTHER READING

Lankshear A, Brown J, Thompson C 1996 Practice placement project. Mapping the nursing competencies required in institutional and community settings in the context of multi-disciplinary healthcare provision: an exploratory study. English National Board for Nursing, Midwifery and Health Visiting, London.
This is a detailed report which deals with complex issues of where to observe and develop competencies in clinical settings as well as having significant chapters on the methodology of competence observation and its conceptual relevance to nursing.

Jenkins-Clarke S, Carr-Hill R 1996 Measuring skill mix in primary care. Dilemmas of delegation and diversification. Discussion paper 144. Centre for Health Economics, University of York
This is a discussion paper which outlines the issues informing the measurement of skill mix in primary care settings and the consequent difficulties that may emerge.

Thompson T, Mathias P 1998 Standards and learning disability, 2nd edn. Baillière Tindall in association with RCN, London
This is the second edition of a leading textbook in the area of learning disability. It takes an innovative approach to the discussion of interprofessional standards and competencies in complex issues associated with learning disability. It particularly emphasizes the implications for professional roles and their interrelationships.

Modernising health and social services – developing the workforce
This is a health circular of 1999 which is also a local authority circular issued in May 1999 and it provides an overview of the government's key objectives and outputs for health and social services.

Clinical governance in the new NHS
This significant health service circular of 1999 sets out what the government programme of modernization of the NHS is intended to achieve. It explains and identifies quality as a driving force for the development of health services and explains why the clinical governance agenda is central to the quality agenda. It sets out the principles and processes that will develop clinical governance. It covers in a very detailed way issues such as integrated planning, staff support and development, workforce solutions, adopting good practice and addressing aspects of poor performance.

1997 National occupational standards – professional activity in health promotion and care. An introductory guide.
This is an excellent introduction to national occupational standards developed and published for the care sector consortium in 1997. It can be obtained from the local government management board. These standards marked a significant step forward and they captured not only the complexity of professional activity but the important principles of values which underpin all multidisciplinary and multiagency working.

REFERENCES

Bicknell J 1988 The mental handicap service – modern concepts of care. In: Sines D, Bicknell J (eds) Caring for mentally handicapped people in the community. Harper and Row, London

Department of Health 1993 Training for the future: training and development guidance and support. HMSO, London

Department of Health 1997 The new NHS: modern, dependable. The Stationery Office, London

Department of Health 1998 Partnerships in action. The Stationery Office, London

Department of Health 1999 Once a day: a primary care handbook for people with learning disabilities. The Stationery Office, London

Shaw I 1998 Learning together – social work and nursing, health and social care. Department of Social Policy, University of York, pp 255–262

Thompson J, Saunders M 1999 Audit in teams. APLD Publications, York

The Stationery Office 1999 The Health Act. The Stationery Office, London

Training Organisation in Personal and Social Services (TOPSS) 2000 Education and training the workforce. TOPSS, London

Weinstein J 1998 The professions and their interrelationships. In: Thompson T, Mathias P (eds) Standards and learning disability, 2nd edn. Baillière Tindall, London

Index

A

Abbreviated progressive
  relaxation (APR), 256
Access pathways, 19
Access to healthcare, 37–38,
  59–60, 223–224
Accessing health information,
  Acorn Group study,
  101–102, 158–168
  case studies, 163–164
  current position of group,
  165–166
  defining information,
  162–164
  formation of group, 160
  giving information,
  methods, 164–165
  practicalities, 166–167
  reason for study, 159–160
  recommendations, 167–168
  running group, 160–162
  starting out, 159
Accountability, 108, 322
Accreditation, 16
Acheson Report, 95
Achievements, value of, 290
Acorn Group see Accessing
  health information,
  Acorn Group study
Action areas
  Northern Ireland, 9
  Scotland, 10
  Wales, 11
Action plan, health needs
  assessment, 121
Activity plans, individual,
  208
Addresses, useful, 319
Adjustment to change, 266,
  276
Adolescent Behaviour
  Checklist, 243
Adolescents
  mental health problems,
  250–252
  case study, schizophrenia
  and challenging
  behaviour, 248–249
  peer support, 54
  transition to adulthood, 272
Adult training centres, 198
Advertisers and health, 29
Advisory groups, 181
Advisory roles, clinical
  governance, 322

Advocacy, 12, 109, 161, 216
  citizen advocacy, 105, 312,
  317
  self–advocacy, 161, 167,
  311–312, 317
Affective disorders, 240, 252
  see also Depression
Age
  of consent, homosexual sex,
  225
  influence on health, 43–44,
  75–77, 97
  mental health problems,
  252–254
  life transitions, 271–274
Ageing, premature, 68
Agendas and initiatives, 3–23
  changing agendas, 14–18
  Conservative legacy, 4–7
  further reading, 20–21
  future direction, 18–19
  policy across UK, 7–13
  public health see Public
  health agenda
Alcohol consumption, 81
All Wales Strategy (AWS),
  10–11, 300
Alliances, strategies for
  building, 313
Alma Ata declaration, 223
Alzheimer's disease
  diagnosing, 254
  Down's syndrome, 68–69,
  237, 253
Amenities, use of, 310
American Psychiatric
  Association, mental
  disorder definition,
  236
Amhara tribe, Ethiopia, 31
Anal intercourse, 218
Analysis of information,
  health needs
  assessment, 120
Anger management, Novaco's
  model, 256
Annual health screening, 152,
  153
Antiracism, 51
Anxiety, 236, 249
  relaxation training, 256
Appetite control,
  abnormalities, 183
Appointments, clinic, 59,
  130

Arthritis, degenerative cervical,
  68
Arthropathy, 76
Asexual label, impact of, 46,
  215
Asker role, circles of support,
  316
Assessment
  health needs, 93, 113–125
  approaches, 115
  case studies, 121–122,
  122–123
  collating public health
  data, 94–95
  conducting an
  assessment, 116–123
  coping mechanisms for
  change, 280
  further reading, 123–124
  in practice, 115–116
  health promotion, 137–143
  community (collective)
  need, 138–139
  individual need, 139–143
  mental health problems,
  240–249
  case study, 246–248
  challenging behaviour
  and diagnosis,
  248–249
  practical approaches,
  241–245
  sexual health, 215–218
  personal and professional
  perspectives, 217–218
Assimilation approach
  for learning disabled people
  see Normalization
  race relations strategy, 50
Atlantoaxial instability,
  Down's syndrome, 68,
  98
Attitudes
  definition, 222
  to disability, 34–35, 184
  learning disabled people's
  to other disabled
  people, 190–191
Audio–taped material, 165
Audit design, evaluative
  research, 151–152
Auditing progress, health
  needs assessment, 121
Autoimmune disorder, Down's
  syndrome, 66

Autonomy, 4, 129, 201–202, 221
Awareness of learning disability, 191

B
Beattie's model of health promotion, 133–136
Beck Depression Inventory, 243
'Before-and-after' design, evaluative research, 152
Behaviour
    challenging see Challenging behaviour
    drive-initiated, 223
    ill health, 34
    inappropriate, 223, 226
    masculine/feminine, 45
    observing, mental health assessment, 245
    routine and quasiroutine, 218
    social class groups, 53
Behaviour relaxation training (BRT), 256
Behaviour therapy, 255–256
Belief system, influence on sexual health, 220–221
    see also Health beliefs
Benefits system see State benefits
Bereavement, 99, 166
    personal account, 175
    see also Death
Betts Committee, 17
Biological factors
    gender differences, 45
    genetic inheritance, 42–43
Birth of sibling, 267–268
Black Report, 26, 52, 95
Body
    importance of, 182, 183
        body size case study, 180
    perceptions of, 184
Body Mass Index (BMI), 79
    Down's syndrome, 70
Boredom, 173, 176
British Institute of Learning Disabilities (BILD), 158, 166
British Sign Language, 217
Building alliances, strategies for, 313
Building expectations, Mental Health Foundation, 155, 180

C
Cancers, 73, 74
    Down's syndrome, 69–70
Cardiovascular disease, 74
    Down's syndrome, 67, 98
Care notes, interprofessional, 328

Care packages, consultation, 167
Care Standards Commission, 108
Care workers, 7
Caregiving trajectory, 294
Carers
    dealing with minor illness, 161
    and health promotion, 129, 131
    interviewing, client's mental health problems, 244
    needs assessment, 300, 302
    recognition of client's mental health problems, 250
    see also Family caregiving
Carers Act 1995, 300, 301
Caring about carers report, 301
Caring, contructions of, 293
Case conference, mental health assessment, 245
Case management, family-oriented, 302
Case study research design, single embedded, 138–139
Cataracts, Down's syndrome, 70–71
Categorizing information, health needs assessment, 120
Central Council for Education and Training in Social Work (CCETSW), 15
Cervical screening, 129, 174, 216, 219
    case studies, 163–164, 224
Challenging behaviour, 236, 238, 239–240
    case studies
        interplay with schizophrenia and adolescence, 248–249
        multidisciplinary assessment, 246–248
    as coping mechanism, 277
    diagnosis in presence of, 248
Change, 264, 265, 266
    analysing life transitions, 278–279
    coping with, 276–278
    further reading, 281–282
    implications for service delivery, 281
    models for managing, 280
    personal change, 266–267
        change in role, 267–271
        change in status, 271–274
        reactions to, 274–275
    personal meaning of transitions, 275–276
    in place, 267, 274
    types of, 265

Child Behaviour Rating Form, 243
Child psychotherapy models, 257
Children
    mental health problems, 250–252
    obesity, 78
    transition to adolescence, 272
Children's Depression Inventory, 244
Circles Networks, 198
Circles of support, 315–317
Circulars, LAC (92) (15) and HAG (92) (42), 333
Citizen advocacy, 105, 312, 317
Citizen focus groups, 106, 107
Citizens' juries, 106, 107, 109
Citizenship, 309–310
Civil rights, 310
Cleanliness, 185
Client group-specific assessments, 116
Clinical governance, 322
Clinics
    appointments, 59, 130
    environment, 224
Closure, health promotion project, 149, 150
Cognitive coping strategies, families, 299
Cognitive deterioration, dementia, 254
Cognitive therapy, 256
Collaboration with service users, 324–325
Collective authoritarian quadrant, Beattie's model, 134, 135
Collective health promotion need, assessment, 138–139
Collective identity, 49
Collective needs assessment, 138–139
Collective negotiated quadrant, Beattie's model, 134, 135–136
Colleges, integration into HEIs, 16
Commission for Health Improvement, 108
Common Foundation Programme (CFP), 18
Communication, 105
    difficulties, learning disabled clients, 129, 130, 163, 167, 227, 250, 311
    and expressed need, 216
    non-verbal people, assessing mental health problems, 240, 244
    reciprocity, 295

undermined confidence,
case study, 275–276
speech patterns, 56–57
staff, interpersonal skills,
109
Communities, working with,
306–319
concept of community,
307–310
further reading, 318
strategies for developing
inclusive communities,
310–317
circles of support,
315–317
citizen advocacy, 312
community connections,
310–311
self–advocacy, 311–312
social networks, 314–315
useful addresses, 319
Community action, 227
Community building,
103–108, 110, 326
community development,
104–106
health promotion,
135–136
practitioner skills
required, 110
direct participation of users,
106
informed views of citizens,
106–108
scrutinization and
regulation, health
services, 108
Community care policy
England, 11, 12, 13
Northern Ireland, 7–8, 9
Scotland, 9–10
Wales, 10
Community learning disability
team (CLDT), mental
health needs
assessment case study,
121–122
Comparative approach,
health needs
assessment, 115
Comparative need, 216–217
Compensating aspects,
problems and
difficulties in life,
237–238
Competence, 202
Composition of family, coping
ability, 297–298
Comprehensive schools, 55
Concepts, health and
disability, 24–39
attitudes to disability,
superimposition of
health and ill health
constructs, 34–35
defining health, 24–28

further reading, 39
health as evolutionary
concept, 28–30
modern constructs,
influence on health
education and
promotion, 32–34
pluralist perspectives of
health, 30–32
quality of life, 36–38
Confidence, undermining, case
study, 275–276
Congenital heart disease,
Down's syndrome,
67, 98
Consent see Informed consent
Conservative administration,
3
legacy, 4–7
issues, 6–7
trends, 4–6
Consumer society, growth of,
266
Contraception, 215, 227
Control
lack of at work, 58
locus of, 221
Coping strategies
change management,
276–277
families
family resilience,
289–291, 294–296
lifespan perspectives,
293–294
mediating factors and
family coping,
296–298
recognizing knowledge
and expertise,
299–300
strengthening coping
mastery, 301–302
stress-coping theory,
288–289
Corporate approach, health
needs assessment, 115
Coterminosity in planning,
332
Council for Health
Professions, 15
Council for the Professions
Supplementary to
Medicine (CPSM), 15
Counselling
health promotion, 134–135
mental health problems,
257
supporting life transitions,
281
Countertransference, 257
Credit rating, 266
Credit-based initiatives, staff
training, 16–17
Culture
culture clash at school, 57

family resilience, 290
influences on health, 48, 49,
99
health beliefs and
experience, 31–32
sexual health, 220
public health roles, 100
tailoring health promotion
interventions, 131
and valued occupation,
203–204

D
Dahlgren and Whitehead,
determinants of health,
97, 100
Down's syndrome case
study, 97–99
Data, health needs assessment
health needs assessment
data, 119–120
organizational data,
118–119
service, team or
practice-based data,
118
Dearing Report, 17
Dearing review, 55
Death
psychological reconstruction
of, 277
of significant person, 268
case study and
discussion, 268–269
see also Bereavement;
Mortality
Decision-making, involving
service users, 5, 106
Deferred gratification, 57, 60
Deliberative opinion polls,
106, 107
Demand, 114
Dementia, 76, 253
diagnosing, 253–254
Down's syndrome, 68–69,
237, 253
Dental health, 75
Department of Health support
system priorities, 329
Depression, 236, 237, 240,
249
diagnostic instruments,
243–244
elderly people, 252
Descriptive design, evaluative
research, 150, 151
Determinants of health,
Dahlgren and
Whitehead, 97, 100
Down's syndrome case
study, 97–99
Developmental stages, 266
change in status, 266–267,
271–274
mental health assessment,
251

Developmental/disability
    trajectory, 294
Devolution, 3, 4
Diagnostic Assessment for the
    Severely Handicapped
    (DASH) scale, 243
Dieting, 184
Disability, 25, 26, 185–186
    attitudes to, 34–35, 184
        learning disabled clients
        to other disabled
        people, 190–191
    consequences, research
        findings, 185
Disability lobby, 13
Discharge letter, long–stay
    hospitals, 159, 162
Discrimination, employment
    issues, 271
Discussions
    group, 119
    involving clients, 106
        action points, 107–108
Disease-specific assessments,
    116
Divorce, 270
Dohrenwend and
    Dohrenwend, 'life
    events' approach to
    stress, 288
Donabedian, structure,
    process, outcome
    evaluation, 153
Down's syndrome, 43, 63, 64,
    65–71, 82
    cancers, 69–70
    case studies, 67–68, 97–99
    heart and congenital
        disorders, 67, 68
    infections and immune
        deficiencies, 65–67
    leg muscle strength, 80
    neurological disorders,
        68–69, 237, 253
    obesity, 70
    personal account, health
        and illness experience,
        171–178
    plastic surgery, 37, 58, 177
    testing for, 177
    vision and hearing
        problems, 70–71
Downstream action, public
    health agenda, 101
Drives, 222–223
Dyskinesia, 76

E
Education action zones, 325
Education Acts
    1944, 54
    1970, 54
    1981, 57
Education consortia, 17
Education Reform Act 1988,
    55

Education system, 54–58
Education of workforce see
    Training and education
Educational interventions,
    mental health
    problems, 258
Elaborated code, 56–57
Elderly people, mental health
    problems, 252
    see also Dementia
Eleven plus exam, 54–55
Emancipatory model, 160
Embedded case study research
    design, 138–139
Emotional arousal and
    self–efficacy, 136
Emotional changes, dementia,
    254
Employer-determined training,
    16–17
Employment
    female/male work roles,
        45–46
    influence on health, 58–59
    learning disabled people,
        13, 46, 96, 99,
        270–271
        personal account,
        172–173
    supported schemes, 198
    work opportunities,
        205
    see also Valued occupation
England, policy, 11–13
English National Board
    (ENB), key areas
    learning disability
    nursing skills, 13
Environment, 99
    clinic, 224
    community, 308–309
    effect on health, 30
    public health roles, 100
Epidemiological approach,
    health needs
    assessment, 115
Epidemiological information
    health needs assessment,
        118–119
    planning health promotion,
        137–138
Epigenetic instructions, 42–43
Epilepsy
    Down's syndrome, 69, 76
    fragile X syndrome, 72
Equal opportunities
    legislation, 220, 223
Ethical grid, Seedhouse,
    229–230
    case study, 230–231
Ethical issues
    dilemmas in valued
        occupation, 201–202,
        209
    sexual health, 129, 229–232
Ethnic minorities, 64

family resilience, 290
    and health promotion,
        126–127, 130, 131
    valued occupation, 203–204
Ethnicity, influence on health,
    31, 48–49
Ethnocentrism, 50
Evaluation, health promotion,
    150, 151–153
Ewles and Simnett, planning
    health promotion
    flowchart, 144–145
Exercise, awareness of
    importance, 188
Exercise programmes, 80
    Down's syndrome clients,
        98
    see also Fitness gain
        intervention, devising
Expectations
    about healthcare, 30
    about learning disability,
        167
        role identified by society,
        191
    clients and carers, 5, 10
Expertise in family caregivers,
    recognising, 299–300,
    302
Exposure corneal disease, 75
Expressed need, 216
External locus of control, 221

F
Facilitator role, circles of
    support, 316–317
Family caregiving, 287–305
    constructions of caring, 293
    discussion, 301–302
    family resilience, 289–291
        practice issues, 294–296
    family systems theory,
        291–293
    further reading, 302–303
    lifespan perspectives,
        293–294
    mediating factors and
        family coping,
        296–298
    practice gaps, families'
        views, 300–301
    recognising knowledge and
        expertise, 299–300
    stress-coping theory,
        288–289
Family life cycle, 294
Fashion
    ideas about clothes, 189
    influence of, 185, 186
Fatness, significance, 184
Feasibility phase, health
    promotion project,
    148, 149
Felt need, 216
Feminine behaviour, 45
Findings, sharing, 120–121

First class service, DoH, 181
*Fit for the future – a new
        approach*, DHSS, 9
Fitness gain intervention,
        devising, 79
Fitness for practice, UKCC,
        18, 20
'Flow experiences', 203, 209
Focus groups, 106, 107
Food
    buying, 53
    knowledge of healthy, 188
Foot disorders, 76
Formative evaluation *see*
        Process evaluation
Fragile X syndrome, 63, 64,
        71–72, 237
Friends, 98, 175, 176, 308
    building relationships, 313
    circles of support, 315–317
    importance of, 314
        personal account, 173
    lack of, 308
    maintaining friendships,
        314
    mutuality, 190
Funding, sexual health
        promotion, 228
Future caregiving, families'
        anxieties, 300

G
Gastrointestinal tract
        disorders, 76
    cancer, 73, 74
    Down's syndrome, 68
Gender
    and coping ability, 296–297
    influence on health, 44–47
    and social class, 54
General practice
    health information
        availability, 161
    health needs assessment
        case study, 122–123
General practitioners (GPs),
        14, 37, 59, 81
    clinic appointments, 59,
        130
    communication difficulties
        with learning disabled,
        250
    discharge letter, long–stay
        hospitals, 159, 162
    experience of, personal
        account, 175
    learning disabled clients
        register, 128
    referral and prescribing
        rates, 116
General Social Care Council,
        15
Generation, influence on
        health, 43–44
Generic assessment, health
        needs, 115

Generic health promotion,
        138
Generic workers, 6–7
Genetic inheritance and
        biology, 42–43, 97
    mental illness, 236, 237
Genitourinary medicine
        (GUM) services, 224
Germ cells, 44
Gnau of Papua New Guinea,
        31
Going to the doctor, booklet,
        160
Gratification experiences,
        family caregivers, 289,
        290
Greater Glasgow Joint
        Learning Disability
        Project, 9–10
Grief, inability to express,
        238
Group identities, construction
        of, 190–192
Group polarization, 50

H
Habitualized behaviour, 218
Hamilton Rating Scale for
        Depression, 243–244
Health
    constructs of
        influence on health
            education and
            promotion, 32–34
        superimposition on
            disability, 35
    defining, 24–28, 38
        component parts, 28
        within public health
            agenda, 92
    as evolutionary concept,
        28–30
    impact on people who
        have learning
        disability, 29–30
    and occupation, 200
    pluralist perspectives of,
        30–32
    promoting positive,
        101–103
    and quality of life, 36–38
    states of, 203
    staying healthy, 171–175
    see also Inequalities of
        health; Influences on
        health; Mental health
Health action model, Tones
        and Tilford, 218, 219,
        222, 223, 224–225
Health Action Zones, 12, 102,
        103, 325, 326
Health authorities, 330, 331
Health beliefs, 200
    influence of culture, 31–32
Health Care Needs Assessment
        series, 119

The health divide, 52
Health education, 32, 38, 93,
        132, 133
Health Improvement
        Programmes, 12, 101,
        103, 111, 117, 325,
        326, 330, 331
Health of the nation, DoH,
        32
*A strategy for people with
        learning disabilities*,
        82, 162
    sexual health objectives,
        211–212
Health needs, 5, 63–88, 114
    assessment *see* Assessment:
        health needs
    Down's syndrome, 65–71
    fragile X syndrome, 71–72
    further reading, 82–83
    implications for practice,
        81–82
    problems not related to
        cause of learning
        disability, 72–77
    risk factors and lifestyle,
        77–78
    staff training, 19
Health persuasion, 134
Health promotion, 32, 38, 60,
        93, 126–157
    access and availability,
        problems with,
        126–129
    approaches, 133–136
    assessing need for, 137–143
        community (collective)
            need, 138–139
        individual need, 139–140
        individual needs
            assessment tool,
            141–143
    barriers to, overcoming,
        129–131
    design and implementation,
        144–146
    elements of, 132–133
    evaluation, 150–152
    further reading, 154–155
    and healthy alliances, 147
    project management,
        147–150
    self-efficacy, importance of,
        136–137
    setting the scene, 132
Health protection, 93, 133
Health screening *see* Screening
Health Services Select
        Committee, 14, 20
Health Survey for England, 81
Health visiting, retention of,
        15
Healthcare needs, 114
Healthy alliances, project
        management,
        147–150, 154

Healthy Living Centres, 102
The healthy way, DoH, 33
Hearing problems, 75, 76
    Down's syndrome, 70–71
    fragile X syndrome, 71
Heart disorders
    Down's syndrome, 67, 98
    fragile X syndrome, 71
Help-seeking/help-giving
        theory, 292, 295
Hepatitis virus infection, 73
    Down's syndrome, 65, 66
Higher education institutions
        (HEIs), 16
Hip abnormalities, 67, 68
History review, mental health
        assessment, 241,
        242–243
HIV/AIDS, 211, 220–221
Homosexual relationships,
        218, 225, 226
Hopson and Adams model,
        impact of transitions
        on self-esteem, 280
Hospital
    inpatient experience,
        175–176
    see also Long-stay
        hospitals
Housing conditions, 55
Human ecology theory,
        291–292
Humanism, 198
Hysteria, 46

I
Id, 222
Ill health constructs,
        superimposition on
        disability, 35
Illness
    defining, 27–28, 38
    as deviation from construct
        of health, 33–34
    and getting well, personal
        account, 175–177
Image, 182–183
Immunological deficiencies,
        Down's syndrome,
        66–67
Impairment, coming to terms
        with, 185
Inappropriate behaviour, 223,
        226
Incontinence, 76
*Independent Inquiry into
        Inequalities in Health*,
        52
Independent sector, 3, 5, 18
    see also Private sector;
        Voluntary sector
Individual authoritarian
        quadrant, Beattie's
        model, 134
Individual definition of health,
        32, 33

Individual health promotion
        need
    assessment, 139, 140
        assessment tool, 141–143
        tailoring to individual,
            140
Individual negotiated
        quadrant, Beattie's
        model, 134–135
Individual plan (IP) of care,
        300
Individuality, expression of,
        182
Inequalties of health, 41,
        95–101
    see also Influences on health
Infections, 72–73
    Down's syndrome, 65, 66
Influences on health, 41–62
    access to health care, 59–60
    age and generation, 43–44
    education system, 54–58
    further reading, 61
    genetic inheritance and
        biology, 42–43
    occupation, work
        environment and
        unemployment, 58–59
    race, ethnicity and culture,
        48–51
    sex and gender, 44–47
    social class, 51–55
    socialization and lifestyle,
        47–48
Information
    access to *see* Accessing
        health information,
        Acorn Group study
    carers' and professionals'
        control over, 188
    for citizens, community
        building, 106–108
Information systems
        development, 327–328
Informed consent, 38, 59–60,
        129, 216
    pictorial form, 160
Initiation phase, health
        promotion project,
        148, 149
Initiatives and agendas *see*
        Agendas and initiatives
Institute of Health Services
        Management,
        community building,
        103–104
Institutional racism, 51
Institutions
    impact on experience of
        community, 308–309
    see also Long-stay
        hospitals; Residential
        care
Intelligence, measuring, 55
Interconnectedness, things in
        life, 196

Internal market, 3, 14, 205
Internet, 165
Interprofessional and
        multi-agency working,
        320–335
    effective teamwork,
        328–329
    framework for
        strengthening helping
        systems, 331–334
    new services and
        understandings,
        332–334
    further reading, 334–335
    need for, 320–324
    partnerships between
        statutory
        organizations,
        322–324
    the quality agenda,
        321–322
    realities of, 324–328
        collaborating wih service
            users, 324–325
        community inclusion,
            326
        developing partnerships,
            325
        individual health needs,
            327
        information systems
            development, 327–328
        primary care services,
            326–327
        support systems, interface
            between, 329–331
Intervention-specific
        assessments, 116
Interventions, complex
        healthcare, 37–38
Interviews, health needs
        assessment, 119
'Inverse care law', 59, 228
Involving clients in processes
        and procedures, 5,
        10
    consultation for NHS
        Charter, 12
    decision-making, 5, 106

J
Jarman Index, 139
Jay Report, 10
JM Consulting, 15
Joint investment plans (JIPs),
        103
Journal of Insanity, 197

K
Keratoconus, Down's
        syndrome, 71
Keratopathy, 75

L
Labour administration, 3, 4,
        181, 205, 321

Language
  use of, social class
      differences, 56–57
  user friendly, 161, 167
      plain English, 104, 105
Lay representation, health
      service regulation, 108
Lazarus and Folkman,
      transactional model,
      288, 289
Leadership skills, project
      managers, 147
League tables, school, 55
Learning Disability Awards
      Framework (LDAF),
      17, 18
Learning disability nurses, 13
  changes in practice, 331
  communication skills, 130
Legal issues, sexual health,
      229–232
Legislative action, health
      promotion, 134, 135
Leisure, 53, 205, 308
Lesch–Nyhan syndrome, 237
Leukaemia, Down's syndrome,
      69–70
Life events, 43, 267–274
  change in place, 267, 274
  change in role, 267–271
  change in status, 271–274
  influence on mental health,
      238, 247, 248
  and stress, 288
'Life events' approach, stress
      management,
      Dohrenwend and
      Dohrenwend, 288
Life expectancy, 52
Life transitions, 264
  analysis, 278–279
  and change, 265–266
  implications for service
      delivery, 281
  life events, 43, 267–274
  models for managing, 280
  personal meaning of,
      275–276
Lifespan perspectives, family
      caregiving, 293–294,
      298
Lifestyle and health, 29, 30,
      47–48, 53
  making decisions about,
      187–189
  peer pressure, 98
  public health roles, 100
  risk factors, 77–81
Literacy, 48, 55, 163
Live running phase, health
      promotion project,
      148, 150
Living conditions, 55, 99, 174,
      175
  public health roles, 100
  rise in standards, 41

Local advocacy groups, 105
Local authorities
  demographic data, 118–119
  learning disabled clients
      register, 128
Local knowledge and interest,
      building on, 117
Locus of control, 221
Lone carers, 297
Loneliness, 173
Long-stay hospitals, 9
  closure, 5–6, 11, 323
  discharge letter to GPs, 159
  reduction in beds, 8, 9
  research evidence on health,
      64
  see also Residential care

M
Makaton signs, 217
Making a difference, DoH, 18,
      20
Male menopause, 272–273
Marriage, 269–270
Marxist views, criticizing
      capitalism, 51
Masculine behaviour, 45
Masturbation, 212, 216, 223,
      226
Meaningful life, importance to
      health, 171–173
Media
  interest in service shortfalls,
      38
  representation of health, 29
  transfering information,
      164, 165
Meetings, involving clients,
      106
  action points, 107–108
Memory loss, dementia, 254
Mencap
  disabled people's rights,
      213–214, 226
  importance of self-efficacy,
      221
  The NHS – health for all?,
      228
Menopause, 272, 273
Menstruation, 46
Mental health, 235–263
  assessment of problems,
      240–249
      diagnosis in presence of
          challenging behaviour,
          248–249
      multidisciplinary
          assessment, case study,
          246–248
      Walkington CLDT case
          study, 121–122
  case recognition, 249–250
  defining mental illness,
      235–236
  prevalence of problems,
      238, 239

problems across lifespan,
      250–254
  ageing and age-related
      problems, 252–254
  children and adolescents,
      250–252
  psychiatric disorders and
      challenging behaviour,
      238, 239–240
  risk factors for mental
      illness, 236–238
  treatment, 254–258
Mental Health Foundation,
      Building expectations,
      155, 180
'Micro-institutionalization',
      309
Mid-life transitions, 272–273
Migrant workers as labour
      army, 51
Mini PAS-ADD, 243, 250
Minimum wage, 271
Miscarriage, 45
Mobility, social, 52
Mood charts, 245, 252
Mortality, 47
  gender differences, 44, 45
  learning disabled people,
      44, 76, 82
      cancers, 69–70, 73, 74
      cardiovascular disease,
          67, 74
      infections, 65, 66, 72–73
      work-related, 46
Motivation, 222, 223
Movement disorders, 76
Moving home, 267, 274
Multi-agency working *see*
      Interprofessional and
      multi-agency working
Multi-infarct dementia, 253
Multimodal treatment, mental
      health problems, 258
Muscular strength and
      endurance, 80, 98
Mutualism, 190

N
National Census data, 119
National Curriculum, 55
National estimates, health
      needs assessment, 119
National health technology
      assessment
      programmes, 114
National Institute for Clinical
      Excellence (NICE),
      114, 323, 331
National Service Framework
      on Mental Health,
      332
National training organizations
      (NTOs), 17
National Vocational
      Qualifications
      (NVQs), 18

Natural selection, 53
Neurological disorders,
    Down's syndrome,
    68–69, 237, 253
*New NHS: modern,
    dependable*, DoH, 20,
    181, 321
NHS Charter, consultation, 12
NHS and Community Care
    Act 1990, 14, 127,
    137, 180, 205
NHS Confederation,
    community building,
    103–104
NHS Executive, community
    building, 103–104
Normalization, 129, 180, 191,
    192, 198, 202
Normative need, 215
Normative system, influence
    on sexual health
    decisions, 220
Northern Ireland, policy, 7–9
Novaco, anger management
    model, 256
Numeracy, 48, 55
Nurse consultant, 18
Nurse specialists, 13
Nurses
    changes in practice, 331
    communication skills, 130
    education, 16–17
    preparation and practice,
        18
Nursing accommodation,
    clients, 5
Nursing, regulatory reviews,
    15

O
Obesity, 76, 82, 183–184
    Down's syndrome, 70
    as risk factor, 77–80
    weight loss and fitness gain
        intervention, 79
Obsessive–compulsive
    disorder, 240
Occupation, concept of, 197,
    200
    see also Valued occupation
Odds ratios, 64–65
Old age, 273–274
Older learning disabled
    people, family
    caregiving, 298
Once a day, NHSE, 37, 127
Opinion polls, 106, 107
'Opted out' schools, 55
Organizational data, health
    needs assessment,
    118–119
Ottawa Charter, 223, 225,
    227, 228
Our healthier nation, White
    Paper, 12, 95, 102,
    110, 111

Outcome evaluation, 153,
    228, 229

P
Paranoid psychoses, 252
Parents who have learning
    disability, 215, 270
Parkinsonism, 76
Parkinson's disease, Down's
    syndrome, 69
Partnership in Action, 205
Partnership approaches, 6, 93,
    101, 102–103, 181
    difficulties in achieving,
        268–269
    health promotion, 132
    health and social services,
        London example,
        11–12
    initiatives, 19
    skills required, 109–110
    supporting families, 290,
        291, 301–302
    valued occupation, 204–206
    see also Communities,
        working with;
        Interprofessional and
        multi-agency working
PAS-ADD checklist, 243, 250
Paternalism, 201–202
Patient's Charter, 161
Peer pressure, 98
Peer support, adolescents, 54
People First, 48, 105, 167,
    173
Perceptions
    of body, 184–186
    of health, 29
    of learning disabled by
        society, 191
    of others, societal values,
        199
Performance of services, 322
    variations in, 323
Person-centred planning, 198,
    327
    and cultural diversity,
        203–204
    enabling valued occupation,
        207–209
Personal account, health and
    illness experiences,
    171–178
    health and staying healthy,
        171–175
    illness and getting well,
        175–177
Personal change, 264,
    266–267
Personal counselling, health
    promotion, 134–135
'Personal tragedy' model of
    disability, 185
Personhood, concept of, 201
Phobias, anxiety management
    techniques, 256

Photographs, 165
Physical fitness, 80
Physiological arousal and
    self-efficacy, 136
Pictorial guides, 165
Pilot schemes, joint working,
    12
Place, change of, 267, 274
Planning
    care packages, 167
    fieldwork, health needs
        assessment, 119
    health promotion project,
        144–145
    project management,
        147–150
Policy, 7–14, 99, 225,
    330–331, 331–332
    disability lobby, 13–14
    England, 11–13
    Northern Ireland, 7–9
    Scotland, 9–10
    Wales, 10–11
Political agendas
    impact on learning disabled
        clients, 99
    public health role
        influencing, 93
Political rights, 310
Population level assessments,
    115
Positive discrimination, 51
Poverty, 45, 53, 55–56, 59,
    95, 96–101
Practice–based data, health
    needs assessment, 118
Prader-Willi syndrome, 183
Pregnancy, 46
    starvation during, 43–44
Premature ageing, 68
Presbyacusis, Down's
    syndrome, 71
Preschool children, parents'
    ability to cope, 298
Prescribing practices, 81, 116
Prevalence
    of disease, 63
        studies of, 64–65
    of learning disability in UK,
        128
Prevention, 133
Primary care, 5, 326–327
    access to, 59
    clinic appointments, 59, 130
    evolving professional
        relationships, 14–15
    health promotion, 128–129
    prescribing practices, 81,
        116
    screening services, 37
    see also General
        practitioners (GPs)
Primary care groups/teams/
    trusts, 14, 128, 321,
    323, 329, 330–331,
    332

Primary prevention, 133
Private sector, 3
    workforce, training and
        education, 17–18
Process evaluation, 153, 228,
    229
Professional boundaries, 5
    working across *see*
        Interprofessional and
        multi-agency working
Professional relationships,
    evolving, 14
Project 2000, 16
Project management approach,
        healthy alliances,
        147–150, 154
    case study, 149–150
    stages, 148–149
Project SHaRE, 298
Prompt sheet, health
        promotion, 131
Protect, need to, 215
Psychiatric Assessment
        Schedule for Adults
        with a Developmental
        Disability (PAS-ADD),
        243
Psychological sense of
        community, loss of,
        307
Psychopathology Instrument
        for Mentally Retarded
        Adults, 243
Psychopharmacology, 254–255
Psychotherapy, 257–258
Public health agenda, 91–112
    assessment data, collating,
        94–95
    building community
        participation, 103–108
    defining public health,
        92–94
    roles, 93–94
    developing skills, 108–110
    further reading, 110–111
    health inequalities and
        causes of ill health,
        95–101
    promoting positive health,
        101–103

Q
Qualitative information, 144
    analysis, 120
    health promotion data, 153
Quality of life, 36–38, 91, 92,
        101
    and mental health, 236–237
Quality of services, 321–322,
        333
Quantitative information, 144
    health needs assessment,
        119
    analysis and presentation,
        120
Quasiroutine behaviour, 218

Questionnaire for learning
        disabled, 162
Quilting, concept of, 313

R
Race, 48, 49
Racism, 49, 50–51, 130, 131
Raising awareness, 94, 96
Randomized controlled trials,
        144, 151, 152
Reciprocity and
        communication
        difficulties, 295
Referral
    for mental health
        assessment, 241
    rates of, 116
Reflective thinking, 209
Reformation, health and social
        care, 321
Regeneration schemes, 103,
        326, 330
Registers, learning disabled
        clients, 128
Registration and Inspection
        teams, 108
Regulation of health services,
        lay representation, 108
Regulatory bodies, change, 15
Regulatory roles, clinical
        governance issues, 322
Reiss screen, 243
Relationships, 186–187,
        189–190
    marriage, 269–270
    sexual, 218, 225, 226
    see also Friends
Relaxation
    tapes, 165
    training, 256
Religious beliefs and sexual
        expression, 220, 222
Renewal, directing change, 277
Reorientation of health
        services, 227–228
Reports and papers, health
        needs assessment, 119
Reproductive organs, cancer
        of, 74
Residential care, 5
    decisions about staying in
        or leaving, 96
    health of those living in, 63
    impact on experience of
        community, 308–309
    lay inspectors, 108
    same-sex relationships, 218
    see also Long-stay hospitals
Resilience in coping strategies,
        289–291, 301
    practice issues, 294–296
Resistance to change, 276
Resources, 330
    health needs assessment, 117
    and identifying urgent need,
        268

Respiratory infection, 72–73
    Down's syndrome, 65, 66
Restricted code, 56, 57
Retirement, 266, 273–274
    transformational view, 277
Review, health promotion
        project, 149, 150
Right employment, 198
Rights
    of citizenship, 310
    disabled people and sexual
        health, 213–214, 226
Risk
    and discussing personal
        relationships, 232
    and valued occupation,
        202–203, 209
Robinson, 'stimulus–response
        model', 288
Role identification by society,
        191
Role transitions, 266
    change in role, 267–271
    as carers age, 292
Routine behaviour, 218

S
Safer sex practices, 218, 221,
        222
Salaries, 46
Same-sex relationships, 218,
        225, 226
    age of consent, 225
*Saving lives: our healthier
        nation*, White Paper,
        12, 32, 132, 154–155
Schizophrenia, 236
    in adolescence
        challenging behaviour
        case study, 248–249
        misdiagnosing, 251–252
School, 54–58
    atmosphere and values, 57
    encouragement of children,
        56
    learning about other
        cultures, 50
    learning disabled child in
        mainstream, 57–58
    special school, 54
        personal experience, 172
School-age children, parents'
        coping ability, 298
'Scientific racism', 49
Scotland, policy, 9–10
*Scottish Health Authorities
        review of priorities for
        the eighties and
        nineties* (SHARPEN),
        9
Screening, 37, 60, 93
    annual health, 152, 153
    cervical, 129, 174, 216, 219
    case studies, 163–164,
        224
    heart valve dysfunction, 67

Secondary prevention, 133
Seedhouse
  definition of health, 27
  ethical grid, 229–230
Self-advocacy, 311–312
  groups, 105, 161, 167, 317
Self-concept, 179–194
  further reading, 193
  group identities,
    construction of,
    190–192
  issues of, 181–190
    image, 182–183
    obesity, 183–184
    perceptions of body,
      184–186
    relationships, 186–190
  legislation, implication of,
    180–181
Self-efficacy, 221
  importance of, 136–137,
    154
Self-esteem, 57, 267, 311
  impact of transitions,
    Hopson and Adams
    model, 280
Self-help groups
  'supporting', 227
  see also Self-advocacy:
    groups
Self-injurious behaviour, 237,
    240, 246, 247, 248
Self-reflection, planning
  valued occupation,
    208
Self-report of symptoms, 81
Separatism, ethnic and racial,
    51
Service provision maps, 19
Service trajectory, 294
Service users
  collaboration with,
    324–325
  participation in
    decision-making, 106
Sex differences, influence on
    health, 44–47
Sex education, 174, 220
Sex in public environments,
    225
Sexist attitudes, 220
Sexual abuse, case studies
  ethical dilemmas, 230–231
    discussion, 231–232
  sexualized and
    self-injurious
    behaviour, 246–248
Sexual health, 98, 211–234
  assessing need, 214–218,
    226
    matching personal and
    professional
    perspectives, 217–218
  case study, health action
    model, 224–225
  defining, 211–213

factors influencing decisions
    about, 219–224
  further reading, 233
  health promotion
    interventions, 225–228
    evaluating, 228–229
  health promotion
    programmes, 146
  legal and ethical issues,
    229–232
  personal experience,
    173–174
  and rights, 213–214
  staying sexually healthy,
    218–219
Sexuality, 46, 98, 212, 213,
    226
Shared values, 180
Shaw Trust, 198
Short-term breaks, 205
Siblings, birth of, 267–268
Signposts for success, NHSE,
    3, 13, 20, 111, 228,
    309
Single-time choice, health
    action model, 218,
    219
Skeletal problems, fragile X
    syndrome, 71
Skills
  development of public
    health, 108–110
  learning disability nurses, 13
    development of, 19, 106
  project managers, 147
  skill mix, 5
Skinfold thickness, 79
Slimness, associations, 184
Smoking, 81
  cessation, 166
    health promotion project
    case study, 149–150,
    151
Social care workforce,
    training, 17–18
Social class
  and education system, 54,
    55
  and health promotion,
    126–127
  influence on health, 48,
    51–54
  and poverty, 59
  and relationship with
    professional services,
    59
Social and community
    influences, 98–99
  public health roles, 100
Social exclusion, 60, 102–103,
    105–106
Social Exclusion Unit, 102
Social inclusion, 105
Social networks
  assessment for support
    during change, 280

circles of support, 315–317
developing inclusive
    communities, 313–314
families of preschool
    children, 298
importance, 98, 102–103,
    314
impoverished, 252, 253
shrinkage over time, 293
support network theory,
    291
understanding, 314–315
Social races, 49
Social rights, 310
Social risk factors, mental
    illness in late life,
    252–253
Social role valorization, 36,
    103, 180, 191, 198,
    208
Social skills training, 227
Social work, regulatory
    bodies, 15
Socialization, 47–48, 54
Somatic symptoms, 240, 247,
    248
Specialist health promotion,
    138
Specialist learning disability
    services, 332
Specialist nurse practitioner,
    4–5, 6, 18
  private residential sector, 18
Speech patterns, social class,
    56–57
Standards, 321, 322
Standing citizens' panels, 106,
    107, 109
State benefits, 52, 56, 96
  benefit trap, 271
  eligibility, 64
  proof of incapacity, 26
Statementing, 57
Status
  change in, 266–267,
    271–274
  devalued, learning disabled
    people, 199
Statutory organizations,
    partnerships between,
    322–324
Stereotypes and labelling,
    gender issues, 46–47
Stigma, 186, 190
  stigmatization and
    depression, 237
Stillbirth, 45
'Stimulus–response model',
    Robinson, 288
Stress, 60, 166
  coping theory, 288–289,
    301
Structure, process, outcome
    evaluation, 153
Suffering, disability perceived
    as, 35

Summative evaluation *see* Outcome evaluation
Superego, 222
Supply, 114–115
Supporting families, 290, 291, 302
  practice gaps, 300–301
  recommendations, 301–302
Surgery, Down's syndrome, 37, 58, 177
Surveys, health needs assessment, 119

T
T cell abnormalities, Down's syndrome, 66
Teamwork, multidisciplinary, 12, 328–329
  health assessment team, 117
Technological developments and health, 30
Television, 30, 164
Temper tantrums, family coping example, 294–295
Tertiary prevention, 133
Thalidomide, 43
'Third places', 308
Thyroid disorders, Down's syndrome, 66–67
Time considerations, health needs assessment, 117, 119
Tones and Tilford, health action model, 218, 219, 222, 223, 224–225
Traditional medicines, 31
Training and education, 4, 5, 209
  future direction, 19
  increasing numbers of staff, 17–18
  joint and shared, 12, 331
  lifelong learning, 333
  nurse, 16–17, 18–19
Training Organization for Personal Social Services (TOPSS), 17, 20–21
Training pack, sexual health, 217
Transactional model, Lazarus and Folkman, 288, 289
Transcedence, 278
Transference, 257
Transformational change, 277–278

Transition *see* Life transitions
Tribe, sense of, 307
Trisomy 21, 43
Tuberculosis, 73

U
UKCC
  replacement, 15
  specialist training, 18–19
Understanding, learning disabled clients, 163, 164, 167
Unemployment, 55, 58–59, 96, 266, 271
United Nations
  community development, 104
  rights of disabled people, 213, 226
Upstream action, public health agenda, 101
Useful addresses, 319

V
Valued occupation, 195–210, 270–271
  concepts of health and occupation, 200
  cultural diversity, 203–204
  defining, 198–200
  discussion, 206–207
  enabling, 207–209
  ethical dilemmas, 201–202
  further reading, 210
  historical perspectives, 197–198
  psychosocial aspects, health and occupation, 203
  risk, 202–203
  service options and partnerships, 204–206
Values
  definition, 222
  shared, 180
  see also Social role valorization
Verbal persuasion, 136, 137
Vicarious experience, 136
Vicarious liability, 322
Videos
  health promotion, 165
  sexual health training pack, 227
Villaging, concept of, 313
VISION (employment scheme), 198
Visual problems, 75, 76
  Down's syndrome, 70–71
  fragile X syndrome, 71
Voluntary sector, 10

W
Waiting times, 59
Wales, policy, 10–11
Walkington Community Learning Disability Team case study, 121–122
Weight problems, 71, 82, 98, 183–184
  attitude to importance of weight loss, 187
  devising intervention, 79
  Down's syndrome, 70
  knowledge, healthy diet and lifestyle, 188
  motivation for weight loss, 184
  obesity as risk factor, 77–80
  personal account, 172, 177
  see also Body size; Obesity
Welfare state *see* State benefits
Welsh Health and Community Care Survey
  obesity, 77
  smoking and alcohol consumption, 81
Work roles, male/female, 45–46
Workforce, 4–7, 320
  education *see* Training and education
  'integrated workforce planning', 15
  workforce profiles, 19
  see also Interprofessional and multi-agency working
World Health Organization (WHO)
  community development, 104
  components of sexual health, 212
  definitions
    of health, 26–27, 34–35
    of health promotion, 132
  diagnosing dementia, 253–254
  traditional medicines, 31

Y
York People First 2000, 46
You and your health, booklet, 165

Z
Zung Self–Rating Depression Scale, 243